EXPANDING MINDSCAPES

EXPANDING MINDSCAPES

A Global History of Psychedelics

EDITED BY ERIKA DYCK
AND CHRIS ELCOCK

The MIT Press
Cambridge, Massachusetts
London, England

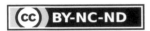
The MIT Press would like to thank the anonymous peer reviewers who provided comments on drafts of this book. The generous work of academic experts is essential for establishing the authority and quality of our publications. We acknowledge with gratitude the contributions of these otherwise uncredited readers.

This book was set in Adobe Garamond and Berthold Akzidenz Grotesk by Westchester Publishing Services. Printed and bound in the United States of America.

Library of Congress Cataloging-in-Publication Data

Names: Dyck, Erika, editor. | Elcock, Chris, editor.
Title: Expanding mindscapes : a global history of psychedelics / edited by
    Erika Dyck and Chris Elcock.
Description: Cambridge, Massachusetts : The MIT Press, [2023] | Includes
    bibliographical references and index.
Identifiers: LCCN 2022059916 (print) | LCCN 2022059917 (ebook) |
    ISBN 9780262546935 (print) | ISBN 9780262376907 (epub) |
    ISBN 9780262376891 (pdf)
Subjects: LCSH: Hallucinogenic drugs—History—20th century. |
    LSD (Drug)—History—20th century.
Classification: LCC RM324.8 .E97 2023 (print) | LCC RM324.8 (ebook) |
    DDC 615.7/883—dc23/eng/20230601
LC record available at https://lccn.loc.gov/2022059916
LC ebook record available at https://lccn.loc.gov/2022059917

10   9   8   7   6   5   4   3   2   1

Contents

DIFFUSION OF SCIENTIFIC RESEARCH ON

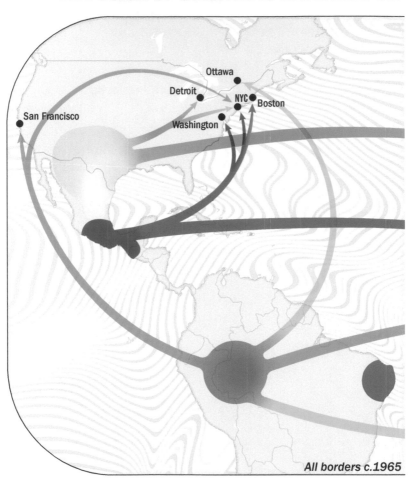

Ottawa
Detroit
San Francisco
NYC
Boston
Washington

All borders c.1965

PEYOTE
(MESCALINE)
4000 BCE - EARLIEST EVIDENCE   1800 - 1880: REGIONAL CULTURAL DIFFUSION

PSILOCYBIN MUSHROOMS
(PSILOCYBIN/PSILOCIN)
2000 BCE - EARLIEST EVIDENCE

AYAHUASCA
(DMT)
2700 BCE - EARLIEST EVIDENCE   1931-1960: SYNTHESIS (OTTAWA, 1931)

MAJOR NATURALLY-DERIVED PSYCHEDELICS

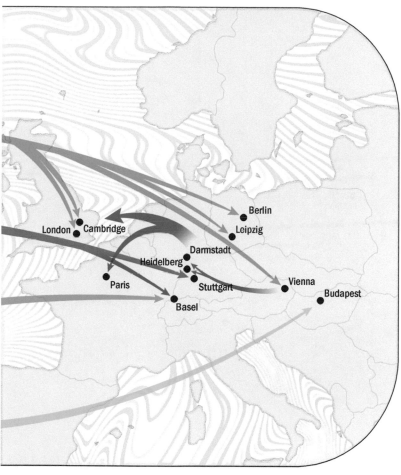

1880 - 1918: EARLY EXPERIMENTS

1919-40: SYNTHESIS (VIENNA, 1919) AND FURTHER DIFFUSION

1900 - 1955: EARLY EXPERIMENTS

1956-1960: SYNTHESIS (BASEL, 1955) AND FURTHER DIFFUSION

AND EARLY EXPERIMENTS*

1961-1990: FURTHER DIFFUSION

* FIRST DELIBERATE INGESTION OF SYNTHESIZED DMT IN BUDAPEST, 1956

DIFFUSION OF SCIENTIFIC RESEARCH

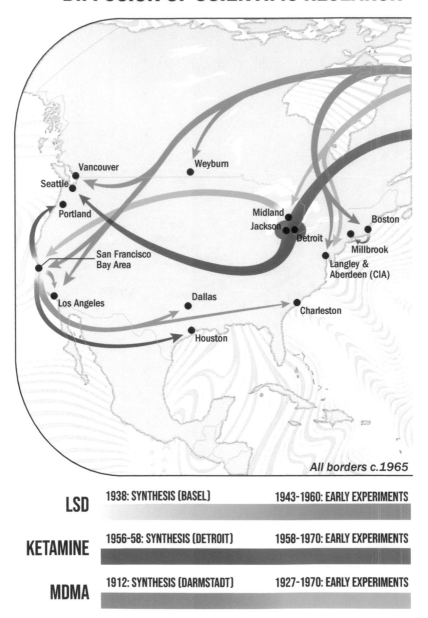

All borders c.1965

LSD	1938: SYNTHESIS (BASEL)	1943-1960: EARLY EXPERIMENTS
KETAMINE	1956-58: SYNTHESIS (DETROIT)	1958-1970: EARLY EXPERIMENTS
MDMA	1912: SYNTHESIS (DARMSTADT)	1927-1970: EARLY EXPERIMENTS

ON MAJOR SYNTHETIC PSYCHEDELICS

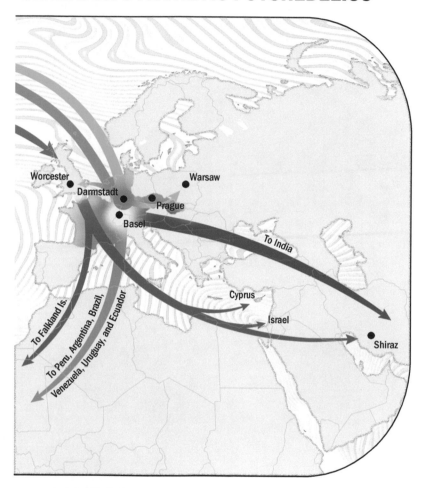

Worcester
Darmstadt
Prague
Basel
Warsaw
To India
Cyprus
Israel
Shiraz
To Falkland Is.
To Peru, Argentina, Brazil,
Venezuela, Uruguay, and Ecuador

1960-1970: FURTHER DIFFUSION

1971-2000: FURTHER DIFFUSION

1970-2000: FURTHER DIFFUSION

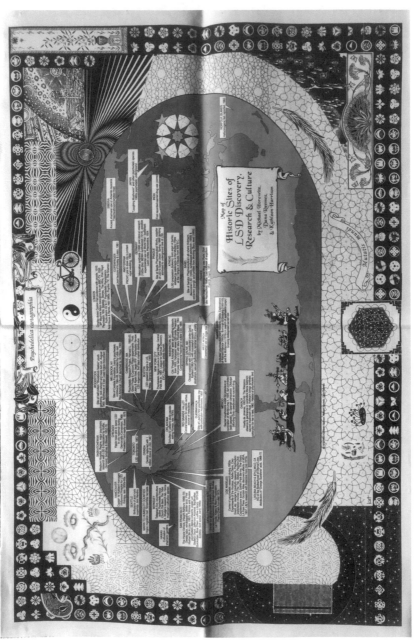

This 1993 map celebrated fifty years since Albert Hofmann's discovery of LSD. Illustrated by Kathleen Harrison and researched by the archivist and book dealer Michael Horowitz, the map was distributed as a newspaper with LSD trivia, stories, and a tribute to its effects around the world. Ringed with images of samurai blotter acid, the image pays homage to Mayan influences, ergot, and Hofmann's notorious bicycle trip. Reprinted with permission from Kathleen Harrison and Michael Horowitz.

INTRODUCTION

Chris Elcock and Erika Dyck

On October 20, 2020, Timothy Leary would have turned 100. A popular media outlet ran a quick synopsis of his life and times while asking friends, former colleagues, and other commentators to reflect on the "High Priest" of LSD twenty-four years after his death in 1996. Predictably, the reviews were mixed. He was described as a charismatic leader, a reckless proselytizer, a bad father, the maker of Charles Manson, an iconoclastic academic, "an asshole," and "a shaman."[1] Leary was a polarizing and controversial figure, to be sure, but it seems almost impossible to read about the history of LSD and psychedelics without forever bumping into him—an ironically fitting legacy for this megalomaniac and narcissistic psychologist. As a result of his towering presence, we are sometimes left with the impression that the bulk of this fascinating and complex history was set in the US during the "psychedelic sixties." But there is a lot more to this story.

Historians like their decades neatly compact, and the 1960s, which have their own academic journal (e.g., the *Global Sixties*, an interdisciplinary journal) and which have drawn a colossal amount of scholarly and lay interest, are perhaps the most fitting illustration of this attention to precise timelines. This might be why Leary continues to exert such a unique influence on this history. Indeed, the Harvard professor encountered psilocybin in 1960 and LSD the year after. After these life-changing experiences, his scientific investigations into both became increasingly idiosyncratic (and unethical by today's standards), and in 1963, his employers chose not to renew his contract after he went AWOL and neglected his teaching duties.

In late 1965, he and his family were arrested at the Texas-Mexico border and charged with smuggling cannabis. To challenge his case, he aggressively promoted these drugs as religious sacraments and explicitly courted baby boomers for support. But after two subsequent marijuana arrests, the law finally caught up with him, and by 1970, the same year that LSD and psychedelics became Schedule I drugs in the US, Leary was behind bars. And that, so it seemed, was the end of the psychedelic sixties.[2]

A different reading of this brief overview reveals that Leary's involvement with these drugs was in fact quite short and perhaps less remarkable than we might think. LSD had arrived in the US just after World War II, and scientists conducted groundbreaking studies into LSD and mescaline in the 1950s.[3] Soon Americans began to experiment with these drugs, along with peyote, ololiuqui, and ibogaine,[4] years before Leary even knew they existed. Even after the 1960s, a small number of clinical trials carried on into the 1970s in spite of tighter regulations.[5] Outside the clinics and research centers, Americans continued to use LSD and psychedelics,[6] and by the 1990s, research into these drugs and a younger generation of lay popularizers were offering a new window into the world of psychedelics.[7] Could it be, then, that the psychedelic sixties lasted almost half a century?

The fascination with the 1960s can also be explained by the cultural context of postwar America. In its best-remembered manifestation, psychedelia appeared at a time when the entire country was going through an unprecedented wave of progressive, radical, and conservative activism that cemented the significance of the 1960s in American history. Leary's vocal promotion of LSD allowed this psychedelic movement to be retrospectively considered alongside the various social movements of the time, even though some historians and commentators found his idea of chemical revolution downright preposterous.[8] Although many of these protest movements have been deemed far more significant, it has been hard to ignore Leary and LSD in the US when reflecting on that turbulent decade. Combined with the coverage of the San Francisco acid culture, as well as the 1969 Woodstock festival, the history of the American psychedelic sixties certainly looms large in the scholarship and the popular mind.

However, psychedelics have a much deeper and broader history that challenges both the chronology and geography of that particular location and time frame. The ritual use of psychoactive plants can be traced to precolonial times in most parts of the world, and scientific, cultural, and intellectual inquiries into these drugs were certainly not confined to the US. By bringing together historians and histories from all over the world, this book is the first attempt to look at the story of psychedelics in a global perspective, in a set of papers that moves the discussion beyond the US and Canada, which has already benefited from scholarly attention.[9]

The contemporary scientific reappraisal of psychedelic compounds like LSD, psilocybin, and DMT, along with interest in Indigenous plant medicines like ibogaine and ayahuasca, has been widely documented to a point where it is now colloquially known as the "psychedelic renaissance."[10] Since 2020, a growing list of American states have now decriminalized these drugs, and Health Canada has created exemptions for the medical use of psychedelics for managing end-of-life anxiety. Ayahuasca is a legal substance in several jurisdictions, including Brazil, Costa Rica, and Peru, leading to the growth of drug tourism in Latin America, accompanied by the proliferation of psychedelic retreat centers or resorts in these jurisdictions, which often combine claims of religious, ceremonial, and healing benefits.

In Portugal and the Netherlands, clinics are now offering psychedelic-assisted therapy using ibogaine and psilocybin, respectively, while several research groups are conducting clinical trials into psychedelics across the European continent. Some scientists are promoting psychedelics as an effective treatment option for a growing list of psychiatric disorders, at a time when the entire field of psychopharmacology is suffering from a lack of breakthrough models for the treatment of mental illness. Much of the enthusiasm for a psychedelic renaissance is forward facing and often deliberately ignores or rejects a more nuanced history that might reveal a more complex past that decenters American activities, whether scientific inquiry or "Leary-ism," and also might point to complicated challenges ahead. This collection confronts a longer and more diverse array of histories that take psychedelics beyond the realms of science and medicine and embed them in cultural phenomena.

Over the past years, several historians have enriched our knowledge about psychedelic history, but very few have considered its global dimension or examined the way that research teams and sociocultural networks have shared knowledge and resources between them transnationally.[11] More recently, others have moved away from North America,[12] but the overwhelming focus has remained on Euro-American historical developments, which are largely framed within Western models of science, religion, and culture.[13] Earlier historical literature on psychedelics created an image of psychedelia as a product of the Cold War, a story of experiments associated with mind control and covert drug testing,[14] and naturally established the US as the main focal point. While this book acknowledges the impact of Cold War mentalities on psychiatric research, it moves beyond the US-dominated narrative of CIA operatives using psychedelics as interrogation tools and mass-incapacitating compounds. Instead, it considers how this period of heightened ideological conflict influenced scientific research and intellectual exchanges across geopolitical borders.

In this way, our collection examines multiple regions and looks at different social, cultural, and scientific histories. It explores how various psychedelic cultures have developed and coexisted, and the authors scrutinize how ideas have moved between spaces and how experiments evolved out of different cultural and political contexts, while also considering how several psychedelic encounters ultimately cohered around shared ideas of consciousness-raising experiences that bring benefits. The language of benefit is not always shared, as it is parsed into medical, cultural, and spiritual discourses, but the human interest in psychedelics and what they represent as tools, teachers, or spiritual guides is part of an enduring quest for mental clarity that has historically operated at the intersection of science, spirituality, politics, and culture.

The rest of this book considers psychedelics in Africa, Asia, the Middle East, Europe, and North and South America. The chapters coalesce around a discrete set of substances that introduced new terminologies, methodologies, and expressions, stretching from ancient ideas in India through the colonial botanical extractions in the nineteenth century and concentrating on twentieth-century developments in botany, science, philosophy, and culture.

Most of these chapters are situated in the postwar period, during the golden age of pharmacology,[15] during which psychedelics emerged as a new category of promising psychoactive compounds in Western clinical science. This moment coincides with the emergence of transnational social movements, and we suggest that the rising enthusiasm for psychedelic research during the Cold War is not coincidental. This period is critical for understanding major shifts in power on an international and interdisciplinary scale.

The relationship between psychedelic experiences and intellectual breakthroughs has been widely known for some major figures, including the philosopher Jean-Paul Sartre's mescaline trip, the writer Aldous Huxley's many psychedelic experiments, and the maverick psychiatrist R. D. Laing's LSD trials in the 1970s, after psychedelic drugs had more or less fallen out of respectability. In 2019, Simeon Wade even revealed that Michel Foucault had enjoyed LSD in 1975 during a trip to California.[16] Far beyond the ivory towers, the introduction of psychedelics into mainstream culture coincided with a number of significant cultural and political shifts in power: a baby boom in the West, crumbling empires, and challenges leveled at colonial structures, whether expressed as independence in African nation-states or ideological coalitions in the Soviet bloc. These dramatic power shifts on the international stage set the course for domestic activism, such as labor strikes in Europe, feminist and gay liberation marches in North America, and environmental activism in South America. A global reckoning of a burgeoning set of social movements was poised to challenge the existing order of things, whether in the workplace, in the bedroom, or at the United Nations. Psychedelics did not cause this moment, of course, but they have been indelibly woven into this history either as culprits or stimulants for exercising new expressions of power and realigning identities away from older, traditional forms of power.

By paying closer attention to these dimensions, this collection makes broad inquiries into the psychedelic past of several countries, but it is also interested in moments of transnational and transcultural contacts, such as the way that Western science has interacted with Indigenous plant medicines and cultural knowledge specific to particular regions. In this way, some of the following chapters examine networks of psychedelic knowledge, some of which operate in shared linguistic and disciplinary spaces, and others that challenge our understanding of mainstream knowledge and scientific evidence. Some authors examine ideas that place Indigenous and local knowledge alongside Western science and the way that some healing frameworks inspired Western scientists who encountered foreign rituals and struggled to make sense of them.

More broadly, some of these chapters illustrate how psychedelics freely circulated through transnational networks, but they also reveal that they were not confined to the clinic or the academy. In many instances, several influential individuals had life-changing experiences with these drugs, and they used these insights to fuel a decidedly rebellious or revolutionary outlook on the world around them. These understandings rarely, if ever, stayed confined within state borders, and in some cases they could influence like-minded communities in other parts of the globe. By adopting such a perspective, this book adds to the histories of how countercultural and radical leftist groups regularly benefited from each other during transnational moments of cooperation and exchange.[17]

With the emphasis on the international circulation of radical psychedelia, and by moving away from Leary and the US, this book also advances a bold proposition: there was an international movement to promote psychedelics as the cure for the ills of humanity if they were freely distributed to everyone.[18] While the American side of this movement is now well documented,[19] we hope that some of the chapters in this book will make a case for a psychedelic movement beyond borders, and that subsequent historical inquiries will strengthen this idea. In this particular instance, it appears that Leary's influence extended beyond his country, and as a writer and figure of international prominence, he might appear in various countercultural locations; but in no way did that make him the leader of such a movement. What transpires instead is that Huxley's early essays, which were translated into dozens of languages, formed the early basis for an international psychedelic culture that occasionally used a more radical rhetoric of psychedelic revolution.

Before offering an overview of the collection, we would like to stress that this book does not have the ambition of being comprehensive. By shifting focus away from North America, we have brought together several histories set in Europe, and this should not come as a surprise, given that that continent has hosted a great deal of scientific research into psychedelics, which quickly spilled into intellectual, artistic, and countercultural settings. However, we compensate for this somewhat lopsided focus by introducing original topics and approaches, including moments of transnational history. But we were unable to gather contributions examining psychedelic history in Pacific countries like Australia and Japan, so this book only touches upon ethnohistory in some rare instances and does not feature in-depth accounts from Indigenous people. This book is a starting point for a global history of psychedelics, and we hope that it will help stimulate future research.

The chapters in this book highlight the exchange of ideas, people, and substances, revealing a fluid history of psychedelics that has stretched around the globe. National and regional priorities continue to shape how psychedelics have moved through space and across time, but our authors show that these boundaries are porous. This collection emphasizes regional differences to underscore diverse ways of thinking about psychedelics and how those ideas have shaped this past in significant and subtle ways. While we do not offer a direct comparison with histories in North America, our authors help us better appreciate how the local specificity of psychedelic experiments generated their own cultural expressions in various contexts, where the influence of the US may have loomed large or where colonial empires and European networks exerted more subtle influences on the local reception of psychedelics in botanical and pharmaceutical pursuits.

Beyond the contributions to global and transnational history, this collection breaks new ground by adopting perspectives currently lacking in the historiography of psychedelics. Historical inquiries into psychedelic science have dominated the scholarship, and the early literature was mostly concerned with chronicling postwar research into LSD and mescaline,[20] while other historians became interested in the way that these drugs influenced society and culture.[21] Others have broadened our understanding of psychedelic history still more through original perspectives like spirituality,[22] creativity,[23] native-newcomer relations,[24] music,[25] architecture,[26] and visual arts.[27] The rest of this book adds to this burgeoning field by offering important discussions on hitherto underexplored or untouched topics such as gender, agriculture, parapsychology, anarchism, and technological innovations.

Our book is divided into three parts: "Evaluating Evidence/Experience"; "Global Networks of Psychedelic Knowledge"; and "Psychedelics as Cultural Phenomena." In many cases, chapters could fit into all three parts, but we group them in the way we chose to encourage subtle comparisons across different settings. The first part pulls readers behind the scenes into a variety of locations that are shaped by different ideological and cultural priorities. The part opens with chapter 1, by Ian Baker, who transports us in time and place in an ethnohistorical account of *soma*. Interrogating the edges of religion, ritual, and philosophy, where psychedelics are concerned, Baker anchors his study into a highly personalized account of historical intrigue and a search for consciousness guided by Eastern philosophy. He aptly reminds readers that this quest for mind alteration is deeply rooted in ancient traditions, spiritual explorations, and an abiding curiosity for seeking deeper truths.

Following Baker's lead, Gautier Dassonneville in chapter 2 reveals another layer in this history of mind alteration and depicts an understanding of plants, consciousness, and the human condition, as attempted by French philosophers. Dassonneville walks readers through Jean-Paul Sartre's flirtations with mescaline, and in so doing illuminates a botanical knowledge network that informed Sartre's and Simone de Beauvoir's phenomenological explorations into French philosophy. In chapter 3, Zoë Dubus retains our focus on France and the famous Sainte-Anne Hospital, where chlorpromazine—hailed as one of the blockbuster pharmacological introductions of the twentieth century—was first discovered. She shows readers that chlorpromazine was not the only drug being experimented with at this facility, and indeed, that story has overwhelmed the history of LSD research taking place at the same time. By looking closely at patient files and hospital records, Dubus highlights the subtleties and idiosyncrasies in this experimental context that revealed differences in how gender and class were interpreted in the psychiatric and psychedelic research environment, while simultaneously placing France on the map for psychedelic research in this moment.

While psychedelic research in France has received very little scholarly attention, Czechoslovakia had been identified as a major site of LSD activity during the Cold War. Ross Crockford's detailed study of LSD behind the Iron Curtain in chapter 4 illuminates subtle differences in how patients were diagnosed in communist-era Czechoslovakia, as well as how psychedelics were adapted to suit particular ideological principles of what constituted pathological behavior. Meanwhile in the UK, the psychiatrist Ronald Sandison was trying to carve out his own place in Western psychedelic psychiatry, as Wendy Kline examines in chapter 5. Reluctant to go along with trends in Canada and the US, Sandison, working at Powick Hospital in Worcestershire, tried to forge his own ideas about psycholytics and how to test, describe, and apply hallucinogens in a psychiatric setting.

But if Sandison was attempting to forge his own path with hallucinogens, researchers in Switzerland had a competitive edge. In chapter 6, Magaly Tornay takes us to the birthplace of LSD in the 1940s and examines how Swiss psychiatrists applied this new hallucinogen, synthesized from ergot, in a region already famous for psychiatric research and cutting-edge pharmacological experimentation. And, as Tornay shows, psychedelics had an appeal that quickly moved beyond the realm of scientific inquiry.

Part II traces global networks of knowledge, reinforcing the idea that psychedelics have diverse roots and both substances and ideas have transgressed political boundaries. Timmy Vilgiate initiates this discussion in chapter 7, beginning with botanical explorations in the nineteenth century where Westerners stumbled across sacred plants but overlooked their meaning since they could not imagine a ready-made commercial opportunity. In a clash of colonial economics with an ignorance of local flora and fauna, he shows how ibogaine was somewhat late to join the psychedelic lexicon despite knowledge of its presence in colonial Africa for over 100 years. Julien Bonhomme's discussion in chapter 8 responds to that historical context by showing how ibogaine became part of Western approaches to psychedelic medicine in the 1950s as a treatment for addiction. He explains that ibogaine, a plant that mainly grows in Gabon, found its way into clinics in Europe and North America as psychiatrists in these places theorized its use while excising it from its cultural and botanical roots.

The agricultural and botanical knowledge has long fed the international pursuit of plant-based substances, medicinal and otherwise. In chapter 9,

Beat Bächi tackles this agricultural-pharmaceutical complex directly in a deft analysis of ergot production in Switzerland, and he explains how it became part of a Swiss pharmaceutical campaign to harness its psychoactive properties in the midst of a looming food crisis. He shows that psychedelics in the context of agriculture were linked to a range of international and ideological priorities that intersected after World War II, related to a ballooning pharmaceutical industry and a desire to invest in a green revolution amid heighted neo-Malthusian concerns about global food shortages. Switzerland was uniquely poised to inherit some of the German advances in agri-biotech and pharmaceutical industries after German facilities were bombed during the war. Swiss firms seized this competitive advantage, but they did not stop there. He shows that Sandoz, the manufacturer of LSD, and Albert Hofmann, its discoverer, used this position to explore new botanical environments, including those in Mexico, where chemists encountered psilocybe mushrooms.

In the twenty-first century, South American destinations have cropped up as spaces for psychedelic tourism, but in chapter 10, authors Hernan Scholten and Gonzalo Salas show us that in 1950s Spanish-speaking South America, psychiatrists and researchers were more inclined to look to North America for guidance on how to study psychedelics. In a review of publications in Chile, Argentina, Colombia, Uruguay, and Ecuador, Scholten and Salas examine how Latin American researchers responded to developments in psychedelic psychiatry and how other influences, notably from North America, shaped how psychedelics were understood and applied in South America. Meanwhile, in chapter 11, Vincent Verroust complicates the idea that Western ideas also flowed south and into unconventional ways of thinking. He explores the French biologist Roger Heim's interest in hallucination-causing mushrooms. Unlike Hofmann, who was interested in their pharmacological and psychoactive properties, Heim became fascinated by the way that mushrooms seemed to open up new divinatory insights, and he stepped well outside his regional and disciplinary boundaries to incorporate insights from parapsychologists, mycologists, and spiritualists in an effort to understand the wide-reaching applications of psychedelics, especially mushrooms.

On the other side of that spiritual coin, in chapter 12, Andrew Jones follows the trajectory of the Christian missionary Florence Nichols, whose work took her to Canada, India, and England in a spiritual quest to heal, a journey that ultimately led her to psychedelics. Blending missionary principles with a cognitive lust for consciousness and healing, Jones reveals a story in which travel, gender, and Christian spirituality blend into an examination of a young woman's journey to understand religion and pathology in her own psychedelic adventure. The final chapter in this part explores another dimension of psychedelic thinking, this time focusing on how psychedelics came to radicalize political movements anchored in the UK but fed from abroad. In chapter 13, Hallam Roffey shows us that British communes and political leaders wrestled with how to incorporate psychedelics into political movements on the left, particularly as these drugs moved into criminal categories in the 1970s.

The last part of this collection features essays that explore how psychedelics have been used to push cultural boundaries or to enhance creativity—whether in the clinic or in society. Peter Collopy opens this discussion in chapter 14 with a vibrant examination of psychedelics at the intersection of technology and visual art. Taking readers through the emergence of Silicon Valley, he shows how psychedelics appealed to engineers and artists interested in transforming visual art and expression, and how they influenced artists working with a new invention—the portable video camera. Bringing us back into the clinic in chapter 15, Stephen Snelders shows us how Dutch psychiatrists in the 1950s and 1960s drew inspiration from a variety of psychedelic research concepts before developing another application through the figure of Jan Bastiaans. Bastiaans's unique use of psychedelics for treating trauma opened up new channels of psychiatric theories about trauma and how to treat it. Despite this particular application, Snelders shows that psychedelic studies attracted volunteers who later moved LSD beyond clinical applications, drawing influence from other Western researchers and challenging the idea that LSD causes a model psychosis, with limited clinical application, in pursuit of an understanding of LSD as a more powerful tool for exploring consciousness that defies linguistic and political differences.

Those themes continue in Henrique Carneiro and Julio Delmanto's study of LSD in Brazil in chapter 16. Here too, the authors examine how LSD moved from the clinic to the streets, but this time in the context of a Brazilian dictatorship that is heavily influenced by American political ideas on drug policy and left-leaning activism. Carneiro and Delmanto highlight how the perhaps-familiar trajectory of LSD from the clinic to the streets played out in a very different political context when it comes to understanding the impact of psychedelics in fuelling social and political activism in 1960s Brazil. Meanwhile, in chapter 17, Ido Hartogsohn and Itamar Zadoff take these ideas to yet another region, in Israel, exploring how psychedelics moved from medical spaces into Israeli society and culture in the 1960s. American influences once again loom large here, but Israel is a different site for cultural and political contests over nationalism, militarism, and religious pilgrimages. Hartogsohn and Zadoff examine literary, musical, and artistic expressions of an Israeli bohemia that blended outside influences with hashish, psychedelics, and trance music scenes. They show how Israel became a cultural destination for American psychedelic leaders, who recognized Israel as a cultural trading zone for Eastern and Western ideas. Rather than explore this environment through the eyes of Timothy Leary or Allen Ginsberg, Hartogsohn and Zadoff situate the emergence of an independent Israeli psychedelic scene within the history of the region.

In chapter 18, Mark Gallagher retains our focus on some of the medicopolitical contexts in which psychedelics were studied, and indeed, contexts that psychedelics themselves were reforming. In his examination of experiments in Britain's Kingsley Hall, Gallagher brings politics and psychiatry together through figures like R. D. Laing and Robin Farquharson, whose interest in psychedelics dovetailed with anti-psychiatry sentiments. Here, psychedelics became part of a political experiment, and Gallagher urges us to question concepts of liberalism, communism, and libertarianism by tracing how some participants adopted psychedelics as a means of enhancing political ideas.

Then, in chapter 19, Alex Gearin moves us forward in space and time, arriving at a perhaps unlikely location for ayahuasca ceremonies: downtown in a major city in China. He shows us another set of transnational exchanges of ideas, psychedelic substances, and Indigenous philosophies. However, it went far beyond simply importing a foreign practice into China. Gearin highlights the cultural significance of bringing ayahuasca and Indigenous knowledge into a hyperurban space, one with strong antidrug policies, as a feature of confronting alienation and improving efficiency for Chinese business elites. Finally, chapter 20 takes us to Pakistan, where Manal Khan explores how psychedelics intersect with expressions of gender, feminist activism, and queer identity in a patriarchal society shaped by Islamic and colonial forces. In a forward-looking inquiry, she reminds us of the generative qualities of psychedelic experiences that blend therapy with personal discovery in an intimate exploration of queer identities. These studies, like Baker's opening chapter, remind us that psychedelics have long represented a historical desire to tap into an unquenched curiosity about consciousness and belonging that are often inspired by these drugs, their associated rituals (whether clinical or spiritual), and their potential to change minds.

NOTES

1. Ed Prideaux, "Timothy Leary Turns 100: America's LSD Messiah, Remembered by Those Who Knew Him," *Vice*, October 23, 2020. https://www.vice.com/en/article/epdg3k/timothy -leary-lsd-acid-history.

2. Robert Greenfield, *Timothy Leary: A Biography* (Orlando, FL: Harcourt, 2006); John Higgs, *I Have America Surrounded: The Life of Timothy Leary* (Fort Lee, NJ: Barricade Books, 2006).

3. Matthew Oram, *The Trials of Psychedelic Therapy: LSD Psychotherapy in America* (Baltimore: Johns Hopkins University Press, 2018); Ido Hartogsohn, *American Trip: Set, Setting, and the Psychedelic Experience in the Twentieth Century* (Cambridge, MA: MIT Press, 2020).

4. Martin A. Lee and Bruce Shlain, *Acid Dreams: The Complete Social History of LSD: The CIA, the Sixties, and Beyond* (New York: Grove Weidenfeld, 1985); Alexander S. Dawson, *The Peyote Effect: From the Inquisition to the War on Drugs* (Oakland: University of California Press, 2018).

5. Oram, *The Trials of Psychedelic Therapy*.

6. Leigh A. Henderson and William J. Glass, eds., *LSD: Still with Us after All These Years* (New York: Maxwell Macmillan International, 1994); Morgan Shipley, "'This Season's People': Stephen Gaskin, Psychedelic Religion, and a Community of Social Justice," *Journal for the Study of Radicalism* 9, no. 2 (2015): 41–92; Jesse Jarnow, *Heads: A Biography of Psychedelic America* (Philadelphia: Da Capo Press, 2016); J. C. Greer, Angel-Headed Hipsters: Psychedelic Militancy in Nineteen-Eighties North America (PhD diss., University of Amsterdam, 2020).

7. Chris Elcock, "From Acid Revolution to Entheogenic Evolution: Psychedelic Philosophy in the Sixties and Beyond," *Journal of American Culture* 36, no. 4 (2013): 296–311.

8. Jill Jonnes, *Hep-Cats, Narcs, and Pipe Dreams: A History of America's Romance with Illegal Drugs* (New York: Scribner, 1996); Camille Paglia, "Cults and Cosmic Consciousness: Religious Vision in the American 1960s," *Arion* 10, no. 3 (January 1, 2003): 57–111; Gerard DeGroot, *The Sixties Unplugged: A Kaleidoscopic History of a Disorderly Decade* (London: Pan, 2009).

9. Erika Dyck, *Psychedelic Psychiatry: LSD from Clinic to Campus* (Baltimore: Johns Hopkins University Press, 2008); Marcel Martel, "Setting Boundaries: LSD Use and Glue Sniffing in Ontario in the 1960s," in *The Real Dope: Social, Legal, and Historical Perspectives on the Regulation of Drugs in Canada*, ed. Edgar-André Montigny (Toronto: University of Toronto Press, 2011), 197–218; Erika Dyck and Tolly Bradford, "Peyote on the Prairies: Religion, Scientists, and Native-Newcomer Relations in Western Canada," *Journal of Canadian Studies/ Revue d'études Canadiennes* 46, no. 1 (2012): 28–52; Patrick Barber, *Psychedelic Revolutionaries: Three Medical Pioneers, the Fall of Hallucinogenic Research and the Rise of Big Pharma* (London: Zed Books, 2019); Jesse Donaldson and Erika Dyck, *The Acid Room: The Psychedelic Trials and Tribulations of Hollywood Hospital* (Vancouver: Anvil Press, 2022).

10. Nicolas Langlitz, *Neuropsychedelia: The Revival of Hallucinogen Research since the Decade of the Brain* (Berkeley: University of California Press, 2013); Ben Sessa, *The Psychedelic Renaissance: Reassessing the Role of Psychedelic Drugs in 21st Century Psychiatry and Society* (London: Muswell Hill Press, 2012); Michael Pollan, *How to Change Your Mind: What the New Science of Psychedelics Teaches Us about Consciousness, Dying, Addiction, Depression, and Transcendence* (New York: Penguin Press, 2018).

11. An outstanding exception to this trend is Nicholas Schou's fascinating account of an international network of LSD, marijuana, and hashish dealers. See *Orange Sunshine: The Brotherhood of Eternal Love and Its Quest to Spread Peace, Love, and Acid to the World* (New York: Thomas Dunne Books, 2010).

12. Stephen Snelders and Charles Kaplan, "LSD Therapy in Dutch Psychiatry: Changing Socio-Political Settings and Medical Sets," *Medical History* 46, no. 2 (2002): 221–240; Sarah Marks, "From Experimental Psychosis to Resolving Traumatic Pasts. Psychedelic Research in Communist Czechoslovakia, 1954–1974," *Cahiers du Monde Russe* 56, no. 1 (2015): 53–75; Zoë Dubus, "Utiliser les psychédéliques pour 'guérir' des adolescents homosexuels? Essai de thérapie de conversion, France, 1960," *Annales Médico-psychologiques, revue psychiatrique* 178, no. 6 (2020): 650–656; Petter Grahl Johnstad, "A Dangerous Method? Psychedelic Therapy at Modum Bad, Norway, 1961–1976," *History of Psychiatry* 31, no. 2 (2020): 217–226; Beat Bächi, *LSD auf dem Land: Produktion und kollektive Wirkung psychotroper Stoffe* (Konstanz, Germany: Konstanz University Press, 2020). In addition, some collections include a range of authors, primarily anthropologists, who publish in English and whose writings are often based on fieldwork in Spanish and Portuguese-speaking communities. See Beatriz Caiuby Labate, Clancy Cavnar, and Alex K. Gearin, eds., *The World Ayahuasca Diaspora: Reinventions and Controversies* (London: Routledge, 2017); Beatriz Caiuby Labate and Clancy Cavnar, eds., *Peyote: History, Traditions, Politics, and Conservation* (Santa Barbara, CA: ABC-Clio/Praeger, 2016).

13. There is even less scholarship about psychedelics in Asia, and it tends to recount interactions with Western actors rather than exploring Asian contexts explicitly. For example, see Yoshihiro Matsushima, Fumio Eguchi, Tadahiro Kikukawa and Takahide Matsuda, "Historical Overview of Psychoactive Mushrooms," *Information and Regeneration* 29, no. 1 (2009): 47–58.

14. Lee and Shlain, *Acid Dreams*; John Marks, *The Search for the "Manchurian Candidate"* (New York: Norton, 1991).

15. David Healy, *The Creation of Psychopharmacology* (Cambridge, MA: London: Harvard University Press, 2004); Harry M. Marks, *The Progress of Experiment: Science and Therapeutic Reform in the United States, 1900–1990* (Cambridge: Cambridge University Press, 2000).

16. Simeon Wade, *Foucault in California: [A True Story—Wherein the Great French Philosophy Drops Acid in the Valley of Death]* (Berkeley, CA: Heyday, 2019).

17. Eric Zolov, *Refried Elvis: The Rise of the Mexican Counterculture* (Berkeley: University of California Press, 1999); Jeremi Suri, "AHR Forum The Rise and Fall of an International Counterculture, 1960–1975," *American Historical Review* 114, no. 1 (2009): 45–68; Lindsey Blake Churchill, *Becoming the Tupamaros: Solidarity and Transnational Revolutionaries in Uruguay and the United States* (Nashville: Vanderbilt University Press, 2014); Patrick Barr-Melej, *Psychedelic Chile: Youth, Counterculture, and Politics on the Road to Socialism and Dictatorship* (Chapel Hill: University of North Carolina Press, 2017).

18. A fitting illustration of such an international movement can be found in Schou's *Orange Sunshine.*

19. Also see the aforementioned biographies by Greenfield and Higgs, as well as Devin R. Lander, "Start Your Own Religion: New York State's Acid Churches," *Nova Religio: The Journal of Alternative and Emergent Religions* 14, no. 3 (February 1, 2011): 64–80; Elcock, "From Acid Revolution to Entheogenic Evolution"; Devin R. Lander, "'Legalize Spiritual Discovery': The Trials of Dr. Timothy Leary," in *Prohibition, Religious Freedom, and Human Rights: Regulating Traditional Drug Use*, ed. Beatriz Caiuby Labate and Clancy Cavnar (Heidelberg, Germany, and New York: Springer, 2014), 165–187; Chris Elcock, "The Fifth Freedom: The Politics of Psychedelic Patriotism," *Journal for the Study of Radicalism* 9, no. 2 (2015): 17–40.

20. Steven J. Novak, "LSD before Leary: Sidney Cohen's Critique of 1950s Psychedelic Drug Research," *Isis* 88, no. 1 (1997): 87–110; Dyck, *Psychedelic Psychiatry.*

21. Lee and Shlain, *Acid Dreams*; David Farber, "The Intoxicated/Illegal Nation: Drugs in the Sixties Counterculture," in *Imagine Nation: The American Counterculture of the 1960s and '70s*, ed. Peter Braunstein and Michael William Doyle (New York: Routledge, 2002), 17–40; Andy Roberts, *Albion Dreaming: A Popular History of LSD in Britain* (London: Marshall Cavendish, 2008).

22. Robert C. Fuller, *Stairways to Heaven: Drugs in American Religious History* (Boulder, CO: Westview Press, 2000); Lander, "Start Your Own Religion,"; Morgan Shipley, *Psychedelic Mysticism: Transforming Consciousness, Religious Experiences, and Voluntary Peasants in Postwar America* (Lanham, MD: Lexington Books, 2015).

23. Milana Aronov, "(Micro-) 'Psychedelic' Experiences: From the 1960s Creativity at the Workplace to the 21st Century Neuro-Newspeak," *Ethnologie Française* 176, no. 4 (October 1, 2019): 701–718, https://doi.org/10.3917/ethn.194.0701.

24. Dyck and Bradford, "Peyote on the Prairies"; Alexander S. Dawson, "Salvador Roquet, Maria Sabina, and the Trouble with Jipis," *Hispanic American Historical Review* 95, no. 1 (2015): 103–133, https://doi.org/10.1215/00182168-2836928.

25. Nicholas Knowles Bromell, *Tomorrow Never Knows: Rock and Psychedelics in the 1960s* (Chicago: University of Chicago Press, 2000).

26. Alastair Gordon, *Spaced Out: Radical Environments of the Psychedelic Sixties* (New York: Rizzoli, 2008); Erika Dyck, "Spaced-out in Saskatchewan: Modernism, Anti-Psychiatry, and Deinstitutionalization, 1950–1968," *Bulletin of the History of Medicine* 84, no. 4 (2010): 640–666, https://doi.org/10.1353/bhm.2010.0041.

27. Scott B. Montgomery, "Radical Trips: Exploring the Political Dimension and Context of the 1960s Psychedelic Poster," *Journal for the Study of Radicalism* 13, no. 1 (2019): 121–54, https://doi.org/10.14321/jstudradi.13.1.0121.

BIBLIOGRAPHY

Aronov, Milana. "(Micro-) 'Psychedelic' Experiences: From the 1960s Creativity at the Workplace to the 21st Century Neuro-Newspeak." *Ethnologie Française* 176, no. 4 (October 2019): 701–718. https://doi.org/10.3917/ethn.194.0701.

Bächi, Beat. *LSD auf dem Land: Produktion und kollektive Wirkung psychotroper Stoffe.* Konstanz, Germany: Konstanz University Press, 2020.

Barber, Patrick. *Psychedelic Revolutionaries: Three Medical Pioneers, the Fall of Hallucinogenic Research and the Rise of Big Pharma.* London: Zed Books, 2019.

Barr-Melej, Patrick. *Psychedelic Chile: Youth, Counterculture, and Politics on the Road to Socialism and Dictatorship.* Chapel Hill: University of North Carolina Press, 2017.

Bromell, Nicholas Knowles. *Tomorrow Never Knows: Rock and Psychedelics in the 1960s.* Chicago: University of Chicago Press, 2000.

Churchill, Lindsey Blake. *Becoming the Tupamaros: Solidarity and Transnational Revolutionaries in Uruguay and the United States.* Nashville: Vanderbilt University Press, 2014.

Dawson, Alexander S. *The Peyote Effect: From the Inquisition to the War on Drugs.* Oakland: University of California Press, 2018.

Dawson, Alexander S. "Salvador Roquet, Maria Sabina, and the Trouble with Jipis." *Hispanic American Historical Review* 95, no. 1 (2015): 103–133. https://doi.org/10.1215/00182168-2836928.

DeGroot, Gerard. *The Sixties Unplugged: A Kaleidoscopic History of a Disorderly Decade.* London: Pan, 2009.

Donaldson, Jesse, and Erika Dyck. *The Acid Room: The Psychedelic Trials and Tribulations of Hollywood Hospital.* Vancouver: Anvil Press, 2022.

Dubus, Zoë. "Utiliser les psychédéliques pour 'guérir' des adolescents homosexuels? Essai de thérapie de conversion, France, 1960." *Annales Médico-psychologiques, revue psychiatrique* 178, no. 6 (2020): 650–656.

Dyck, Erika. *Psychedelic Psychiatry: LSD from Clinic to Campus.* Baltimore: Johns Hopkins University Press, 2008.

Dyck, Erika. "Spaced-out in Saskatchewan: Modernism, Anti-Psychiatry, and Deinstitutionalization, 1950–1968." *Bulletin of the History of Medicine* 84, no. 4 (2010): 640–666. https://doi.org/10.1353/bhm.2010.0041.

Dyck, Erika, and Tolly Bradford. "Peyote on the Prairies: Religion, Scientists, and Native-Newcomer Relations in Western Canada." *Journal of Canadian Studies/Revue d'études Canadiennes* 46, no. 1 (2012): 28–52.

Elcock, Chris. "From Acid Revolution to Entheogenic Evolution: Psychedelic Philosophy in the Sixties and Beyond." *Journal of American Culture* 36, no. 4 (2013): 296–311.

Elcock, Chris. "The Fifth Freedom: The Politics of Psychedelic Patriotism." *Journal for the Study of Radicalism* 9, no. 2 (2015): 17–40.

Farber, David. "The Intoxicated/Illegal Nation: Drugs in the Sixties Counterculture." In *Imagine Nation: The American Counterculture of the 1960s and '70s*, edited by Peter Braunstein and Michael William Doyle, 17–40. New York: Routledge, 2002.

Fuller, Robert C. *Stairways to Heaven: Drugs in American Religious History*. Boulder, CO: Westview Press, 2000.

Gordon, Alastair. *Spaced Out: Radical Environments of the Psychedelic Sixties*. New York: Rizzoli, 2008.

Greenfield, Robert. *Timothy Leary: A Biography*. Orlando, FL: Harcourt, 2006.

Greer, J. C. Angel-Headed Hipsters: Psychedelic Militancy in Nineteen-Eighties North America. PhD diss., University of Amsterdam, 2020.

Hartogsohn, Ido. *American Trip: Set, Setting, and the Psychedelic Experience in the Twentieth Century*. Cambridge, MA: MIT Press, 2020.

Healy, David. *The Creation of Psychopharmacology*. Cambridge, MA: Harvard University Press, 2004.

Henderson, Leigh A., and William J. Glass, eds. *LSD: Still with Us after All These Years*. New York: Maxwell Macmillan International, 1994.

Higgs, John. *I Have America Surrounded: The Life of Timothy Leary*. Fort Lee, NJ: Barricade Books, 2006.

Jarnow, Jesse. *Heads: A Biography of Psychedelic America*. Philadelphia: Da Capo Press, 2016.

Johnstad, Petter Grahl. "A Dangerous Method? Psychedelic Therapy at Modum Bad, Norway, 1961–1976." *History of Psychiatry* 31, no. 2 (2020): 217–226.

Jonnes, Jill. *Hep-Cats, Narcs, and Pipe Dreams: A History of America's Romance with Illegal Drugs*. New York: Scribner, 1996.

Labate, Beatriz Caiuby, and Clancy Cavnar, eds. *Peyote: History, Traditions, Politics, and Conservation*. Santa Barbara, CA: ABC-Clio/Praeger, 2016.

Labate, Beatriz Caiuby, Clancy Cavnar, and Alex K. Gearin, eds. *The World Ayahuasca Diaspora: Reinventions and Controversies*. London: Routledge, 2017.

Lander, Devin R. "'Legalize Spiritual Discovery': The Trials of Dr. Timothy Leary." In *Prohibition, Religious Freedom, and Human Rights: Regulating Traditional Drug Use*, edited by Beatriz Caiuby Labate and Clancy Cavnar, 165–187. Heidelberg, Germany, and New York: Springer, 2014.

Lander, Devin R. "Start Your Own Religion: New York State's Acid Churches." *Nova Religio: The Journal of Alternative and Emergent Religions* 14, no. 3 (February 2011): 64–80. https://doi.org /10.1525/nr.2011.14.3.64.

Langlitz, Nicolas. *Neuropsychedelia: The Revival of Hallucinogen Research since the Decade of the Brain*. Berkeley: University of California Press, 2013.

Lee, Martin A., and Bruce Shlain. *Acid Dreams: The Complete Social History of LSD: The CIA, the Sixties, and Beyond*. New York: Grove Weidenfeld, 1985.

Marks, Harry M. *The Progress of Experiment: Science and Therapeutic Reform in the United States, 1900–1990*. Cambridge: Cambridge University Press, 2000.

Marks, John, and Geheimdienst-und Terrorismusexperte. *The Search for the "Manchurian Candidate."* New York: W. W. Norton, 1991.

Marks, Sarah. "From Experimental Psychosis to Resolving Traumatic Pasts. Psychedelic Research in Communist Czechoslovakia, 1954–1974." *Cahiers du Monde Russe* 56, no. 1 (2015): 53–75.

Martel, Marcel. "Setting Boundaries: LSD Use and Glue Sniffing in Ontario in the 1960s." In *The Real Dope: Social, Legal, and Historical Perspectives on the Regulation of Drugs in Canada*, edited by Edgar-André Montigny, 197–218. Toronto: University of Toronto Press, 2011.

Matsushima, Yoshihiro, Fumio Eguchi, Tadahiro Kikukawa, and Takahide Matsuda. "Historical Overview of Psychoactive Mushrooms." *Information and Regeneration* 29, no. 1 (2009): 47–58.

Montgomery, Scott B. "Radical Trips: Exploring the Political Dimension and Context of the 1960s Psychedelic Poster." *Journal for the Study of Radicalism* 13, no. 1 (2019): 121–154. https://doi.org /10.14321/jstudradi.13.1.0121.

Novak, Steven J. "LSD before Leary: Sidney Cohen's Critique of 1950s Psychedelic Drug Research." *Isis* 88, no. 1 (1997): 87–110.

Oram, Matthew. *The Trials of Psychedelic Therapy: LSD Psychotherapy in America*. Baltimore: Johns Hopkins University Press, 2018.

Paglia, Camille. "Cults and Cosmic Consciousness: Religious Vision in the American 1960s." *Arion* 10, no. 3 (January 1, 2003): 57–111.

Pollan, Michael. *How to Change Your Mind: What the New Science of Psychedelics Teaches Us about Consciousness, Dying, Addiction, Depression, and Transcendence*. New York: Penguin Press, 2018.

Prideaux, Ed. "Timothy Leary Turns 100: America's LSD Messiah, Remembered by Those Who Knew Him." *Vice* (October 2020). https://www.vice.com/en/article/epdg3k/timothy-leary-lsd -acid-history. Accessed January 19, 2023

Roberts, Andy. *Albion Dreaming: A Popular History of LSD in Britain*. London: Marshall Cavendish, 2008.

Schou, Nicholas. *Orange Sunshine: The Brotherhood of Eternal Love and Its Quest to Spread Peace, Love, and Acid to the World.* New York: St Martin's Press, 2010.

Sessa, Ben. *The Psychedelic Renaissance: Reassessing the Role of Psychedelic Drugs in 21st Century Psychiatry and Society.* London: Muswell Hill Press, 2012.

Shipley, Morgan. *Psychedelic Mysticism: Transforming Consciousness, Religious Experiences, and Voluntary Peasants in Postwar America.* Lanham, MD: Lexington Books, 2015.

Shipley, Morgan. "'This Season's People': Stephen Gaskin, Psychedelic Religion, and a Community of Social Justice." *Journal for the Study of Radicalism* 9, no. 2 (2015): 41–92.

Snelders, Stephen, and Charles Kaplan. "LSD Therapy in Dutch Psychiatry: Changing Socio-Political Settings and Medical Sets." *Medical History* 46, no. 2 (2002): 221–240.

Suri, Jeremi. "AHR Forum: The Rise and Fall of an International Counterculture, 1960–1975." *American Historical Review* 114, no. 1 (2009): 45–68.

Wade, Simeon. *Foucault in California: [A True Story—Wherein the Great French Philosophy Drops Acid in the Valley of Death].* Berkeley, CA: Heyday, 2019.

Zolov, Eric. *Refried Elvis: The Rise of the Mexican Counterculture.* Berkeley: University of California Press, 1999.

I EVALUATING EVIDENCE/EXPERIENCE

In this part, the authors peel back some of the common assumptions about the history of psychedelic research by transporting us into different kinds of experimental settings, reminding us that there are many ways to interpret psychedelic origin stories and that experience matters. Driven by personal and clinical curiosity, hallucinogenic experiences and the quest for nonordinary states of consciousness have attracted thinkers and scholars across disciplinary, linguistic, religious, ideological, and therapeutic traditions. Evidence generated from psychedelics has often had a very personalized quality, making it intimate and difficult to describe in a meaningful way. These challenges have long complicated the categorization of psychedelic experiences. Are these medicines harnessed to treat deficiencies or pathological conditions? Should psychedelics be reserved for spiritual encounters, often separated from medicinal applications? Are these mind-altering experiences indeed windows into other ways of thinking, better suited for creative pursuits permitting insights into different ways of organizing and understanding human experience?

The authors here reveal that there was no consensus on who was most qualified to investigate nonordinary states of consciousness, and perhaps even less agreement on who should benefit from hallucinogens. Is meaning generated from personal insight, mediated through guides anchored in intellectual traditions? Or are psychedelic substances simply another tool in a medical arsenal, with doses and outcomes filtered through a more traditional doctor-patient relationship, reminiscent of a set of power dynamics that sifts experience into clinical categories of meaning? What happens when those clinical settings are themselves shaped by ideological contexts that further impregnate descriptions of experience with meanings associated with individualism or collectivism? How do these contexts help us to appreciate the murky ethical landscape that psychedelics operated in during the post–World War II period?

Despite having vast differences in how such experiences were interpreted and mobilized, the authors in this part show us that psychedelic encounters have attracted enthusiastic drug seekers and help us to ask important questions about the role of personal experience in producing objective evidence. Contrary to trends with competing blockbuster pharmaceuticals like chlorpromazine, personal experience with psychedelics has been cherished as much as contested as a valid method of interpretation and a source of generalizable insight. Isolating experience as a variable also highlights important differences in intellectual traditions that were used to interpret hallucinations—both organic, pathological, and unwanted hallucinations, and those acknowledged as insightful gifts conveying wisdom and even cultural, social, and economic capital. Putting these diverse experiences into the same category involved some professional risk and walking a delicate line between madness and enlightenment. But for some, it was worth the personal risk.

Harnessing the power to learn from nonordinary states of consciousness animated this history long before the introduction of the formal "psychedelic" concept in 1957; this latter moment merely formalized through a new layer of vocabulary an enduring quest to find legitimacy in nonordinary states of consciousness. This part urges us to think carefully about how psychedelic experiences have been used as evidence for both madness and enlightenment.

1 NECTAR OF THE BLUE GODDESS: A LIVING TRADITION OF *SOMA* CONSUMPTION IN WEST BENGAL, INDIA

Ian A. Baker

We have drunk Soma; we have become immortal; we have obtained the
light; we have found the gods.

ṚG VEDA (8-XLVIII-3)

INTRODUCTION

As evidenced in the *Ṛg Veda*, an archaic Sanskrit text of the late Bronze
Age,[1] *soma* (hereafter Soma) is the first recorded psychedelic (i.e., "mind-
manifesting")[2] substance to be used in both pharmacological and religious
contexts.[3] More than 114 hymns in Book Nine of the *Ṛg Veda* praise Soma as
the favored drink of gods and humans and associate the deified vegetal compound with healing and longevity as well as ecstatic, self-transcendent states
of consciousness.[4] Although sacramental Soma consumption is historically
well established, the psychoactive constituents of this potent, entheogenic
(i.e., "realizing the divine within")[5] libation have been widely contested as
no authentic, living tradition of Soma consumption has been known to
exist. Scholars have sought for two-and-a-half centuries to establish Soma's
identity, with investment banker and amateur mycologist Robert Gordon
Wasson making an influential, if mycocentric, case for the *Amanita muscaria*
mushroom in 1968.[6] However, Wasson's theory did not account for descriptions in the *Ṛg Veda* of pressing and filtering Soma, and consequently, the
sacramental plant potion of the Vedas has remained a botanical enigma.
Although many theories persist as to the original substance or combination
of ingredients that comprised Soma, or even whether it refers to psychotropic

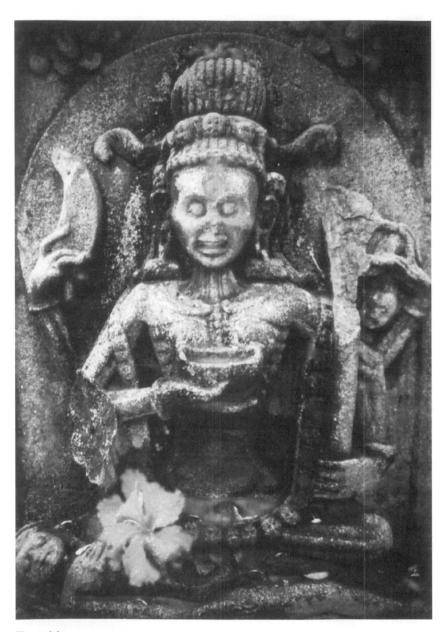

Figure 1.1

Cāmuṇḍā, a fearsome mother goddess (*mātṛkā*) invoked in Tantric rites involving ritual consumption of intoxicants. Kamakhya Temple, Nilachal hills, Assam. Photo by Ian Baker.

endocrinal secretions associated with "accomplishment in yoga" (*yogasid-dhi*),[7] this chapter reveals a living tradition of Soma consumption in an ancient center of Tantric practice in West Bengal, India.[8] It describes the process by which the sacrament is prepared from sixty-four syncretic and complementary ingredients, the yogic practices and beliefs that accompany its use, and the visionary and revelatory experiences said to result from its ritual consumption. The report thus reexamines the long-contested composition of Soma in an entheogenic context analogous to original Vedic-era usage in which Soma was simultaneously revered as a sacrament and phytomorphic deity, while providing new perspectives on the ways in which psychedelic substances have been used across cultural domains for therapeutic and soteriological purposes through their facilitation of rarefied, nonordinary states of conscious awareness.

THE SEARCH FOR SOMA

Since the Vedas first came to the attention of European scholars in the eighteenth century, over fifty botanical substances have been proposed for the plant-derived "elixir of immortality" that was central to Vedic notions of spirituality and the divine.[9] Candidates for Soma have ranged from red and white spotted fly-agaric mushrooms (*A. muscaria*) to telepathine-containing Syrian rue (*Peganum harmala*) to synergetic combinations of *Ephedra sinica*, cannabis, and opium, as well as more potent substances such as the highly toxic hallucinogen jimson weed (*Datura stramonium*).[10] Andrew McDonald, writing in 2004, proposed that the "famous psychotropic of the ancient Aryans" was the ubiquitous eastern lotus (*Nelumbo nucifera*).[11] More recently, Dmitri Semenov has revitalized an earlier hypothesis that the most likely candidate for the original "Soma substance" is "some species of *Ephedra*."[12] He concedes, however, that "no persuasive solution to the problem [has yet been] found."[13]

The anthropologist and professor emeritus Geoffrey Samuel concurs that "Ephedra seems the most plausible current opinion,"[14] but he suggests that knowledge of Soma's identity "was lost at an early stage" and was thus replaced over time by locally available, largely pharmacologically inactive, substances, and that, in the absence of efficacious sacraments, the exalted states of consciousness associated with Soma were gradually compensated for by yogic techniques aimed at psychological and spiritual exaltation.[15] Semenov notes that the *Śathapatha Brāhmana* (4.5-X-2-6), dated to approximately 700 BCE, "mentions substitute plants for extracting Soma-like substances in order of closeness to the original Soma for use in Soma offering."[16] But he also observes that the *Ṛg Veda* (10-LXXXIX-5) itself "says that the state brought about by the [original] Soma substance is to be preferred to those caused by substitutes," and that, as the Veda commentary *Śathapatha Brāhmana* later states, "no similarities deceived [the god] *Indra*,"[17] the chief enjoyer of Soma, the deified state of the imbiber, and a condition of consciousness characterized by ecstasy and illumination.

Although the *Ṛg Veda* (9-LXXIX-5) clearly indicates that Soma is of an "intricate composition," the principal ingredient has remained elusive. Professor Douglas R. Brooks relates that, "[t]he enigmas remain and there are no clear resolutions to the historical questions of identity of the plant that provided the core experience associated with the composition of the *Ṛg Veda*, the ritual use of the substance, the relationship precisely to the deity [Soma], or the allegories associated with it."[18] The Indologist Wendy Doniger O'Flaherty effectively summarized the quest as of 1969: "Handicapped by a rudimentary knowledge of the vernacular and ancient languages of India and by inadequate communication in the academic world, scholars covered the same ground over and over again. Time and again the same ideas reappear, are disproved, and reappear as if they were proven theories."[19] Following O'Flaherty, the Vedic scholar John Brough concluded in 1971 that "the problem is insoluble."[20]

Research on Soma has nonetheless continued, with Dr. Matthew Clark speculating that, in light of the extensive botanical knowledge in Asian cultures, Soma may have been a multiplant, entheogenic analog of Amazonian ayahuasca combining a source of DMT, such as *khadīra* (*Acacia catechu*), with a synergic monoamine oxidase inhibiter (MAOI), such as Syrian rue (*P. harmala*), both of which are widely distributed in India and Central Asia.[21] The cultural historian Mike Jay has also argued for an ayahuasca analog and advanced a theory that Soma, as well as *haoma* used in Zoroastrianism,[22] may have been a combination of *harmal* (Syrian rue) and *Psilocybin cubenis*

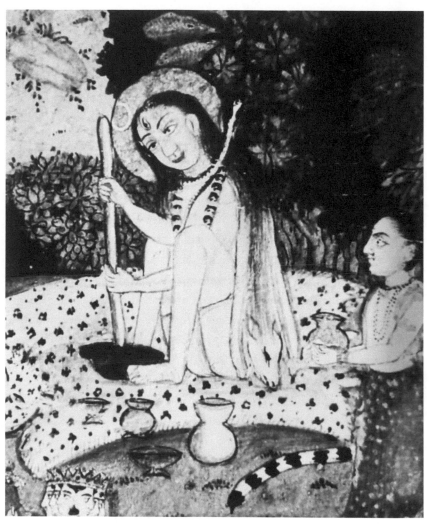

Figure 1.2
Śiva concocting *bhāṇg*, nineteenth century. Academy of Fine Arts and Literature, New Delhi, India.

mushrooms so as to produce "a close chemical analogue with the same pineal interaction of tryptamines and beta-carbolines."[23] The posited sacrament was dubbed by the anthropologist and ethnopharmacologist Christian Rätsch as "somahuasca."[24] More recently, Meena Maillart-Garg and Michael Winkelman have presented archaeological and iconographical evidence to support Wasson's original claim that Soma was derived from a mushroom,[25] while a reputedly Vedic tradition of Soma consumption in North America, active until thirty years ago, combined peeled, roasted, and powdered *A. muscaria* skins with frozen, crushed Syrian rue and fermented mare's milk.[26]

Although Soma's composition may have varied across time and geographies depending on the local availability of pharmacologically active plants, this preliminary ethnographic report establishes the persistence of the ritual use of Soma as a highly psychoactive substance at one of India's preeminent sites of Tantric practice, connected with the evocation of a salvific goddess known as Nīlakaṇṭha (or "blue-throated") Tārā. Although her neck color recalls the bluing reaction on the stems of freshly harvested psilocybin mushrooms, entheogenic fungi may or may not be included among the sixty-four synergetic ingredients of the Soma formula found in Tārāpīṭh, a pilgrimage town in the Birbhum district of West Bengal, India.[27]

A LIVING TANTRIC TRADITION

In November 2018, while I was in Tārāpīṭh investigating the use of psychotropic[28] plants in Vajrayāna Buddhism, I was fortunate to meet a Tantric adept named Ānanda Tīrthanāth who revealed a living tradition of Soma preparation and consumption connected with a "blue-throated" form of the Tantric goddess Tārā.[29] The meeting took place at Tīrthanāth's home above the banks of the Dwaraka River, which borders Tārāpīṭh's highly renowned Tārā Maa temple. He agreed to meet me as a fellow initiate of the esoteric Yoginī Kaula tradition of Hindu Tantra which venerates the procreative energy (*śakti*) underlying existence in the form of ten knowledge-bestowing goddesses (*dasmahāvidyā*).[30] The Yoginī Kaula source text, *Jñānanirṇaya Mahāyoginīkaula*, dating to the ninth or tenth century, makes specific reference to Soma as an offering to the Yoginīs within the *cakras,* or focal centers, of the human body so as to attain supernatural powers (*siddhi*) and liberating knowledge (*mokṣa*).[31] The meeting had been arranged by Maitreyi Brahmachari, the daughter of one of Ānanda Tīrthanāth's former colleagues, who explained to me that only Tīrthanāth knew the complete procedure for preparing and imbibing the esteemed elixir.[32]

Ānanda Tīrthanāth, whose name means "Blissful Lord of the Crossing Place,"[33] greeted us in red cotton robes offset by a necklace of *rudrākṣa* (*Elaeocarpus ganitrus*) beads. His sitting room was filled with Sanskrit texts, and paintings of the ten wisdom-bestowing goddesses of the *mahāvidyā* adorned the walls. "The essence of Tantra is *gyān*, or knowledge," Tīrthanāth explained. "And in our tradition, it is Śakti [the female principle], not Śiva [her male consort], who bestows liberating nondual gnosis (*mokṣa*)." He added that this was not to transcend the world, as in Buddhist ideology, but to inhabit the world more fully and joyously.

THE BLUE GODDESS

The name Tārā derives from the Sanskrit verbal root *trī*, to "overcome or liberate,"[34] connoting her ability to free the mind from inhibiting illusion (*māyā*).[35] She is conventionally represented in Mahāyana Buddhism as a compassionate savior. In one Buddhist manifestation, she appears as Khadīravanī Tārā, "Tārā of the Acacia Grove," adorned in the bark of the *khadīra* tree, an Indian variety of mimosa and a phytochemical source of DMT also known in India as *somasara*, literally "essence of soma" or "soma power."[36]

In the Kaula tradition, Tārā is esteemed as the bestower of life and immanent ground of being.[37] She presents herself dynamically, and is typically shown as skirted in tiger skins, her disheveled hair braided with serpents, and laughing wildly as her third, spiritual eye transmits liberating knowledge (*gyān*).[38] She is commonly depicted as pressing her left foot against the navel of a supine Śiva, while her right foot cradles a snake with bared fangs. A crescent moon in her tiara symbolizes *Candradvīpa*, the "Island of the Moon," whence the Yoginī Kaula teachings are said to have originated.[39] Tīrthanāth specified that Nīlakaṇṭha ("blue-throated") Tārā is the most important of eight Tārās, or Śaktis, revered in the Kaula tradition, and that her dark blue

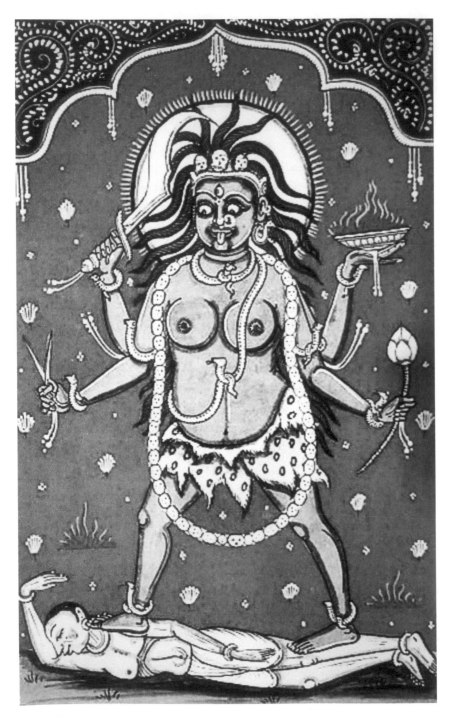

Figure 1.3
A variant form of Nīlakaṇṭha ("Blue-throated") Tārā. Tārāpīṭh votive image.

body, garlanded in severed heads and brandishing a scimitar, skull bowl (*kapāla*), and blue lotus (*nīlotpala*), signifies the transformation of inhibiting mental states concordant with her dedication to liberate beings from the thrall of phenomenal appearances and to introduce them to the "pure light" of their essential being.[40]

Tīrthanāth explained that Nīlakaṇṭha Tārā's forename derives from her mythic role in rescuing Śiva from the debilitating effect of deadly poisons that arose when *devas* and *asuras* (powerful demigods) used a venomous serpent to churn the primordial ocean to produce an immortality-bestowing nectar (*amṛta*) from the juices of myriad plants and trees.[41] According to the *amṛta-manthana* narrative, the churning process produced lethal by-products, which, out of his supreme beneficence, Śiva consumed lest they contaminate the world. As he succumbed to their effects, his throat swelled and turned blue. But the goddess Śakti, manifesting as Tārā, nourished him with milk from her breasts to antidote the poisons, during which his blue cast transferred to his redeemer.[42]

As Tārā's nectariferous breast milk revived Śiva from the toxic side effects involved in the production of Soma, she became intimately associated with the primal sacrament that the *Ṛg Veda* praises as the "milk of heaven" (9-LI-2) and which, in Kaula practice, bestows both sensory exhilaration and an entheogenic recognition of the inseparability of the human and the divine, and thus of the adept and the cosmos.[43]

THE PRIMORDIAL ELIXIR

Tīrthanāth explained that Nīlakaṇṭha Tārā is specifically associated with transforming toxins into deifying nectar (*paramamṛta*) and intoxication into liberating knowledge (*gyān*).[44] He clarified that, in imbibing Soma, initiates partake in the ecstasy of celestial divinities, in particular the nondual gnosis of Śiva-Śakti and the associated state of *turiya*, a transcendent fourth state of consciousness beyond waking, dreaming, or sleeping characterized by *sahajānanda*, or self-existing bliss beyond temporal delimitation.[45] He indicated that, for humans, *turiya* is not meant to be a continuous state of consciousness, but an insight acquired in the realm of the gods that infuses and

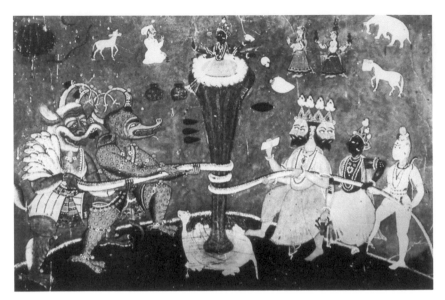

Figure 1.4
Churning the Cosmic Ocean (*Samudra Manthana*), a seventeenth-century watercolor, Pahari school of art. San Diego Museum of Art.

informs all subsequent mental states. Tīrthanāth said that when consumed in a ritual context, Soma promotes epiphanic insight (*prājña*), leading the *sādhaka,* or spiritual aspirant, to existential freedom (*mokṣa*) and immortality, not in the sense of endless duration but in the fullness of life.[46]

According to Tīrthanāth, ritual ingestion of Soma continues in the Yoginī Kaula lineage at Tārāpīṭh, although few initiates know the formula for its preparation. Tīrthanāth, who learned it from his teacher, explained that the elixir's sixty-four botanical and mineral ingredients are blended with fermented rice and buried in a clay vessel underground for at least one month. During this lunar cycle, initiates embark on a meditative rite known as *manoj pūjā,* which involves unification with Śiva and Śakti and offering them various substances by ingesting them oneself. Leaves of cannabis, for example, are offered to lineage gurus and are also consumed by the assembled devotees. Once the Soma has ripened underground, initial observances are performed before the *soma-ras,* or liquified Soma, is distributed in nine or eleven portions to the gathered celebrants who then commence the full *sādhana*, or religious rite, of Soma.

Tīrthanāth said that he no longer consumes Soma as he no longer needs it at this stage of his practice.[47] With regard to the recipe, he clarified that it was passed down orally in both Vedic and Kaula traditions, and later written on palm leaves and parchment. He copied one such manuscript from his guru. As Tīrthanāth explained, all Kaula initiates previously consumed Soma, but it was especially necessary for beginners to attain transcendental awareness (gyān). He further noted that those who consume Soma merely as a recreational intoxicant, rather than to establish an ecstatic, self-transcendent sensibility, are known as somapa, or abusers of Soma, and they invite the wrath of the Blue Goddess in the form of madness and psychosis.

Tīrthanāth carefully shared the basics of his Soma recipe for he was, to the best of his knowledge, the last person in Tārāpīth who knew how to make it properly, and he was concerned that the knowledge might not outlive him if it wasn't recorded. The complex recipe uses sixty-four ingredients, an auspicious number based on a multiplication of the eight Vedic mother-goddesses (aṣṭamātrikā). Ingredients include roots of various nonpsychoactive herbs and spices, such as cardamom and curcumin, as well as dried and powdered seeds of highly intoxicating dhattūra (white thornapple), a species of flowering nightshade (Solanaceae) whose seeds contain tropane alkaloids that produce powerful visionary and deliriant (anticholinergic/antimuscarinic) effects.[48]

Some of the sixty-four substances are beneficial for health and others, besides dhattūra, are highly psychoactive including, according to Tīrthanāth, "old and rotten" rice to which bananas and other fruits are blended with unpasteurized milk before fermenting the mixture underground. Nonpsychoactive, yet medicinal, ingredients include śilājīt, a mineral-rich extrusion from Himalayan rockfaces, and gul, a kind of molasses. Aśvagandhā (Withania somnifera)[49] is also added, as is rauwolfia (Rauvolfia serpentina), which reduces blood pressure raised by alkaloids, such as atropine and scopolamine, contained in dhattūra. According to Tīrthanāth, the formula for Soma includes neither opium (Papaver somniferum)[50] nor alchemically processed cinnabar, a mercurial ingredient in Āyurvedic rasāyana and Siddha medicine formulas for rejuvenation.[51] With regard to the potentizing additive of dhattūra, Tīrthanāth noted that it can be replaced with Datura stramonium mother tincture, a nontoxic homeopathic derivative available at specialty pharmacies in Tārāpīṭh.[52]

The key ingredient of the Tārāpīṭh Soma formula is a barely psychoactive forest vine called *somalatā* (or in Sanskrit *somabhalli*). According to Tīrthanāth, it was the fermented juice of *somalatā,* in combination with synergetic substances, that allowed ancient adepts to commune with the gods, just as some contemporary tribal groups in West Bengal use fermented extracts of *somalatā* to invoke meteorological spirits of wind and rain. Tīrthanāth said that the leafless creeper is commonly known in Bengal as *dwijo priyo,* "favorite of the brahmins."[53] He described the vine as having small, creamy white flowers that increase and decrease with phases of the moon. Maitreyi claimed that *somalatā* is known in Latin as *Sarcostemma brevistigma*, although Clark (2021) has shown that, although *somalatā* is currently used in Vedic rites elsewhere in India, it has few if any psychoactive properties, thus making this botanical identification uncertain.[54] According to Tīrthanāth, the lactiferous juice of the crushed *somalatā* vine nonetheless accelerates the fermentation and potentization of Soma's other ingredients, including *D. Stramonium.*

To prepare the Soma, parboiled rice (*chamalmuni*) is cooked with raw molasses (jaggery) and fruit in a Soma *yaga*, a ritual oven fed with leaves and wood from the *bel* tree. The concoction is then transferred to a clay vessel (*kalasá*) and buried underground for a month, during which time the Soma begins to mold and ferment.[55] It gradually becomes *patchai*, or rice liquor, while incorporating the other active ingredients. After the fermentation stage, the liquified concoction (*somaras*) is decanted into a baked clay jar.

Prior to the commencement of the Soma rite and imbibing the *somaras*, a purificatory ritual must be performed to negate a mythical curse placed on Soma—as a Vedic lunar deity[56]—by his disgruntled father-in-law, the *ṛṣi*-king Dakṣa, for marrying twenty-seven of his daughters but favoring only one of them. Adepts must also perform internal *mantra* recitation (*jap*) prior to consuming Soma. Tīrthanāth clarified that the silently recited *mantras* are most effective when combined with *kumbhaka prāṇāyām*, a respiratory exercise in which the breath is held "in a vase" (*kumbhak*) beneath the navel.

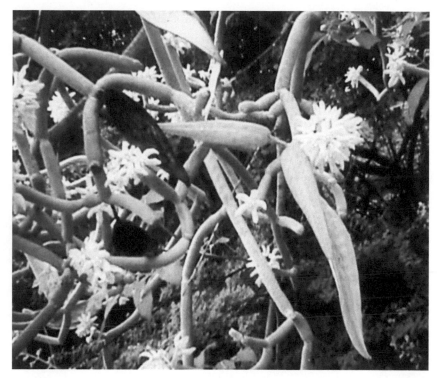

Figure 1.5
Somalatā Vine (*Sarcostemma brevistigma*). India Biodiversity Portal.

Each participant in the nocturnal rite subsequently consumes nine to eleven small clay cups of *somaras* at intervals of sixty to ninety minutes.

THE AZURE TIDE

The initial effects of ingesting Soma, Tīrthanāth explained, are dizziness and a sensation of bees buzzing in one's head, similar to the effects of consuming *Datura* and cannabis in the form of *bhāng*. But he clarified that, after 108 *mantra* recitations dedicated to one's spiritual mentor, the dizziness abates.[57] After subsequent servings of *somaras* and silent recitation of one's personal *mantra*, an intangible luminescence beyond the mind arises like "bright moonlight." He explained that one typically sees visions of the goddess Tārā amid radiant multihued lights, and sometimes a writhing snakelike figure appears (as in ayahuasca ceremonies). He said that light is sometimes seen emanating from a *sādhaka's ājñā cakra* (third eye), indicating the arising of *kuṇḍalinī*, Śakti's somatic expression in the human body, or the presence of Śiva, as luminous awareness.[58] If the ritual is practiced properly, glowing heat (*tapas*) arises in the body, Tīrthanāth said. And, as suggested in the *Ṛg Veda*, a "blue tide" appears in one's field of vision as the effulgence of divine energy (*kula*).[59] As the numinous nectar is absorbed and digested, the *Ṛg Veda* effuses that the body becomes "ever-shining," with currents of vital airs "clothed in melodies."[60]

Tīrthanāth stated that the Soma ceremony is most effective when performed in a cremation ground, as commonly found in Tārāpīṭh, or at least, in an unwalled *mandapa*, or ritual pavilion. He related how, during one occasion of consuming Soma, he saw the light before him transform into a person, and he felt a transcendent happiness characterized by warmth, bliss, and incorporeality associated with the arising of *gyān*, or transcendental knowledge. He also described watching the lips of a statue of the goddess Kālī begin to move, although he could not make out the words.

As Tīrthanāth described, Soma is ingested throughout an entire night devoted to the veneration of Śiva-Śakti, an anthropomorphic representation of dyadic unity that can alternately elicit terror and joy. He maintained that Soma supports mental concentration and the awakening of *kuṇḍalinī*, a bio-electric energy conceived as a yogini-goddess who normally lies dormant at the base of the spine. If one feels sleepy during the ritual, an additional cup of *somaras* will "brighten the mind." According to Tīrthanāth, *kuṇḍalinī*, as an internal expression of the blue-throated goddess Tārā, manifests somatically as rapture (*ānand*) and heat (*tapas*), experienced like a "tingling of ants crawling up the spine," or auditorily as a "buzzing of bees" and the *bīja* ("seed") *mantra Hūm*. When *kuṇḍalinī* rises, the *sādhaka* dissociates from the outer world and senses a "glow of moonlight" in the *ājñā cakra*, linked to the arising of a transcendent form of knowledge (*gyān*), beyond the immersive meditative states of *samādhi* and *mahāsamādhi*.

Both male and female initiates perform Soma rituals, which may occur several times a year. During the nocturnal rite, *sādhakas* typically ingest the

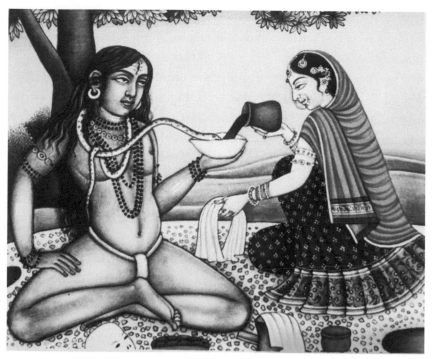

Figure 1.6
The goddess Parvatī offering Śiva *bhāṅg*, Pahari school of art. Wiki Commons.

equivalent of nine to eleven clay tumblers of *somaras*.[61] The first four cups of Soma are dedicated to the guru, the spiritual preceptor, and thus protect from any potential ill effects of subsequent consumption. (Like all psychedelic medicine, Soma holds both power and danger.) If female practitioners participate in the circle of *sādhakas*, they drink first on the fifth serving of *somaras* and then they pass the potion to their male companions, drinking from the same clay tumbler. The subsequent six to nine servings of *somaras* awaken *kuṇḍalinī* and produce intensified psychalia, emotional states characterized by auditory and visual hallucinations. The rite continues from sunset until dawn. Between repeated cups of the liquid Soma, *sādhakas* may consume legumes, meat, and other nourishing substances.

Somaras provides a powerful, long-lasting visionary experience, Tīrthanāth said, and the decoction may sometimes be replaced in the ritual with a milder substitute (*pratinidhi*) such as cannabis mixed with milk, honey, and mashed bananas. Tīrthanāth emphasized, however, that the rapture (*ānand*) and transcendent gnosis (*gyān*) that result from Soma consumption far surpass the psychoactive effects of cannabis, a view reflected in the *Ṛg Veda*.[62] Tīrthanāth also noted that some ignorant people might skip the essential process of fermenting *somalatā*, a variety of the Sarcostemma vine, and the seeds of *dhattūra* underground or might even replace the resultant fermented mash with locally available Old Monk triple-x rum. This is the "sad demise" of Tantra, Tīrthanāth lamented, when careful formulas for inducing insight and ecstatic transcendence devolve into mere intoxication.[63] "That's why we invoke Nīlakaṇṭha Tārā," Tīrthanāth clarified, while elaborating on the somatic alchemy symbolized by the liberating nectar issuing from her breasts.[64] "Soma relieves both suffering and delusion (*avidya*)," Tīrthanāth asserted, equating the sacramental intoxicant with the ambrosial milk of the blue-throated goddess.

Before leaving Ānanda Tīrthanāth's home, I told him that I hoped to return to Tārāpīṭh the following year to learn from him how to prepare Soma and to be guided through the stages of psychosensory inebriation intrinsic to its consumption. "Come when the moon is full," Tīrthanāth said, "that's when Tārā confers her blessings."[65] As I descended the narrow staircase leading back to the street and the dwindling waters of the Dwaraka River, I reflected on the cosmic waters from which Soma is said to have first arisen. Whatever its ingredients Soma was ultimately a state of mind, a "nectariferous tide" that, as medical science defines psychedelics, "seems to expand the consciousness and enlarge the vision,"[66] annihilating the limited perceptions that commonly obscure our original nature (in Kaula terms, a luminescent cognizance beyond the mind). As Tīrthanāth suggested, rapture is an essential component of human experience, and Soma is an intrinsic aspect of our biochemistry. When ingested as a communal sacrament—as prefigured in humanity's oldest known religious text, the *Ṛg Veda*—Soma elevates the mind and heart and promotes the realization of an experiential dimension beyond personal identity that, according to the revelations of the nectarous, blue-throated goddess of Tārāpīṭh, is paradoxically the essence of self-knowledge.

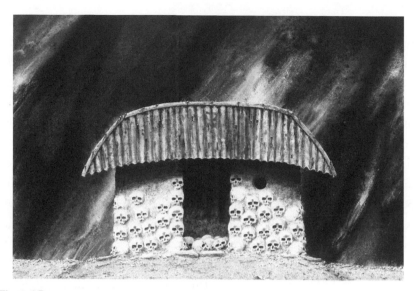

Figure 1.7
Meditation *kutī* at Tārāpīṭh, constructed of human skulls. Detail of a watercolor painting by Robert Powell.

CONCLUSION

More than twenty years ago, Mike Jay observed, "There is no consensus about which plant it was that provided the elixir of the gods. The botanical identity of *soma* remains one of the great unsolved mysteries of the ancient world."[67] As reviewed in this chapter, Vedic scholars, entheobotanists, ethnographers, and historians have debated the subject for centuries, but an encounter in Tārāpīṭh, India, in November 2018 revealed a living tradition of Soma production and consumption that validates arguments for a synergetic combination of psychotropic plant substances, rather than a single botanical source for the sacramental potion.[68] Although further fieldwork has yet to fully document what is clearly an endangered legacy, the preliminary research recounted in this report establishes a living heritage of Soma consumption commensurate with the "sacred wisdom" of the *Ṛg Veda,* which presents Soma as a phytochemical key to an "immortal, unfading world" and a realm of "inextinguishable light" surpassing in vastness both Earth and sky.[69]

This chapter has also demonstrated the ways in which contemplative practices, respiratory techniques, and spiritual exercises are used in the context of contemporary Soma consumption to both enhance and mitigate the self-transcendence and dissociative states accompanying ecstatic intoxication. In this context, psychedelically enhanced ritual consciously disrupts consensual reality and actualizes latent psychophysical states within a process of empowerment and transformation. As Tīrthanāth recounted, sacramental Soma consumption entails embodied transactions of matter, energy, and light in which fear transforms into possibility and unknowing into illumination. From this perspective, Soma evokes nothing less than the divine ground of being. As Robert Calasso writes in his philosophical reflections on the Vedas, "Only in rapture can gods and men communicate. Only in *soma* do they meet."[70]

It's hoped that this account of contemporary Soma consumption in West Bengal, India, will stimulate further investigation of the confluences of pharmacology, religion, and transformational states of consciousness. Soma reputedly conferred on its original celebrants "a life that—for a while—is divine . . . a passing into another order of things."[71] This chapter has presented a case for Soma's continued relevance as a visionary, "mind-manifesting" (psychedelic) sacrament up to the present day, with ceremonial, spiritual, medicinal, and therapeutic applications.[72]

NOTES

1. The *Ṛg Veda*, literally "Praise of Sacred Knowledge," was committed to writing between 1200 and 900 BCE and consists of 1,028 Sanskrit hymns, 120 of which are dedicated to the hallucinogenic potion Soma. See Stephanie W. Jamison and Joel P. Brereton, trans., *The Rigveda: The Earliest Religious Poetry of India* (Oxford: Oxford University Press, 2017). See also Christopher Partridge, *High Culture: Drugs, Mysticism, and the Pursuit of Transcendence in the Modern World* (Oxford: Oxford University Press, 2018), 298.

2. The word "psychedelic" derives from the Greek *psychē*, meaning "soul or mind," and *dēloun*, meaning "to manifest," and refers to substances whose actions "seem to expand the consciousness and enlarge the vision." See *Stedman's Medical Dictionary*, 28th ed. (Baltimore: Williams and Wilkins Company, 1996), 1321. For a discussion of Soma as a psychedelic, see Claudia Müller-Ebeling, Christian Rätsch, and Surenda Bahadur Shahi, *Shamanism and Tantra in the Himalayas* (Rochester, VT: Park Street Press, 2002), 178.

3. For accounts of Soma in Vedic ritual, see Wendy Doniger O'Flaherty, "The Post-Vedic History of the Soma Plant," in *Soma: Divine Mushroom of Immortality*, edited by R. Gordon

Wasson (New York: Harcourt Brace Jovanovich, 1969), 95–147; Frits Staal, "How a Psychoactive Substance Became a Ritual: The Case of Soma," *Social Research* 68, no. 3 (2001), 745–778; Robert Calasso, *Ardor* (U.K.: Penguin Books, 2015); Matthew Clark, *The Tawny One: Soma, Haoma and Ayahuasca* (London: Aeon Books, 2017); Partridge, *High Culture.*

4. In Book Nine of the *Ṛg Veda*, Soma is specifically referred to as a "food of the gods" (9-CIV-5), a "healer of disease" (1-XXCI-612), a "bestower of wisdom" (9-XII-8), "heightened mental powers" (9-XXVIII-1), "omniscience" (9-LXXVII-3), and "Immortality" (9-XII-1) (Stephanie W. Jamison and Joel P. Brereton. *The Rigveda: The Earliest Religious Poetry of India.* Oxford: Oxford University Press, 2017). See also George Thompson, "Soma and Ecstasy in the Ṛgveda," *Electronic Journal of Vedic Studies* 9, no. 1 (2003), 1–13; George Thompson, "A Brief Anthology of Hymns in the *Ṛgveda* Having to Do with *Soma* (and Shamanism)," in *On Meaning and Mantras: Essays in Honor of Frits Staal,* edited by George Thompson and Richard K. Payne (Moraga, CA: Institute of Buddhist Studies/BDK America, 2016), 557–577.

5. Andrew Weil speculated in 1988 that the word "entheogen" would "wind up on the linguistic trash heap . . . the final resting place of most neologistic inventions." See Andrew Weil, Review of Wasson, *Persephone's Quest: Entheogens and the Origins of Religion* (1986), *Journal of Psychoactive Drugs* 20, no. 4 (1988), 489.

6. R. Gordon Wasson, *Soma: Divine Mushroom of Immortality* (New York: Harcourt Brace Jovanovich, 1968); R. Gordon Wasson, "The Soma of the Rig Veda. What Was It?" *Journal of the American Oriental Society* 91, no. 2 (1971), 169–187. See also Wendy Doniger, "Somatic Memories of R. Gordon Wasson," in *The Sacred Mushroom Seeker: Tributes to R. Gordon Wasson,* edited by Thomas J. Riedlinger (Rochester, VT: Park Street Press, 1997), 55–59; Huston Smith, "Wasson's Soma: A Review Article," *Journal of the American Academy of Religions* 40, no. 4 (1972), 480–499; Jonathan Ott, "The Post-Wasson History of the Soma Plant," *Eleusis,* no. 1 (1998): 9–37; Kevin Feeney, "Revisiting Wasson's Soma: Exploring the Effects of Preparation on the Chemistry of Amanita Muscaria," *Journal of Psychoactive Drugs* 42, no. 4 (2010), 499–506; Stephan Hillyer Levitt, "New Considerations Regarding the Identity of Vedic *Sóma* as the Mushroom Fly Agaric," *Studia Orientalia* 3 (2011), 105–118; Scott Hajicek-Dobberstein, "Soma Siddhas and Alchemical Enlightenment: Psychedelic Mushrooms in Buddhist Tradition," *Journal of Ethnopharmacology* 48, no. 2 (1995), 99–108. See also, Andrew Weil, Review of *Persephone's Quest,* 489–490 and Kevin Feeney, "The Significance of Pharmacological and Biological Indicators in Identifying Historical uses of Amanita muscaria," in *Entheogens and the Development of Culture: The Anthropology and Neurobiology of Ecstatic Experience,* edited by J. Rush (Berkeley, CA: North Atlantic Books, 2013), 279–318.

7. For the relationship of *amṛta* and pineal melatonin, a tryptophan-derived hormone, see William C. Bushell and Neil D. Theise, "Toward a Unified Field of Study: Longevity, Regeneration, and Protection of Health through Meditation and Related Practices," *Longevity, Regeneration, and Optimal Health: Integrating Eastern and Western Perspectives, Annals of the New York Academy of Sciences,* vol. 1172 (2009), 5–19. The chapter describes melatonin's "elixir-like" pleiotropic effects on multiple tissues, organs, and pathologies. See also,

William C. Bushell, "Serum factor that restores youthful function to apparently senescent stem cells is identified by recently developed expert decision tree-guided bioinformatics program," in *Control and Regulation of Stem Cells*, edited by T. Grodzicker et al (LXXIII Cold Spring Harbor Symposium on Quantitative Biology) (Cold Spring Harbor, NY: Cold Spring Harbor Laboratories Press, 2009). The relationship of melatonin's pleiotropy to that of its close chemical (tryptophan-derived) relations, serotonin and DMT, as well as that of other psychedelics, is discussed in Baker, Bushell, Castle, et al (in progress) in the context of secretions of multiple tryptophan-derived substances from the pineal gland that correlate with "inner Soma" and its activation. See also endnote 72, below.

8. The word "tantra" literally means "loom, weave, warp" and denotes esoteric traditions of Hinduism and Buddhism that developed in India from the middle of the first millennium onward.

9. See Mike Crowley, *Secret Drugs of Buddhism: Psychedelic Sacraments and the Origins of the Vajrayāna*. (Hayfork, CA: Amrita Press, 2016), 254; Clark, *The Tawny One*, 61–62.

10. See Andrew Sherrett, "Introduction: Peculiar Substance," in *Consuming Habits: Drugs in History and Anthropology*, edited by Jordan Goodman, Paul E. Lovejoy, and Andrew Sherrett (New York: Routledge, 1995), 29; Christian Rätsch, *The Encyclopedia of Psychoactive Plants: Ethnopharmacology and Its Applications*, trans. John R. Baker (Rochester, VT: Park Street Press, 2005), 792–795; Partridge, *High Culture*, 300.

11. Andrew McDonald, "A Botanical Perspective on the Identity of Soma (Nelumbo nucifera Gaertn.) Based on Scriptural and Iconographic Records," *Economic Botany* 58 (Winter 2004): 147–173. He references psychoactive alkaloids in the lotus, including aporphine and nuciferine, which are structurally similar to the opiate alkaloids morphine, codeine, and thebaine (152).

12. Dmitri Semenov, *Treatise on Soma Hymns of Rigveda* (Idaho Springs, CO: Sattarka Publications 2020), 39. The Ephedra plant is a primary source of the powerful stimulant ephedrine and a principal ingredient in the manufacture of methamphetamine, the initial actions of which include the "exhilaration, intoxication, and delight" identified as the psychoactive properties of Soma. See also N. A. Qazilbash, "Ephedra of the Rigveda," *Pharmaceutical Journal* 26 (1960), 497–501; A. David Napier, *Masks, Transformation, and Paradox* (Berkeley, Los Angeles, and London: University of California Press, 1986), 159; S. Madhihassan, *The History and Natural History of Soma as Ephedra* (Islamabad: Pakistan Science Foundation, 1987); Matthew Clark, *Botanical Ecstasies: Psychoactive Plant Formulas in India and Beyond* (London: Psychedelic Press, 2021), 15.

13. Dmitri Semenov, *Treatise on Soma Hymns of Rigveda* (Idaho Springs, CO: Sattarka Publications 2020), 39.

14. Geoffrey Samuel, *The Origins of Yoga and Tantra: Indic Religions to the Thirteenth Century* (Cambridge: Cambridge University Press, 2008), 97–98.

15. Samuel, *The Origins of Yoga and Tantra*, 98, 340. Eliade similarly holds that Soma's apparent disappearance led to the seeking of other means of ecstasy, namely "ascesis, or orgiastic excess,

meditation, and techniques of yoga and mystical devotion." See Mircea Eliade, *A History of Religious Ideas: From the Stone Age to the Eleusinian Mysteries* (Paris: Payot, 1976): 225–230. See also Clark, *Botanical Ecstasies: Psychoactive Plant Formulas in India and Beyond* (London, U.K.: Psychedelic Press, 2021), 7–10.

16. Semenov, *Treatise on Soma Hymns of Rigveda*, 39.

17. Semenov, *Treatise on Soma Hymns of Rigveda*, 38.

18. Personal correspondence, Douglas Brooks, September 2021. See also Douglas R. Brooks, *The Secret of the Three Cities: An Introduction to Hindu Śakta Tantrism* (Chicago: University of Chicago Press, 1990).

19. O'Flaherty, "The Post-Vedic History of the Soma Plant," 144. Mike Crowley observed more recently that "thousands of pages . . . have been devoted to this contentious issue" (Crowley, *Secret Drugs of Buddhism*, 254–255).

20. John Brough, "Soma and *Amanita muscaria*," *Bulletin of the School of Oriental and African Studies* 34, no. 2 (1971), 331–362.

21. Clark, *The Tawny One*, 198. Amazonian *ayahuasca* is a psychotropic concoction of *Psychotria virdis* leaves, as a source of DMT, and boiled *Banisteriopsis caapi* vine (*yagé*), as a source of MAOIs, which block an enzyme called monoamine oxidase, which is involved in removing the neurotransmitters norepinephrine, serotonin, and dopamine from the brain and inactivating the psychotropic effects of DMT. MAOIs prevent this from happening, which makes more of these brain chemicals available to effect changes in both cells and circuits and potentiating the effects of DMT.

22. Regarding Iranian antecedents, David Napier observes that Soma (as *hoama*) was "mixed with bull's blood to confer both immortality and ecstatic enjoyment to the followers of Mithra" (Napier, *Masks, Transformation, and Paradox*, 147).

23. Mike Jay, *Blue Tide: The Search for Soma* (Brooklyn, NY: Automedia, 1999), 172.

24. Rätsch, *The Encyclopedia of Psychoactive Plants*, 795. Nominal formulations of "Soma"—combining *Peganum harmala* as a serotonin-elevating mono amine oxidase (MAO) inhibiting beta-carboline with DMT containing *Psychotria viridis* (chacruna) and/or *Acacia* or *Mimosa hostilis*—are often used with the addition of local varieties of *Psilocybe cubensis* and *Psilocybe samuiensis* in entheogenic and therapeutic ritual contexts on the islands of Koh Phagnan and Koh Samui in the Gulf of Thailand (personal observation).

25. Meena Maillart-Garg and Michael Winkelman, "The 'Kamasutra' Temples of India. A Case for the Encoding of Psychedelically Induced Spirituality," *Journal of Psychedelic Studies* 3, no. 2 (2019), 81–101; See also Clark, *Botanical Ecstasies*, 13–14; Kevin Feeney, "Revisiting Wasson's Soma: Exploring the Effects of Preparation on the Chemistry of Amanita Muscaria," *Journal of Psychoactive Drugs* 42, no. 4 (2010), 499–506.

26. Max Christensen, personal communication, July 2021. The concoction was reputedly prepared in, and subsequently drunk from, a hoofprint formed by a male horse, ideally on land struck by a meteorite so as to infuse the blend with celestial minerals.

27. At the time of my initial research, I was not able to establish whether the 64 designated ingredients included any form of psychoactive fungi, most notably *Amanita muscaria*. Intended follow-up fieldwork in 2020–2021 was forestalled by the global COVID-19 pandemic.

28. This denotes substances that affect the psyche, from the Greek *trophē*, "a turning."

29. The term "tantra," from the Sanskrit root *tan*, to expand, and *tra*, method, refers to practices for expanding human capacity and imagination through ritualized aesthetic and sensory experience. Tantra developed in both Buddhism and Hinduism from the sixth century onward, although its roots are more ancient than its institutionalized forms. The Tārā Tantra itself asserts that the worship of Tārā was introduced into India from mahācīna (i.e., China and Tibet). See Ian A. Baker, *Tibetan Yoga: Principles and Practices* (London: Thames & Hudson, 2019).

30. The Ten Mahāvidyās are *Kālī, Tārā, Tripura Sundarī, Bhuvaneśvarī, Tripura Bhairavi, Chhinnamastā, Dhūmāvatī, Bagalāmukhi, Mātaṅgī*, and *Kamalatmika*. The tradition is a historical development and subdivision of the Yoginī Kaula, or "divine energy (*kula*) of the yoginīs." See David R. Kinsley, *Tantric Visions of the Divine Feminine: The Ten Mahāvidyās* (Berkeley: University of California Press, 1997); Satkari Mukhopadhaya, *The Kaulajñānanirnaya: The Esoteric Teachings of Matsyendrapāda, Sadguru of the Yoginī Kaula School in the Tantra Tradition* (New Delhi: Aditya Prakashan, 2012).

31. See Mukhopadhyaya, *The Kaulajñānanirnaya*, 173, 201–203.

32. Ānanda Tīrthanāth's teacher's name was Paramānanda, which means "Infinite Bliss." Maitreya's father, Chittaranjan Brahmachari, held the initiate name Brahmānanda, which means "Bliss of Ultimate Being." Brahmānanda's teacher was Sachithanadā and, unlike Tīrthanāth's guru, neither prepared nor consumed Soma. Maitreya conveyed, however, that at the time of sacrificial fire rituals (*homa*), her father and his disciples, who were otherwise abstemious, would dip their fingers into sacramental wine and touch it to their tongues.

33. The term *tīrtha* refers to a fordable passage across the sea of interminable births and deaths, otherwise known as *saṃsāra*. The Sanskrit word *nāth*, or *nātha*, literally means "lord, protector, master," and refers to Adi Nātha, a synonym for Śiva. Initiation into the Nāth tradition includes receiving a name ending in -*nāth*. The Nāth tradition within medieval Hinduism in India combined ideas from Buddhism, Śaivism, and Yoga.

34. Joseph Campbell, *The Mythic Image* (Princeton, NJ: Princeton University Press, 1974), 52.

35. Campbell, *The Mythic Image*.

36. Mike Crowley notes that *khadīra* bark is often referred to as *soma-valka*, or "Soma bark," and he explains that the DMT in acacia bark can be activated through the addition of MAO-inhibiting plants, such as passion fruit or tobacco. He also argues that the absence of *khadīra* in formulations of Soma would have deprived it of its entheogenic power, as anthropomorphically embodied in the seated, bark-wrapped form of Khadiravanī Tārā (See Crowley, *Secret Drugs of Buddhism*, 211, 212, 215, 220–221).

37. See Mukhopadhyata, *The Kaulajñānanirnaya*, 199.

38. The third eye in Indo-Tibetan deities symbolically links physiology with spirituality and correlates with the *ājñā*, or "command," *cakra* at the brow, as well as the light-sensitive pineal gland, the only part of the brain that is not bilaterally symmetrical (See Napier, *Masks, Transformation, and Paradox*, 240n33).

39. See Mukhopadhyaya, *The Kaulajñānanirnaya*, 199–200.

40. Tīrthanāth implied that the Blue Goddess of Soma is less an unaltering iconographic form than a fluent archetype from which all other forms arise, thereby upholding the Kaula view that deities are entities whose nature is emptiness and thus are inherently paradoxical and indescribable while consisting ultimately of pure light.

41. As stated in *Mahābhārata* I, 5, 16, "The many juices of herbs and the manifold resins of the trees flowed into the water of the ocean. And with the milk of these juices that had the power of the Elixir . . . the Gods obtained immortality."

42. The myth draws from earlier Vedic references to Sarasvatī, the lotus-born consort of Brahma, whose breasts flow with the nectar of immortality (*Ṛg Veda* 7-XCI-5–6). See J. Bruce Long, "Life out of Death: A Structural Analysis of the Myth of the 'Churning of the Ocean of Milk'," in *Hinduism: New Essays in the History of Religions*, ed. Bardwell L. Smith (Leiden, Netherlands: E. J. Brill, 1982), 171–207. See also Judit Törzcök for an internalization of the myth in which the *sādakha* imaginatively imbibes the ambrosial breast milk of a terrifying goddess who emerges from the cosmic ocean. Judit Törzcök, "Why Are the Skull Bearers (Kāpālikas) Called Soma?" in *Śaivism and the Tantric Traditions: Essays in Honour of Alexis G. J. S. Sanderson* (Leiden, Netherlands: Brill, 2016), 33–46.

43. See also Mukhopadhyata, *The Kaulajñānanirnaya*, 213, note 84. Tīrthanāth further noted that Nīlakaṇtha Tārā is also known as Sarasvatī, the Indian goddess of learning, whose name literally means "that which flows," and also refers to the Asian medical plant *Bacopa monnier* (Rätsch, *The Encyclopedia of Psychoactive Plants*, 95). In terms of esoteric pharmacology, Tirthanath suggested that the myth speaks to the importance of adding unpasteurized milk to the Soma formula to mitigate distressing gastrointestinal side effects and increase its potency, a process that parallels the decarboxylation of ibotenic acid into more highly psychoactive muscimol in traditional preparations of *Amanita muscaria*. See Kevin Feeney and Trent Austin, "Soma's Third Filter: New Findings Supporting the Amanita muscaria as the Ancient Sacrament of the Vedas" in *Fly Agaric: A Compendium of History, Pharmacology, Mythology & Exploration*, edited by Kevin Feeney (Fly Agaric Press, 2020), 51–62. See also note 64 below for a further account of the symbolism.

44. In the Vedic tradition, Tārā is held to be the daughter of Brahmā and is intimately connected with Soma via an adulterous union with the deity King Soma, who embodies the "strange intoxication that flows from liberty" and the "fluid that penetrates everywhere and makes all desirable" (Calasso, *Ardor*, 4–5, 309, 310).

45. *Turiya*, the "fourth" state, underlies and pervades the three mental states of waking, dreaming, and dreamless sleep, in a scheme first presented in the Hindu *Upaniṣads* but also evident

in the Vajrayāna Buddhist traditions of Mahāmudrā, the "Great Seal," and Dzogchen, the "Great Completion."

46. Douglas Brooks notes that, in the Śākta Tantra, the state that Soma induces is "natural insofar as the plant or the ritual or the substance or the meditation merely wakes it up inside us" (personal correspondence, September 2020.)

47. As Tīrthanāth clarified, an endogenous analog of Soma is produced in the body of a person who reaches a higher state of consciousness. Within an analogous tradition of Datura consumption among Aghori ascetics in Varanasi, adepts consume the potent deliriant until hallucinations resolve in a vision of supernal light equated with Śiva, at which point consumption of Datura is abandoned (personal observation).

48. Tīrthanāth referred also to *dhattūra ghota*, the fruit of Datura, which can be mixed with milk and cannabis and is commonly used during religious festivals to give strength to those carrying icons of the gods on heavy palanquins. It also aids in the worship of Śiva by introducing a state of possession. A similar effect, Tīrthanāth stated, can be achieved using carefully administered venom from an Indian cobra (*Naja naja*).

49. *Aśvagandhā* ("horse-smell") is also known as Indian ginseng, an adaptogenic herb widely used in Āyurvedic and contemporary herbal medicine.

50. Opium was formerly added to *pān*, or betel quids, Tīrthanāth maintained, as was *Datura*.

51. Tīrthanāth referred to naturally occurring "mercury" at the base of the spine, which is drawn upward through the *suṣumṇā nāḍī* in the practice of *kuṇḍalinī* yoga.

52. Diverse cultures have used *Datura* as a plant medicine to treat a variety of ailments, as well as to achieve hallucinogenic and entheogenic effects associated with intense, psychomimetic visions. Although immoderate consumption can cause profound, long-lasting disorientation and potentially fatal outcomes, *Datura* is sometimes added to *ayahuasca* brews in South America to intensify the psychotropic effects of DMT. *Datura* is also used in some Tantric Buddhist rituals (Baker, *Tibetan Yoga*, 231), as well as in initiatory rites by some African and South American groups (Clark, *Botanical Ecstasies*, 104–105).

53. Crowley notes that *soma-vallari*, meaning "Soma creeper," is a cognate with *soma-vallabha*, meaning "beloved" (Crowley, Secret Drugs of Buddhism, 212).

54. *Sarcostemma brevistigma* was first discussed as a candidate for Soma in 1814, in an article in *Hortus Bengalensis* (Clark, *The Tawny One*, 62n236).

55. Considering the recipe's diverse ingredients, the fermentation process may yield additional psychoactive compounds, particularly in connection with the addition of unpasteurized milk. See, e.g., Feeney and Austin, "Soma's Third Filter," 2020.

56. As Calasso writes regarding Soma as a deity, he "has been left in obscurity because many have thought it enough to identify him with the *soma* plant or (later on) with the moon. But being an intoxicating juice, a celestial body, a king, and a god, all at the same time, is not in itself a problem in Vedic thought" (Calasso, *Ardor*, 319).

57. Tīrthanāth clarified that in Kaulamārga, practitioners attune inwardly to a single-syllable *mantra* that is never recited outwardly, thus referencing an ever-present, indwelling state of transcendent reality. He maintained that one who dwells in that heightened vibratory condition is referred to as a *siddha*.

58. According to Tīrthanāth, the principle of Śakti, or primordial female power, within the psychophysical body, is *kuṇḍalinī*, while the essence of *kuṇḍalinī* is *turiya*, the transcendent "fourth state" of consciousness, signified by Śiva.

59. Jay (*Blue Tide*, 34) notes that the color blue is one of the most concrete leitmotifs associated with *ayahuasca* visions. He further writes that *harmaline*, as contained in Syrian rue, produces the same effect—a distinctive blue radiance or glow that also appears when *harmal* is dissolved in alcohol or illuminated under an ultraviolet light. According to the *Ṛg Veda* (9-LXVIII-8cd), the consumption and metabolization of Soma gives rise to a "heavenly wave" in the body's middle channel (*suṣumnā*).

60. Semenov, *Treatise on Soma Hymns of Rigveda*, 49.

61. The Brahmayāmala Tantra specifies that pots for the preparation and consumption of Soma, as a reenactment of the churning of the primordial ocean, be made from clay obtained from cremation grounds. See Törzsök, "Why Are the Skull Bearers Called Soma?", 40.

62. See *Ṛg Veda* 10-LXXXIX-5.

63. Calasso writes that, in traditional contexts, "Soma not only induced intoxication, but encouraged truth" in anyone who received or "receives Soma into the circulation of their mind" (Calasso, *Ardor*, 330).

64. Tīrthanāth explained that Tārā's vivifying breast milk symbolizes the flow of internal Soma from the udder of the "cow of heaven," located at the uvula and pineal gland, to the heart *cakra*, the seat of Śiva as fully awakened consciousness, while the primordial waters from which Soma arose signify the "azure tide" that, in the context of the *Ṛg Veda*, transports consumers of the elixir to the realm of the gods.

65. Sadly, this was not to be, as Ānanda Tīrthanāth passed away in November 2021.

66. *Stedman's Medical Dictionary*, 1321.

67. Jay, *Blue Tide*, 6. In the same year, Dr. Sadie Plant commented that "although there have been many attempts to identify the plant, or the potion, soma has defied even the most determined drug detectives." Sadie Plant, *Writing on Drugs* (New York: Farrar, Straus and Giroux, 1999), 117.

68. See Clark, *Botanical Ecstasies*.

69. See Jay, *Blue Tide*, 3.

70. Calasso, *Ardor*, 331.

71. Calasso, *Ardor*, 331, 335.

72. As for "medicinal and therapeutic applications" of Soma, in the context of psychedelics in general (and following from endnote 7, above), a rapidly emerging body of studies is

demonstrating that a variety of psychedelics, including DMT, possess a considerable range of health and longevity enhancing effects. See, e.g., Ede Frecska, Szabo A., Winkelman M. J., Luna L. E., and McKenna D. J., "A Possibly Sigma-1 Receptor Mediated Role of Dimethyl-tryptamine in Tissue Protection, Regeneration, and Immunity," *Journal of Neural Transmission* (Vienna), 120, no. 9 (2013), 1295–1303; D. E. Nichols, Johnson, M. W., & Nichols, C. D., "Psychedelics as Medicines: An Emerging New Paradigm," *Journal of Clinical Pharmacology and Therapeutics*, 101, no. 2 (2017), 209–219; O. Simonsson, Sexton J. D., and Hendricks P. S., "Associations between Lifetime Classic Psychedelic Use and Markers of Physical Health," *Journal of Psychopharmacology* 35, no. 4 (2021), 447–452. This research is discussed in depth with additional references in Baker, Bushell, Castle, et al, in-progress.

BIBLIOGRAPHY

Baker, Ian A. *Tibetan Yoga: Principles and Practices*. London: Thames & Hudson, 2019.

Brooks, Douglas R. *The Secret of the Three Cities: An Introduction to Hindu Śakta Tantrism*. Chicago: University of Chicago Press, 1990.

Brough, John. "Soma and Amanita muscaria." *Bulletin of the School of Oriental and African Studies* 34, no. 2 (1971): 331–362.

William C. Bushell, "Serum factor that restores youthful function to apparently senescent stem cells is identified by recently developed expert decision tree-guided bioinformatics program." In T. Grodzicker et al (eds.), *Control and Regulation of Stem Cells* (LXXIII Cold Spring Harbor Symposium on Quantitative Biology). Cold Spring Harbor, NY: Cold Spring Harbor Laboratories Press, 2009.

Bushell, William C. and Neil D. Theise. "Toward a Unified Field of Study: Longevity, Regeneration, and Protection of Health through Meditation and Related Practices." In *Longevity, Regeneration, and Optimal Health: Integrating Eastern and Western Perspectives, Annals of the New York Academy of Sciences*, vol. 1172, 2009.

Calasso, Robert. *Ardor*. U.K: Penguin Books, 2015.

Campbell, Joseph. *The Mythic Image*. Princeton, NJ: Princeton University Press, 1974.

Clark, Matthew. *Botanical Ecstasies: Psychoactive Plant Formulas in India and Beyond*. London: Psychedelic Press, 2021.

Clark, Matthew. *The Tawny One: Soma, Haoma and Ayahuasca*. London: Aeon Books, 2017.

Crowley, Mike. *Secret Drugs of Buddhism: Psychedelic Sacraments and the Origins of the Vajrayāna*. Hayfork, CA: Amrita Press, 2016.

Crowley, Mike, and Ann Shulgin. *Secret Drugs of Buddhism: Psychedelic Sacraments and the Origins of the Vajrayana*. Santa Fe, NM: Synergetic Press, 2019.

Doniger, Wendy. "Somatic Memories of R. Gordon Wasson." In *The Sacred Mushroom Seeker: Tributes to R. Gordon Wasson*, edited by Thomas J. Riedlinger, 55–59. Rochester, VT: Park Street Press, 1997.

Eliade, Mircea. *A History of Religious Ideas: From the Stone Age to the Eleusinian Mysteries*. Paris: Payot, 1976.

Feeney, Kevin. "Revisiting Wasson's Soma: Exploring the Effects of Preparation on the Chemistry of Amanita Muscaria." *Journal of Psychoactive Drugs* 42, no. 4 (2010): 499–506.

Feeney, Kevin, and Trent Austin. "Soma's Third Filter: New Findings Supporting the *Amanita muscaria* as the Ancient Sacrament of the Vedas." In Kevin Feeney (ed.), *Fly Agaric: A Compendium of History, Pharmacology, Mythology & Exploration*. Fly Agaric Press, 2020.

Frecska, Ede, Szabo, A., Winkelman, M.J., Luna, L.E., and McKenna, D.J. "A possibly sigma-1 receptor mediated role of dimethyltryptamine in tissue protection, regeneration, and immunity." *Journal of Neural Transmission* (Vienna), 120, no. 9 (2013): 295–303.

Goodall, Dominic, Shaman Hatley, Harunaga Isaacson, and Srilata Raman. *Śaivism and the Tantric Traditions: Essays in Honour of Alexis GJS Sanderson*. Leiden, Netherlands: Brill, 2020.

Hajicek-Dobberstein, Scott. "Soma Siddhas and Alchemical Enlightenment: Psychedelic Mushrooms in Buddhist Tradition." *Journal of Ethnopharmacology* 48, no. 2 (1995): 99–108.

Jamison, Stephanie W., and Joel P. Brereton. *The Rigveda: The Earliest Religious Poetry of India*. Oxford: Oxford University Press, 2017.

Jay, Mike. *Blue Tide: The Search for Soma*. Brooklyn, NY: Automedia, 1999.

Kinsley, David R. *Tantric Visions of the Divine Feminine: The Ten Mahāvidyās*. Berkeley: University of California Press, 1997.

Levitt, Stephan Hillyer. "New Considerations Regarding the Identity of Vedic Sóma as the Mushroom Fly Agaric." *Studia Orientalia* 3 (2011): 105–118.

Long, J. Bruce. "Life out of Death: A Structural Analysis of the Myth of the 'Churning of the Ocean of Milk'." In *Hinduism: New Essays in the History of Religions*, edited by Bardwell L. Smith, 171–207. Leiden, Netherlands: Brill, 1982.

Madhihassan, S. *The History and Natural History of Soma as Ephedra*. Islamabad: Pakistan Science Foundation, 1987.

Maillart-Garg, Meena, and Michael Winkelman. "The 'Kamasutra' Temples of India. A Case for the Encoding of Psychedelically Induced Spirituality." *Journal of Psychedelic Studies* 3, no. 2 (2019): 81–101.

McDonald, Andrew. "A Botanical Perspective on the Identity of Soma (Nelumbo nucifera Gaertn.). Based on Scriptural and Iconographic Records." *Economic Botany* 58 (Winter 2004): 147–173.

Mukhopadhaya, Satkari. *The Kaulajñānanirnaya: The Esoteric Teachings of Matsyendrapāda, Sadguru of the Yoginī Kaula School in the Tantra Tradition*. New Delhi: Aditya Prakashan, 2012.

Müller-Ebeling, Claudia, Christian Rätsch, and Surenda Bahadur Shahi. *Shamanism and Tantra in the Himalayas*. Rochester, VT: Park Street Press, 2002.

Napier, A. David. *Masks, Transformation, and Paradox*. Berkeley, Los Angeles, and London: University of California Press, 1986.

Nichols, D. E., M. W. Johnson, and Nichols, C.D. "Psychedelics as Medicines: An Emerging New Paradigm." *Journal of Clinical Pharmacology and Therapeutics*, 101, no. 2 (2017): 209–219.

O'Flaherty, Wendy Doniger. "The Post-Vedic History of the Soma Plant." In *Soma: Divine Mushroom of Immortality*, edited by R. Gordon Wasson, 95–147. New York: Harcourt Brace Jovanovich, 1969.

Ott, Jonathan. "The Post-Wasson History of the Soma Plant." *Eleusis*, no. 1 (1998): 9–37.

Partridge, Christopher. *High Culture: Drugs, Mysticism, and the Pursuit of Transcendence in the Modern World*. Oxford: Oxford University Press, 2018.

Plant, Sadie. *Writing on Drugs*. New York: Farrar, Straus and Giroux, 1999.

Qazilbash, N. A. "Ephedra of the Rigveda." *Pharmaceutical Journal* 26 (1960): 497–501.

Rätsch, Christian. *The Encyclopedia of Psychoactive Plants: Ethnopharmacology and Its Applications*. Translated by John R. Baker. Rochester. VT: Park Street Press, 2005.

Samuel, Geoffrey. *The Origins of Yoga and Tantra: Indic Religions to the Thirteenth Century*. Cambridge: Cambridge University Press, 2008.

Semenov, Dmitri. *Treatise on Soma Hymns of Rigveda*. Idaho Springs, CO: Sattarka Publications, 2020.

Sherrett, Andrew. "Introduction: Peculiar Substance." In *Consuming Habits: Drugs in History and Anthropology*, edited by Jordan Goodman, Paul E. Lovejoy, and Andrew Sherrett, 17–26. New York: Routledge, 1995.

Simonsson, O., Sexton, J.D., and Hendricks, P.S. "Associations between lifetime classic psychedelic use and markers of physical health." *Journal of Psychopharmacology* 35, no. 4 (2021): 447–452.

Smith, Huston. "Wasson's Soma: A Review Article." *Journal of the American Academy of Religions* 40, no. 4 (1972): 480–499.

Staal, Frits. "How a Psychoactive Substance Becomes a Ritual: The Case of Soma." *Social Research* 68, no. 3 (2001): 745–778.

Stedman's Medical Dictionary, 28th ed. Baltimore: Williams and Wilkins Company, 1996.

Thompson, George. "A Brief Anthology of Hymns in the Ṛgveda Having to Do with Soma (and Shamanism)." In *On Meaning and Mantras: Essays in Honor of Frits Staal*, edited by George Thompson and Richard K. Payne, 557–577. Moraga, CA: Institute of Buddhist Studies/BDK America, 2016.

Thompson, George. "Soma and Ecstasy in the Ṛgveda." *Electronic Journal of Vedic Studies* 9, no. 1 (2003): 1–13.

Törzsök, Judit. "Why Are the Skull-Bearers (Kāpālikas) Called Soma?" In *Śaivism and the Tantric Traditions*, 33–46. Leiden, Netherlands: Brill, 2020.

Wasson, R. Gordon. *Soma: Divine Mushroom of Immortality*. New York: Harcourt Brace Jovanovich, 1968.

Wasson, R. Gordon. "The Soma of the Rig Veda. What Was It?" *Journal of the American Oriental Society* 91, no. 2 (1971): 169–187.

Weil, Andrew. Review of Wasson, *Persephone's Quest: Entheogens and the Origins of Religion* (1986), *Journal of Psychoactive Drugs* 20, no. 4 (1988).

2 MESCALINE, BETWEEN PSYCHOPATHOLOGY AND PHENOMENOLOGY: SARTRE AND EXPERIMENTATION IN 1930s FRANCE

Gautier Dassonneville

In this chapter, I examine the undocumented history of mescaline in medical and psychiatric circles in France by reconstructing the scientific context in which Jean-Paul Sartre's famous bad trip took place in February 1935.[1] In this way, we can first consider that the very term "bad trip," sometimes ascribed to the experience retrospectively[2] on the basis of accounts by Simone de Beauvoir (1908–1986) in *The Prime of Life*[3] in 1960 and by Sartre himself in 1970,[4] may connote a psychedelic perspective that did not exist yet. At that time, the French writer and philosopher was in the process of formulating a phenomenological theory on the imagination, which he went on to introduce in *The Imagination*[5] (1936) and further develop in *The Imaginary*[6] (1940), when he decided to have himself injected with mescaline under the supervision of the psychiatrist Daniel Lagache (1903–1972), a former colleague from the École Normale Supérieure (ENS) who was then interning at the Sainte-Anne Hospital psychiatric ward. Following these injections, Sartre fell prey to somewhat nightmarish visions, as described by Beauvoir: "He saw umbrella-vultures, skeleton-shoes, monstrous faces; all around him were crawling crabs, octopi, contorted things."[7] During the intoxication, the hallucinogen did not produce the pleasant, dreamlike, kaleidoscopic visions that Sartre was expecting. However, it did have an impact on his psyche: he was then haunted by flashbacks from these hallucinations for several months afterward. Mescaline, according to Sartre, was the "incidental cause"[8] that sent him into a fit of depression that lasted from March 1935 to March 1937. Influenced by his research into psychopathology, Sartre believed that he was suffering from a chronic bout of hallucinatory psychosis during this period. However, he eventually decided to come to his senses and see off his crustaceous hallucinations once and for all.

To understand this legendary episode that Beauvoir's narrative sets in the beginning of French existentialism, Sartre's mescaline experience should be placed in the theoretical and cultural context of French philosophy of the interwar years. Mescaline was then a focal point for a generation of French intellectuals who were searching for inspiration from German schools of thought, including phenomenology, Gestalt psychology, and psychoanalysis. The following pages will highlight the interaction between philosophy and psychiatry in France, first by placing Sartre's mescaline experience in the context of Karl Jaspers's influence on French psychophilosophy, and then by reconstructing the Jacksonian model (discussed later in this chapter),[9] which presided over the initial mescaline research in the mid-1930s at Sainte-Anne, "central Paris's major psychiatric hospital."[10] When Sartre's misadventure may be presented as a countermodel that reveals the importance of set and setting in psychedelic studies, this inquiry will mostly focus on the French contribution to the "model psychoses theory"[11] of psychedelic drug effects.

SARTRE'S EARLY PSYCHOLOGY OF IMAGINATION

It was common knowledge that the young Sartre, with his fellow ENS philosophy students at his side, would rather go to see the psychology professor Georges Dumas present patients at Sainte-Anne than attend the eminent psychologist Pierre Janet's lectures at the Collège de France.[12] Yet, a large part of the analysis that Sartre presented in his graduate thesis (*diplôme d'études supérieures*), entitled *Mental Image in Psychological Life: Role and Nature*,[13] fell within these two authors' theoretical spheres of influence. This was before Sartre became acquainted with the development of phenomenology among German-speaking thinkers, and yet he had already concluded with an original theory of mental imagery as nonrepresentative (i.e., distinct from perception) and described it as a spontaneous creation of the mind. His early work demonstrated a critical appropriation of the theories and tools of scientific psychology. This was particularly manifest in the debate between Sartre and the Würzburg School, which promoted a method of experimental introspection and a theory of pure thinking. It is remarkable that in his graduate thesis, Sartre also used introspection as a basis for his contradictory interpretation of the conclusions of the Würzburg School's key psychological conception of "imageless thought," as well as drawing on the ideas of his fellow students Lagache and Raymond Aron. The former was himself at that time accomplishing his graduate thesis, *Consciousness and Delirium: On Delirious Mental Patients' Belief in their Own Madness*. Thus, it was beginning in the late 1920s that French intellectuals became seriously engaged in a dialogue between psychology and philosophy that focused on the mechanisms of psychological activity and the dialogue between Sartre and Lagache about normal and pathological imagination would continue in the mid-1930s.

Indeed, in his training as a psychiatrist, Lagache looked to the example of Georges Dumas, Pierre Janet, and the French tradition of philosopher-doctors. When the subject of pathological imagination again brought together the two former classmates in 1935, Lagache had just defended his medical dissertation, *Verbal Hallucinations and Speech* (1934),[14] and Sartre had just returned from studying Husserlian phenomenology in Berlin and had been asked to write a philosophical essay on the imagination by his former research director, the psychologist Henri Delacroix (1873–1937). In *The Imaginary*, Sartre describes the mental image as an "irreal object" being observed through what he called, by using a concept he found in the work of Edmund Husserl, an *analogon*—"equivalent to the perception," so to speak—made of knowledge, affectivity, and movement. In this respect, imaginary consciousness is incompatible with perceptive consciousness, as the latter has its origins in the sensory perception of reality. Genuine hallucinations—those with no external, real-world referent—therefore threatened to undermine Sartre's theory, as the hallucinatory images seemed to become indistinguishable from perception. This was why Sartre considered it important to understand the most recent psychopathology data by reading Lagache, and to visit Sainte-Anne to experience mescaline for himself to be subject to its hallucinatory effects. It was this experience that enabled Sartre to write the chapter on the "pathology of the imagination," which he felt was essential to confirm the validity of his hypothesis on the unreal nature of the imaginary consciousness.

Only a little observation from this experiment was exploited in *The Imaginary*,[15] but when his "Notes on Taking Mescaline"[16] were published in 2010, we finally got a better insight into the conditions and the way that it was carried out. Following a brief foreword, in which Sartre documents his state of mind and expectations before receiving two 0.30-g injections of mescaline, his notes convey a sense of the time line and location, taking place in a "small office in the Sainte-Anne mental institution" as well as in "the guard room" during the lunch hour (from 1 to 2 p.m.). The first injection was given at 11:10 a.m., the second at noon, and the last recorded observation was made at approximately 4:30 p.m., at which point Sartre was experiencing only "mild waves of mental confusion."[17] The handwritten manuscript, held at the French National Library, does not mention the moment when the decision was made to end the experiment, and it is hard to say whether some pages have been lost or whether Sartre stopped writing his report partway through.[18] Apparently, Sartre was authorized to go back home when the intoxication was going down but still producing some hallucinatory effects.

Figure 2.1
Original text from Jean-Paul Sartre about early mescaline experience. French National Library, NAF 28405, Copyright Gallimard (authorization of reproduction E2127 NQ).

"Finally, my anguish is translated by a motor agitation. I get up, I take a few steps, I stay standing. The worst of the intoxication is over.

It would be necessary to place here, I believe, a very fast phenomenon of hallucinosis. I looked at the calorifier whose pipes seemed to me very comical. Suddenly I heard singing or walking (I don't remember exactly) in the corridor. I listened to this noise. At that moment three light mists appeared in my visual field. Here the phenomenon of laterality took another form. Without a doubt these forms were seen in the very center of my visual field. But I was not looking. All my attention was absorbed by the noise. And, while I was listening, very quickly and furtively, the impression passed that I had seen three forms. I looked: they were no longer there.

Lagache went out to take a survey. I spoke with Rouault. He seems to me to have become absolutely normal again. A little heavier. Nausea. Apathetic but no more hallucinations.

Around half past four Lagache returns. Slight puffs of psychic troubles. I see the crosses again from time to time. I say to myself: "And if Lagache had a moustache. Immediately I "see" in the half-light Lagache's face adorned with a mustache. Not, in fact, when I look at his upper lip, which appears hairless. Rather, when I take a global perception of the face.""

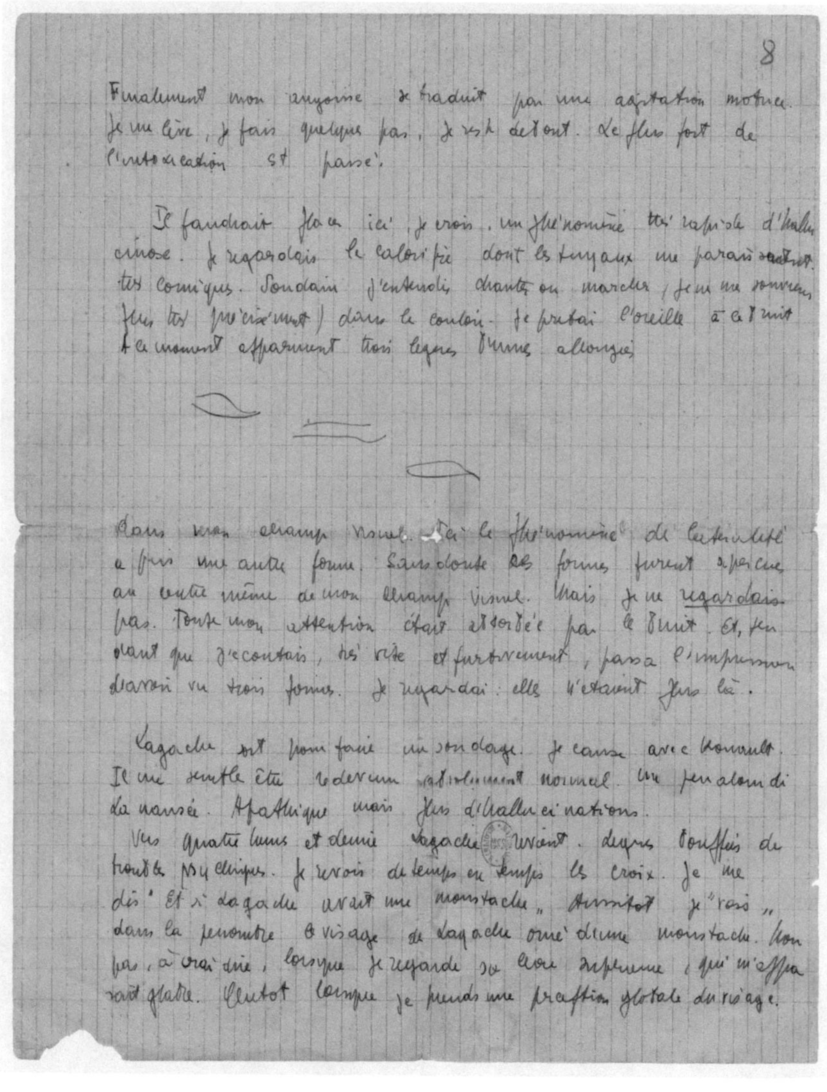
8

Finalement mon angoisse se traduit par une agitation motrice. Je me lève, je fais quelques pas, je reste debout. Le plus fort de l'intoxication est passé.

Il faudrait placer ici, je crois, un phénomène très rapide d'hallucinose. Je regardais le calorifère dont les tuyaux me paraissaient très comiques. Soudain j'entendis chanter ou marcher (je ne me souviens plus très précisément) dans le couloir. Je prêtai l'oreille à ce bruit. À ce moment apparurent trois lignes brunes allongées

dans mon champ visuel. Ici le phénomène de latéralité a pris une autre forme. Sans doute ces formes furent aperçues au centre même de mon champ visuel. Mais je ne regardais pas. Toute mon attention était absorbée par le bruit. Et, pendant que j'écoutais, très vite et furtivement, passa l'impression d'avoir vu trois formes. Je regardai : elles n'étaient plus là.

Lagache sort pour faire un sondage. Je cause avec [illegible]. Il me semble être redevenu absolument normal. Un peu alourdi de nausée. Apathique mais plus d'hallucinations.

Vers quatre heures et demie Lagache revient. Légères bouffées de troubles psychiques. Je revois de temps en temps les croix. Je me dis "Et si Lagache avait une moustache". Aussitôt je "vois" dans la pénombre le visage de Lagache orné d'une moustache. Non pas, à vrai dire, lorsque je regarde sa lèvre supérieure (qui m'apparaît glabre). Plutôt lorsque je prends une perception globale du visage.

Figure 2.1

Sartre's notes contain another discovery—one that contributes more to our understanding of the epistemological context: Lagache was not the only psychiatrist to oversee the experiment. With him was a "Dr. Rouault," who Sartre claims to have met just that morning and who appears to have played an important role in the proceedings. Unlike Lagache, who "was familiar with all the research on the subject," Rouault, "who had previously injected the drug himself," was better placed to share his impressions, in particular at the end of the session. Moreover, Rouault himself appears to have written observations on Sartre's reactions throughout the experiment, while Lagache had to leave the room at one point.[19] As stated in his foreword, Sartre was "fairly convinced that the alterations—if there were any—would occur with the objects within his perception," and he therefore could not "imagine losing himself in a dream, like Dr. Rouault." The precise identity of this Dr. Rouault is therefore of interest. He may be the same individual described in Simone de Beauvoir's account as "one of the housemen" who "was amazed" by the nightmarish turn that Sartre's experience had taken, while he had himself "gone romping through flowery meadows, full of exotic houris."[20] However, to reconstruct the history of these events, a hypothesis is in order: it appears highly likely that the individual whom Sartre called Dr. Rouault was in fact Dr. Julien Rouart (1901–1994), an intern in Professor Henri Claude's neuropsychiatric department at the time.[21] The identification of this new protagonist also completes the backdrop against which we can now examine the epistemological issues surrounding the collaboration between the as-yet unknown philosopher and the psychiatrists conducting research using mescaline on the imagination and its pathological forms.

MESCALINE AND *ERLEBNIS* ("LIVED EXPERIENCE")

From this fresh perspective, Sartre, Lagache, and Rouart all shared an interest in the phenomenological approach developed in the field of psychiatry by Karl Jaspers (1883–1969) at the beginning of the twentieth century, which was influenced by the work of Husserl. Sartre's youthful enthusiasm for Jaspers is well known, in particular due to his collaboration with his comrade

Paul Nizan (1905–1940) on the first French version of Jaspers's *Allgemeine Psychopathologie,* published by Alcan in 1928.[22] The treatise introduced a key distinction between *explaining* physical causality in nature and *understanding* psychical connection in the human mind. It became clear that French psychiatrists were adopting this approach in their methodology with the 1933 republication of the translation in an extremely detailed report on Jaspers's *Psychopathologie générale,* signed off by Lagache and Rouart in the *Journal de Psychologie Normale et Pathologique* (November–December 1935).[23] In this report, the two authors presented an extensive and meticulous synopsis of the treatise's nine chapters and made the case for its great "educational value."[24]

At the same time as Husserl and Martin Heidegger's respective phenomenological theories were being discussed by 1930s French philosophers, Jaspers's incorporation of phenomenological ideas into theories of psychopathology inspired a resurgence in French psychiatry. This movement found a following at Sainte-Anne in Claude's department, whose clinical director was the young Henri Ey (1900–1977). This period of emulation and clinical and experimental research was marked by the publication of several dissertations on mental health: the psychoanalyst and philosopher Jacques Lacan's *On Paranoid Psychosis in Relation to the Personality* (1932),[25] Lagache's *Verbal Hallucination and Speech* (1934)[26] and Rouart's *Manic Depressive Psychosis and Split-Personality Disorder* (1935).[27] These essays all drew inspiration from the categories and methods of German psychopathology, built by thinkers such as Emil Kraepelin (1856–1926), Jaspers, and the pioneering psychiatrist Eugen Bleuler (1857–1939). Paying close attention to the work of his peers, Ey observed that Jaspers's notion of the *expérience délirante* (delusional experience) was central to Lacan, Lagache, and Rouart's work. He defined the *expérience délirante* as "an unusual state of disturbance originating in the mind, in the personality, which manifests itself in the same way as a mescaline experience."[28] Here, Ey is clearly making a connection between Jaspers's comprehensive approach and Kurt Beringer's *Meskal Psychoze* theory, which was long used to define the psychotomimetic action of mescaline. Furthermore, the discussion on the question of the "lived experience" that took place between Drs. Édouard Pichon (1890–1940),[29]

Lacan, Lagache, and Ey following a presentation by Julien Rouart during a 1936 meeting of the *Évolution psychiatrique* group[30] demonstrated how the notion of *Erlebnis* (German for "lived experience") was becoming accepted in French psychopathology at that time.[31] The idea was to "reveal the nature of the instantaneous and concrete elements of [the patient's] consciousness"[32] by following Jaspers's recommendation in the early pages of the *General Psychopathology*: to "gain personal insight into an extensive collection of phenomenological examples using real cases" to develop "guidelines and comparative scales to examine new cases."[33] Hence, it was important for Jaspers to gather this information from patients. He documented these revelations in many patient autobiographies, compiling accounts from those suffering from mental disorders, as well as the experiences of healthy individuals who had taken psychotropic drugs. One of his sources was the Slovenian psychiatrist Alfred Šerko (1879–1938),[34] whose self-observations of *Meskalinrausch* ("mescaline rush")[35] provided several descriptions of altered perception of "object consciousness," which were included in a section of Jaspers's 1913 treatise, "Aspects of Abnormal Psychological Experience."[36] In his 1935 notes about his own mescaline experience, Sartre claimed to know nothing of this previous research on mescaline; yet his involvement in the first French translation of *Allgemeine psychopathologie* would have led him to discover descriptions of the twisted world of experimental schizophrenia as early as 1927. Sartre was not so much in search of a trip as he was looking for a specific type of *Erlebnis*–the delusional one–which would give him a better understanding of both the intentionality of the hallucinatory consciousness and the individual's hallucinatory experience.

THE JACKSONIAN MODEL

Despite Sartre's interest in Jaspers's comprehensive phenomenological approach, it was not the only conceptual tool that he used to develop a phenomenological description of hallucinatory consciousness. He also drew on the ideas of the English neuropsychiatrist John Hughlings Jackson (1835–1911), who had developed principles of what he called the evolution and dissolution of structures, and his theories emphasized biopsychological functionalism.[37] In his description of neurological and brain functioning in hierarchical form, lower levels see their functions released inappropriately when higher levels of control fail. Julien Rouart adopted this approach and collaborated with Henri Ey to write an article called "Trial Application of Jackson's Principles to a Dynamic Conception of Neuro-psychiatry" (1936),[38] in which they noted the descriptive value of experimentation with psychotropics: "Mescaline sometimes allows us to observe fairly profound dissolution (confusion) and signs of positivity which are at times fairly intense (oneirism) and at times less so (mere feelings of depersonalization, mild disturbances in perception). Both Moreau de Tours (Hashish) and Jackson (*Solanaceae*) had been struck by the experimental importance of this dissolution."[39]

There is continuity between Ey's initial research on hallucination and delusions[40] (1934) and his mammoth "Treatise on Hallucinations"[41] (1973), which presents a general overview of hallucinogenic drugs, with separate sections on hashish, LSD, and mushrooms, before providing an extensive summary of existing studies on peyote and mescaline.[42] As his career progressed, Ey became a proponent of a form of neo-Jacksonism[43] that aimed to incorporate psyche and consciousness into a theory of the dynamic structure of the nervous system. Ey's doctrine can be summarized as

a general theory of psychopathology, of organic dynamism, a system which is intended to go beyond pure psychodynamic theory (and above all Freudian psychoanalysis) and organistic (mechanistic) ideas in order to encapsulate the subconscious and the cerebral organ (in the biological sense) within the workings of psychological mechanisms whereby the hallucination brings to light the hierarchical structure of the brain—and thus the domination of the conscious over the subconscious—as it reveals the disorder.[44]

Due to Ey's early interest in hallucinatory phenomena, he became one of the main instigators of clinical and experimental research into mescaline and, along with Henri Claude (1869–1945), defined it as a hallucinogenic substance.

Indeed, in 1932, Claude and Ey joined forces to develop a dynamic theory of hallucinatory psychosis in which a distinction was made between the notion of *hallucinosis* and that of *hallucination*, thus allowing for varying levels of belief in the hallucinatory phenomena. According to Claude, hallucinosis was a hallucination that the subject recognized as such, while Ey insisted on the role of belief in the reality of the hallucinatory object, which makes the individual experiencing the hallucination behave as though it were real. Following in the footsteps of Jackson and Moreau de Tours, a nickname of French psychiatrist and pioneering researcher of hashish Jacques-Joseph Moreau (1804–1884), Claude and Ey's joint efforts aimed to demonstrate that "the personal hallucination-belief of perceiving an object which is not there must arise from a significant disturbance in psychological and perceptive activity."[45] From 1933 onward, experimentation with mescaline would become a method of choice for developing their understanding of hallucinations, as documented in their 1934 paper "Mescaline: A Hallucinogenic Substance." This very brief but invaluable report pinpoints the moment when research into experimental psychosis first began in Professor Claude's department at Sainte-Anne. The two-page document demonstrated the advantages of mescaline for experimental purposes from a Jacksonian perspective, in terms of the "remarkable deterioration in visual function"[46] generated by the drug. The report contained three sections: first, on the effects of mescaline on the psyche; second, on its effects on the body; and third, on its effects on psychiatric patients. For "an adult of average weight," whether "doctor or patient," the researchers administered 0.45 g of either Merck's mescaline sulfate or Roche's mescaline hydrochloride.

Rouart was involved in these experiments from the beginning, in the context of his research into the "systematic study of the neuro-vegetative system."[47] Finally, Claude and Ey highlighted the therapeutic potential of mescaline, as was documented in the case "of a patient admitted with melancholic depression with feelings of depersonalization who recovered her personality and normal bodily sensations while under the influence of mescaline" and who "left, cured, a few days later."[48] The conclusion of this pioneering article underlined once more the theoretical knowledge acquired through experimentation, which led the clinic to align its views on the role of functional deficits in hallucinations with those of Jackson, in that mescaline "liberates, but does not create, delusions."[49]

THE PROBLEM OF HALLUCINATIONS:
A BERGSONIAN HERITAGE

At the crossroads of psychopathology and philosophy, two other French authors appear to have encouraged Claude and Ey to begin studies on mescaline at Sainte-Anne: Pierre Quercy (1889–1946) and Raoul Mourgue (1886–1950), whose research into hallucinations, published in 1930 and 1932, respectively, served as the starting point for later psychiatrists and philosophers who went on to use phenomenological methods in their work. Both of them are identified as Bergsonian thinkers.[50] As early as 1921, Mourgue highlighted two outstanding features of Jackson's clinical psychology: it was *"phenomenological* (Jaspers, according to Husserl)," and it required "a clear understanding of *functional psychology*."[51] He was also an early commentator on the work of influential Heidelberg psychiatrists, in particular Wilhelm Mayer-Gross's and Kurt Beringer's study of experimental psychosis triggered by Merck's mescaline. In the introduction to *Neurobiologie de l'hallucination* (1932), his *"essay on a particular variety of disintegration of the function"*, Mourgue criticizes their work by highlighting the methodological limitations[52] of this research. Mourgue's work had a big impact on the psychomedical circles of the early 1930s, and Sartre was obliged to mention it in *The Imaginary*[53] to prove that his notion of kinesthetics in the *analogon* was not undermined by the neurobiological approach. Merleau-Ponty also used Mourgue's work in his first book, *The Structure of Behavior* (1942),[54] to highlight the fact that "rather than a perception without an object, hallucination is a global conduct related to a global alteration of nerve functioning."[55] Sartre and Merleau-Ponty were decidedly more critical of Quercy's work, which they thought represented a traditional view of psychology that subdivided our understanding of human beings into abstract ideas. Nevertheless, Quercy's clinical observations provided a source of information that Sartre certainly drew upon and analyzed.

Ey, meanwhile, often expressed admiration for Mourgue's neurobiological work, and in Quercy he found a theoretical adversary who helped him to clarify his own ideas. Moreover, the subjective observations of peyote intoxication documented in Quercy's essay *Études sur l'hallucination* (1930)[56] made a great impression on Ey at a time when he was also investigating the role of belief in "perception without an object"—as hallucinations had traditionally been defined since the early work of the psychiatrist Jean-Étienne Esquirol (1872–1840). In his 1932 report, Ey was enthusiastic about experimenting with hallucinogens to gain personal insight into perception without an object: "Mr Quercy has in fact experimented with peyote and has experienced hallucinations that he describes with great joy. He emphasizes how vivid his impressions were, their complete aesthesia. Ultimately, Mr Quercy's essay is essentially a new testimony—and a very interesting one!— that of a hallucinating individual who tells us 'I saw . . . I believed.'"[57] Ey's initial enthusiasm at reading Quercy's accounts soon prompted the young psychiatrist to begin experimenting with mescaline himself, which in turn led him to steer his students' research in this direction.[58]

THE DISINTEGRATION OF CONSCIOUSNESS

Following this tour through the beginning of French mescaline research, it is unsurprising to see the Jacksonian paradigm appear in Sartre's "Notes on Taking Mescaline." When it came to analyzing the phenomena that he experienced between 2:50 and 3:15 p.m. in more detail, his account even takes its structure from the trials carried out in general psychopathology, placing them into three categories: (1) the world of objects, (2) higher functions, and (3) affectivity. Thus, Sartre's choice of conceptual tools to document his experience was also an allusion to Jacksonian-inspired psychopathology: in particular, the idea of oscillation,[59] which he used to describe the various phases of intoxication and which came from Janet's branch of psychopathology. As the psychiatrist and writer Jean Delay[60] (1907–1987) reminds us, "it is thanks to Pierre Janet that we have a dynamic theory of the mind based on psychological tension and its oscillations. His notion of the hierarchy of behaviors is based on the opposition of automatic actions and synthetic processes: the former are associated with low levels of tension, which facilitates simple operations such as dreaming, and the latter—those involving a conscious effort of concentration—with high levels of tension."[61] Delay understands Janet's ideas as a precursor to the emergence of drug therapy since he was the first person to highlight the psychological tension that the psychotonic and neuroleptic drugs discovered at the turn of the 1950s acted upon. But here we face the second wave of mescaline research at Sainte-Anne, led by Delay—who eventually classified the substance as a "psycho-dysleptic"[62] (a substance that disrupts psychic functioning) in the 1950s before investigating psilocybin and LSD in the 1960s.

When he described the disintegration of the higher functions of his own consciousness in 1935, Sartre was brought closer to the ideas of the French philosopher Henri Bergson, which had found their place in French psychopathology in the interwar years, perhaps especially his concept of a "weakening of the sense of reality"—the equivalent in Janet's work being the "loss of function of reality." Sartre was somewhat conflicted on this matter, as elsewhere he rejected[63] Bergson's explanations relating to a "weakening of attention to life,"[64] thus further developing his critical position to the Bergsonian concept of image that he had maintained since his 1927 graduate thesis. Yet the various phenomenological explanations for the spontaneous degradation of the consciousness—and the resulting organization of the individual consciousness into phenomenological themes according to the theory of *captive consciousness*—emerged from these same theoretical fundamentals of French psychopathology. As for the psychopathological concept of the "morbid consciousness," Sartre attributed a "*functional* role" to hallucinations in connection with a general pattern of behavior: the dialectical adaptation of the patient (the I) to their visions (rebellious spontaneity), which was defined as "hallucinatory conduct."[65] He thereby built upon his 1927 interpretation of schizoid behavior as an adaptation to images through physical conduct.[66]

Ultimately, Sartre's phenomenological account of hallucinations in *The Imaginary* maintained the mutual exclusivity of both perceptive and imaginary consciousness, defending the notion that genuine hallucinations involved acute disintegration of consciousness. In a further development of Janet's ideas, which reduced hallucination to a disorder of belief in which the patient related to the hallucinatory phenomena only retrospectively,[67] Sartre proposed two distinct moments in hallucinatory experience. The first was "the pure experience," which is the consciousness descending into a state of participation in which the subject and object were indistinguishable from one another, followed immediately by a memory of this event (the second moment). Finally, borrowing from Jaspers's psychopathology research, Sartre described this fragmentation of the consciousness as a "twilight state."[68] In the end, he formulated a theory of the pathological imagination that relied upon the absolute and impersonal spontaneity of the consciousness. In his view, the act of hallucinating was proof that the consciousness could forget itself and allow itself to be fooled by its own magical behavior. By distinguishing radically perception and imagination, Sartre emphasized the idea that the imaginative act is relying on the annihilation power of consciousness. Following these ideas, Sartre assigned "bad faith" to the heart of human reality and suspended mental illness as a question of self-deception.

In a way of a short conclusion, we can say that mescaline in France thus found itself caught between psychopathology and phenomenology, at the heart of a debate around the philosophical and metaphysical principles

Figure 2.2
Original text from Jean-Paul Sartre about early mescaline experience. French National Library, NAF 28405, Copyright Gallimard (authorization of reproduction E2127 NQ).

". . . of an approximate localization. From that moment until half past five, I kept distorting Rouault's face and making him wince. But I no longer identified him with C. and B. Around this time, looking at a pulley lamp, as there was one in my grandmother's room (who died three years ago) above my head, I saw it vaguely moving. In reality one would have to speak here of "motionless movements" and of frozen deformations. The lamp seemed to have lines of force running through it.

At the same time, I saw (in the same way as the Egyptian and Assyrian arabesques above) lozenges on the grey ceiling and these lozenges referred me to the marquetry table, the lamp and my grandmother's room presented themselves as the deep meaning of the objects, a reference to my history. But it seemed to me, with a little arbitrariness on my part, a kind of good will in all these constructions.

Perhaps the first great oscillation had just come to an end. It is indeed necessary to imagine the psychic development of the intoxication, more or less like this. It seemed to me that, at the moment of which I speak, a kind of dissociation between the interpretations and the perceptions took place. Thus, considering an umbrella hanging in front of me on a peg, I said to myself that it looked like a vulture. The comparison itself was rather strange. The bent handle of light wood would have been the bare neck and head of the vulture, the black cloth would have represented the body and the wings."

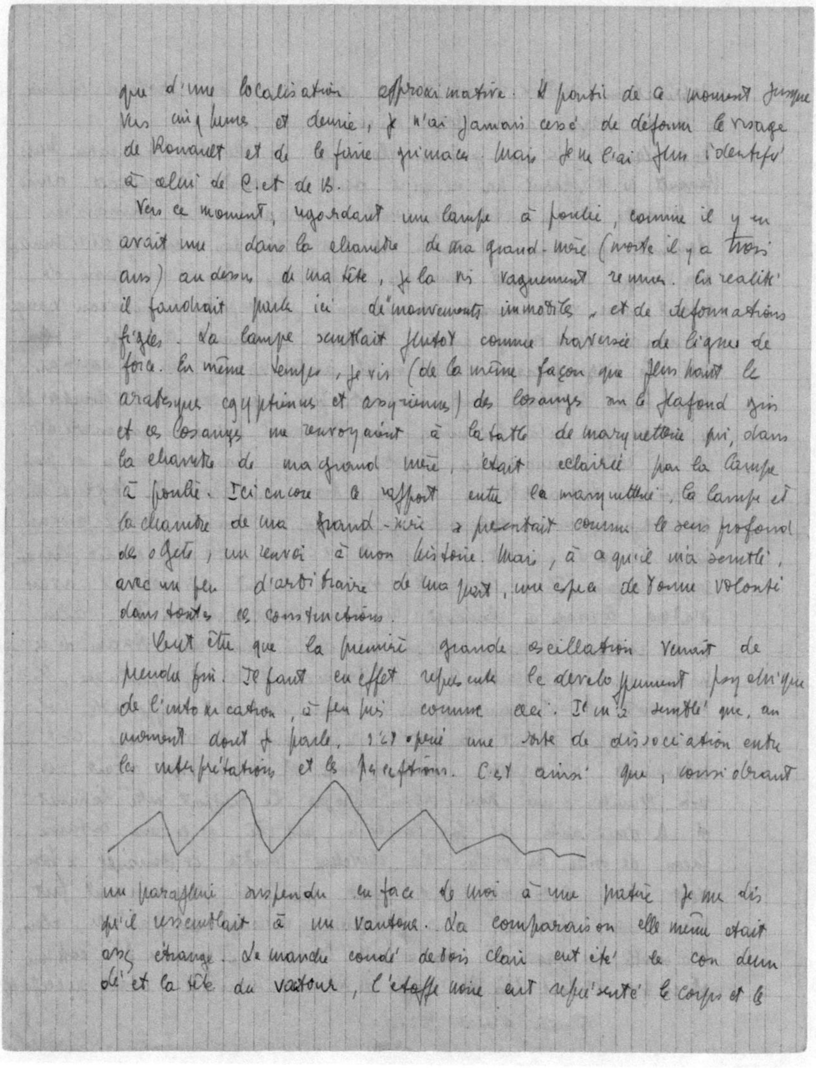

que d'une localisation approximative. A partir de ce moment jusque vers cinq heures et demie, je n'ai jamais cessé de déformer le visage de Renault et de le faire grimacer. Mais je ne l'ai plus identifié à celui de C. et de B.

Vers ce moment, regardant une lampe à poulie, comme il y en avait une dans la chambre de ma grand-mère (morte il y a trois ans) au-dessus de ma tête, je la vis vaguement remuer. En réalité il faudrait parler ici de «mouvements immobiles», et de déformations figées. La lampe semblait plutôt comme traversée de lignes de force. En même temps, je vis (de la même façon que plus haut les arabesques égyptiennes et assyriennes) des losanges sur le plafond gris et ces losanges me renvoyaient à la table de marqueterie qui, dans la chambre de ma grand-mère, était éclairée par la lampe à poulie. Ici encore le rapport entre la marqueterie, la lampe et la chambre de ma grand-mère se présentait comme le sens profond des objets, un renvoi à mon histoire. Mais, à ce qu'il m'a semblé, avec un peu d'arbitraire de ma part, une espèce de bonne volonté dans toutes ces constructions.

Peut-être que la première grande oscillation venait de prendre fin. Il faut en effet représenter le développement psychique de l'intoxication, à peu près comme ceci. Il m'a semblé que, au moment dont je parle, s'est opéré une sorte de dissociation entre les interprétations et les perceptions. C'est ainsi que, considérant

un parapluie suspendu en face de moi à une patère je me dis qu'il ressemblait à un vautour. La comparaison elle-même était assez étrange. Le manche coudé de bois clair eût été le cou dénudé et la tête du vautour, l'étoffe noire eût représenté le corps et les

Figure 2.2

behind the epistemological paradigms used in psychiatry. This can be seen in the discussions held during the Bonneval conference in September 1946 about the *Problem of the Psychogenesis of Neuroses and Psychoses*,[69] where rivaling perspectives went to collide about the conception of mental illness origins, Lacan opposing a new conception of psychical causality of psychosis (psychogenesis) to Ey's view of neurophysiological roots of madness (organogenesis). As for him, Rouart attempted to liberalize the Jacksonian doctrine of dissolutions to give a more significant role to the psychogenetic perspective, in particular by linking up with the Sartrean theory of emotions. In addition, understanding the predominance of Jacksonian epistemology in the first experiments with mescaline at Sainte-Anne in the 1930s will shed light on the direction taken in the research into psychodysleptic drugs led by Jean Delay after World War II and its role in the psychopharmaceutical revolution set in motion by the discovery of chlorpromazine in 1952. The exploration of the epistemological paradigms used to further psychiatric knowledge undoubtedly poses ethical questions that a historical view helps to put into perspective. There, during years when Michel Foucault was an intern in Delay's service at Sainte-Anne, it has been one of his first contributions to criticize radically the Jacksonian model of evolution as a scientific and an ethical myth.[70]

NOTES

1. Here, I follow the chronology provided by Michel Contat and Michel Rybalka in J.-P. Sartre, *Œuvres romanesques* (Paris: Gallimard, "Pléiade," 1980), xxv–civ. January 1935 is occasionally mentioned by biographers.

2. Cf. Carole Hayne-Curtis, "Sartre and the Drug Connection," *Philosophy: Journal of the Royal Institute of Philosophy* 70, no. 271 (January 1995): 87–106; Thomas Smith, "On Sartre and the Drug Connection: A Response to Haynes-Curtis," *Philosophy* 70, no. 274 (October 1995): 590–593; Mike Jay, *Mescaline: A Global History of the First Psychedelic* (New Haven, CT: Yale University Press, 2019), 158; Patrick Farrell, "Mescaline Scribe," *Chacruna* (2020); Stéphanie Chayet, *Phantastica: Ces substances interdites qui guérissent* (Paris: Grasset, 2020), 76–77.

3. Simone de Beauvoir, *The Prime of Life*, transl. Peter Green (Harmondsworth, Midlesex, UK: Penguin Books Ltd; Ringwood, Victoria, Australia: Penguin Books Pty Ltd, 1962), 209–213.

4. John Gerassi, *Talking with Sartre: Conversations and Debates* (New Haven, CT, and London: Yale University Press, 2009), 62–63 (March 1971 interview), 79–80 (April 1971 interview),

and 193–194 (May 1972 interview). These testimonies should be taken with caution: it is noteworthy that the friendly tone of the discussion and Sartre's sometimes fading recollections, which include cuts and transcriptions and translations of old audio recordings, do not seem to match completely with the historical facts.

5.   Jean-Paul Sartre, *The Imagination*, transl. Kenneth Williford and David Rudrauf (Routledge: London, 2012). For references concerning the topic of this chapter, see the "Translators' Introduction," 11–99, particularly n6.

6.   Jean-Paul Sartre, *The Imaginary. A Phenomenological Psychology of the Imagination*, revision and historical introduction by Arlette Elkaïm-Sartre, translation and philosophical introduction by Jonathan Webber (Routledge: London, 2004). Arlette Elkaim-Sartre's revision only concerns an emandation she made to the text because of a line that had seemed to jump in the first edition of *L'Imaginaire* (Cf n34, page 203 and Jonathan Webber's Notes on the translation, page XXX).

7.   Beauvoir, *The Prime of Life*, 209.

8.   *Sartre by Himself: A Film Directed by Alexandre Astruc and Michel Contat with the Participation of Simone de Beauvoir, Jacques-Laurent Bost, Andre Gorz, and Jean Pouillon*, transl. Richard Seaver (New York: Urizen Books, 1978), 37–38.

9.   A neuropsychological model in psychiatry based on the British neurologist John Hughlings Jackson's ideas on brain functions.

10.   Allan D. Schrift, *Twentieth-Century French Philosophy. Key Themes and Thinkers* (Malden, MA: Wiley-Blackwell, 2005).

11.   Link R. Swanson, "Unifying Theories of Psychedelic Drug Effects," *Frontiers in Pharmacology* 9, no. 172 (March 2018): 1–23.

12.   Cf. Daniel Lagache, "Janet au Collège de France," *Évolution psychiatrique* 3 (1950): 417; A. Cohen-Solal, *Sartre. 1905–1980* (Paris: Gallimard, "folio," 2005), 140; Thomas R. Flynn, *Sartre: A Philosophical Biography* (Cambridge: Cambridge University Press, 2014).

13.   Jean-Paul Sartre, *L'image dans la vie psychologique: Rôle et nature, dans Études sartriennes*, "Sartre inédit: le mémoire de fin d'études (1927)," *sous la direction de Gautier Dassonneville* 22 (2019), 43–246.

14.   Daniel Lagache, *Les Hallucinations verbales et la parole* (Paris: Alcan, 1934).

15.   Sartre, *The Imaginary*, 156–157.

16.   J.-P. Sartre, "Notes sur la prise de mescaline," *dans Les Mots et autres écrits autobiographiques* (Paris: Gallimard, "Pléiade," 2010) 1222–1237; 1223; See also the editor Juliette Simont's note, 1606–1611.

17.   Sartre, "Notes sur la prise de mescaline," 1, 237.

18.   Held with the Sartre papers (NAF 28405) at the French National Library, the manuscript comprises seven leaflets printed on both sides (except leaflet 4). A copy of the first leaflet was

published in the library's catalog for the Sartre exhibition, which shows that "the manuscript, written with a strong hand, was given to Merleau-Ponty by Sartre." *Sartre*, ed. Mauricette Berne (Paris: BNF/Gallimard, 2005), 70–71.

19. See, for instance, Sartre, "Notes sur la prise de mescaline," 1229: "'As Rouault then noted, it is common to see complementary colors in these visions.' But then I immediately realize that I *see* neither red nor green," and, further, on 1233: "I'm chatting to Rouault. He seems to have gotten completely back to normal."

20. Beauvoir, *The Prime of Life*, 209. To understand these nightmarish effects, Thomas Riedlinger applied Stanislav Grof's reading grid and suggested that a traumatic abreaction occurred. See "Sartre's Rite of Passage," *Journal of Transpersonal Psychology* 14 (1982): 105–123; "Two Classic Trips. Jean-Paul Sartre and Adelle Davis," *Gnosis Magazine* 34 (Winter 1993): 34–41.

21. This hypothesis is confirmed in David Haziot's biographical sketch, in which we learn that Julien, the son of the painter Ernest Rouart and Julie Manet, was "instructed to supervise Sartre's mescaline experience." See D. Haziot, *Le Roman des Rouart (1850–2000)* (Paris: Fayart, 2012), 347.

22. Karl Jaspers, *Psychopathologie générale*, traduit d'après la 3ᵉ édition par A. Kastler et J. Mendousse, révisée par J.-P. Sartre et P. Nizan (Paris: Alcan, "Bibliothèque de philosophie contemporaine," 1928).

23. Daniel Lagache and Julien Rouart, "La *Psychopathologie générale* de Karl Jaspers," *Journal de Psychologie Normale et Pathologique* 32 (1935): 776–797.

24. Lagache and Rouart, "La *Psychopathologie générale* de Karl Jaspers," 797.

25. Jacques Lacan, *De la psychose paranoïaque dans ses rapports à la personnalité* (Paris: Librairie E. Le François, 1932).

26. Lagache, *Les hallucinations verbales et la parole* (Paris: Alcan, 1934).

27. Julien Rouart, *Psychose maniaque dépressive et folie discordante: Situation nosographique de quelques formes particulières par rapport à ces entités* (Paris: G. Doin, 1935). The foreword is signed off with a dedication: "My friend, Henri Ey, whose ward is so widely open to me, can be assured of my deep gratitude and our strong friendship."

28. Henri Ey, "Paul Balvet, *Le sentiment de dépersonnalisation dans les délires de structure paranoïde* (thèse de Lyon, 1936)," *L'Encéphale, Journal de neurologie et de psychiatrie* 2 (1936): 226–228.

29. A grammarian, pediatrist, and psychiatrist, Pichon cofounded in 1927 the *Société psychanalytique de Paris* [Psychoanalytic Society of Paris].

30. Julien Rouart, "Du rôle de l'onirisme dans les psychoses de type paranoïaque et maniaque-dépressif," *L'Évolution psychiatrique* IV (1936): 61–94.

31. Rouart, "Du rôle de l'onirisme dans les psychoses," 86–89.

32. Rouart, "Du rôle de l'onirisme dans les psychoses," 88, in the words of Ey.

33. Jaspers, *Psychopathologie générale*, 48.

34. Alfred Šerko, "Im Meskalinrausch," *Jahrbücher für Psychiatrie und Neurologie* 34 (1913): 355–366.

35. The translators of Jaspers's *Psychopathologie générale* (1928) proposed at first "*ivresse de mescaline*" (mescaline intoxication), but Henri Ey in the 1930s preferred to speak of "*l'ivresse mescalinique*" ("mescalinic intoxication") or "*l'intoxication mescalinique*" ("mescalinic poisoning"). In doing so, he used the adjective formed by Alexandre Rouhier (*La Plante qui fait les yeux émerveillés*, Part III, chap. V, 1927), who spoke of "peyotlic" or "mescalinic" intoxication. We can notice that in French, *ivresse* refers more to the transformation of the state of mind or mood, while *intoxication* refers more to a biochemical process. In the 1950s, Jean Delay and Henri Michaux preferred the adjective *mescalinienne* ("mescalinian"), which in my opinion has a broader connotation, focusing less on the molecule as such and more on its effects and the world that it gives access to.

36. Jaspers, *Psychopathologie générale*, 50–100.

37. G. E. Berrios, "French Views on Positive and Negative Symptoms: A Conceptual History," *Comprehensive Psychiatry* 32, no. 5 (1991): 395–403.

38. Henri Ey and Julien Rouart, "Essai d'application des principes de Jackson à une conception dynamique de la neuro-psychiatrie," *L'Encéphale: Journal de neurologie et de psychiatrie* 1 (1936): 313–356, and no. 2, 30–60, 96–123. While Rouart turned to a more psychoanalytical approach, Ey developed his take on neo-Jacksonianism using the organodynamic model. One of Ey's rare English texts is "Hughlings Jackson's Principles and the organo-dynamic concept of psychiatry," *American Journal of Psychiatry* 118 (1962): 673–682.

39. Ibid., no. 2, 101–102. See also on p. 117, the mention of "phenomena resembling hallucinations" that are sometimes triggered by the mescaline intoxication.

40. Henri Ey, *Hallucinations et délire: Les formes hallucinatoires de l'automatisme verbal* (Paris: Alcan, 1934).

41. Henri Ey, *Traité des hallucinations*, tome 1 (Paris: Masson et Cie, 1973).

42. Ey, *Traité des hallucinations,* 602–681. In this chapter, Ey uses his unpublished observations from around fifty tests that he carried out between 1934 and 1937 as a basis for his analyses of mescaline intoxication—including one experiment in 1934 in which he self-administered 0.50 g of mescaline sulfate, which he described as producing nothing more than "a few sensory illusions" and "an unpleasant sense of unease."

43. See Philip Evans, "Henri Ey's Concepts of the Organization of Consciousness and Its Disorganization: An Extension of Jacksonian Theory," *Brain* 95 (1972): 413–40; Emmanuel Delille, "L'organo-dynamisme d'Henri Ey: l'oubli d'une théorie de la conscience considéré dans ses relations avec l'analyse existentielle," *L'Homme et la Société* 1–3, no. 167–169 (2008): 203–219.

44. Régis Patrouillard, "L'hallucination chez Henri Ey et sa signification aujourd'hui," *La Revue lacanienne* 1 (2007): 62–67.

45. Henri Claude and Henri Ey, "Hallucinose et hallucination: Les théories neurologiques des phénomènes psycho-sensoriels," *L'Encéphale* 27, no. 7 (1932): 376–621.

46. Henri Claude and Henri Ey, "La mescaline, substance hallucinogène," *Comptes rendus des séances hebdomadaires de la Société de Biologie* 115 (1934): 838–841.

47. Claude and Ey, "La mescaline, substance hallucinogène," 840. Two other individuals are also cited as having taken part in the study: a man named "Caron" (probably meaning the doctor Marcel Caron), and a doctor named "K. Agadjanian." The latter wrote a 1934 memorandum on "Reflexive Methodology in the Study of the Mechanism behind the Appearance of False Images" (*Comptes rendus des séances hebdomadaires de la Société de Biologie*, "22 December meeting," vol. 117, 1934, 1183–1186) and later wrote "Introduction to the Experimental Study of the Issue of Hallucination" (*Archives internationales de neurologie*, Paris, October, November, December 1939—January 1940).

48. Claude and Ey, "La mescaline, substance hallucinogène," 840–841.

49. Claude and Ey, "La mescaline, substance hallucinogène," 841.

50. Pierre Quercy, "Remarques sur une théorie bergsonienne de l'hallucination," *Annales médico-légales* (1925): 242–69; Raoul Mourgue, "Le point de vue neuro-biologique dans l'œuvre de M. Bergson et les données actuelles de la science," *Revue de métaphysique et de morale* 27, no. 1 (1920): 27–70.

51. Raoul Mourgue, "La méthode d'étude des affections du langage d'après Hughlings Jackson," *Journal de Psychologie Normale et Pathologique* 18 (1921): 753. Emphasis in original.

52. Raoul Mourgue, *Neurobiologie de l'hallucination*, 20: "For now, at least, I can't see another way [of using the *Hirnforschung*'s and the clinic's data] and that would explain the relatively poor results that Beringer, among others, has produced as a result of his experiences with mescaline, for example. Indeed, these offer little more than essentially artificial productions and, as I mentioned before, this raw material needs interpreting. It is worth stating once again: nothing is more deceitful than language and, it seems, *phenomenology* makes the mistake of ignoring this fact." Emphasis as per original.

53. Sartre, *The Imaginary*, 200n39.

54. Maurice Merleau-Ponty, *The Structure of Behavior*, transl. Alden L. Fischer with a foreword by John Wild (Boston: Beacon, 1963).

55. Merleau-Ponty, *The Structure of Behavior*, 205.

56. Pierre Quercy, *Études sur l'hallucination*, 2 vols. (Paris: Alcan, 1930).

57. Henri Ey, "La croyance de l'halluciné (À propos des études de M. Quercy sur les hallucinations)," *Annales médico-psychologiques* 11 (1932): 13–37, 21.

58. Ey (1973, 606) mentions the thesis that he suggested to his student Daniel Colomb, Contribution à l'étude pharmacologique de la Mescaline (Paris: Thèse, 1939).

59. Sartre, "Notes sur la prise de mescaline," 1228.

60. Inspired by the teachings of Pierre Janet and Georges Dumas, Delay became an intern in the Paris hospitals in 1927 and defended a medical thesis on the *Astéréognosies* [Astereognosis] in 1935, which was followed by another 1942 thesis in philosophy on *Les Dissolutions de*

la mémoire [The Dissolutions of Memory], which included a preface by Pierre Janet. He then trained with Henri Ey at the Sainte-Anne Hospital, where he was made chair of clinical mental illness and encephala in 1946.

61. J. Delay, "Des médicaments psychologiques," *Revue des Deux Mondes (1829–1971)*, 15 June 1956, 602. Janetian psychopathology left a cultural mark on Sartre during his training years at the ENS, during which he integrated psychasthenia and the idea of successive low- and high-tension periods into his personal representations.

62. Yves Edel, "Expérimentations des psychodysleptiques à Sainte-Anne dans les années 1960," *Annales médico-psychologiques* 175, no. 7 (2017): 653–660; Zoë Dubus, "Le LSD, psychédé- lique ou psychodysleptique," *L'information psychiatrique* 97, no. 9 (2021): 803–808.

63. In particular, see Sartre, *The Imaginary*, 42–43, where the Bergsonian expression that appears in Jean Jacques Lhermitte's *Le Sommeil* [The Sleep] (Paris: Colin, 1925) as part of the study of the creation of hypnagogic images is dismissed as surrendering to the illusions of immanence (i.e., a mistake that considers the image as an object inside the consciousness). However, Sartre is prepared to use it to explain "a hallucinatory renaissance" (42) and he freely uses it to describe the "radical revamping of the conscious attitude toward the unreal" that becomes apparent during hallucination (157).

64. Sartre, *The Imaginary*, 42–43.

65. Sartre, *The Imaginary*, 159.

66. Sartre, *L'image dans la vie psychologique*, 200–1.

67. Pierre Janet, "L'hallucination dans le délire de persécution," *Revue Philosophique de la France et de l'étranger*, tome 113, 1932, 61–98. See also Henri Ey, "La conception de P. Janet sur les hallucinations et les délires," dans *L'Évolution psychiatrique: Hommage à Pierre Janet*, vol. 15 (Aurillac: Poirier-Bottreau, 1950), 437–449.

68. Sartre, *The Imaginary*, 304. See Jaspers, *Psychopathologie générale*, 528–531.

69. Lucien Bonnafé, Henri Ey, Sven Follin, Jacques Lacan, and Julien Rouart, *Le problème de la psychogenèse des névroses et des psychoses* (Paris: Desclée de Brouwer, 1950), 202.

70. Michel Foucault, *Mental Illness and Psychology*, translated by Allan Sheridan with a foreword by Hubert Dreyfus (Berkeley-Los Angeles-London: University of California, 1987), 24–25.

BIBLIOGRAPHY

Primary Sources
Sartre papers (NAF 28405) at the French National Library.

Secondary Sources
Sartre by Himself: A Film Directed by Alexandre Astruc, and Michel Contat, with the Participation of Simone de Beauvoir, Jacques-Laurent Bost, Andre Gorz, and Jean Pouillon. translated by Richard Seaver. New York: Urizen Books, 1978.

Beauvoir, Simone de. *The Prime of Life*, translated by Peter Green. Harmondsworth, Middlesex, UK: Penguin Books Ltd; Ringwood, Victoria, Australia: Penguin Books Pty Ltd, 1962.

Beringer, Kurt. *Der Meskalinrausch: Seine Geschichte und Erscheinungsweise (Monographien aus dem Gesamtgebiete der Neurologie und Psychiatrie)*. Berlin-Heidelberg GmbH: Springer, 1927.

Berríos, Germán Elías. "French Views on Positive and Negative Symptoms: A Conceptual History." *Comprehensive Psychiatry* 32, no. 5 (1991): 395–403.

Bonnafé, Lucien, Henri Ey, Sven Follin, Jacques Lacan, and Julien Rouart. *Le problème de la psychogenèse des névroses et des psychoses*. Paris: Desclée de Brouwer, 1950.

Chayet, Stéphanie. *Phantastica: Ces substances interdites qui guérissent*. Paris: Grasset, 2020.

Claude, Henri, and Henri Ey. "Hallucinose et hallucination. Les théories neurologiques des phénomènes psycho-sensoriels." *L'Encéphale* 27, no. 7 (1932): 576–621.

Claude, Henri, and Henri Ey. "La mescaline, substance hallucinogène." *Comptes rendus des séances hebdomadaires de la Société de Biologie* 115 (1934): 838–841.

Cohen-Solal, Annie. *Sartre 1905–1980* [1985]. Paris: Gallimard, 1999.

Colomb, Daniel. Contribution à l'étude pharmacologique de la mescaline. PhD diss., Faculté de médecine et de pharmacie de Lyon, 1939.

Contat, Michel, Michel Rybalka, and Jean-Paul. Sartre. *Œuvres romanesques*. Paris: Gallimard, "Pléiade," 1980.

Delay, Jean. "Des médicaments psychologiques." *Revue des Deux Mondes (1829–1971)* (1956): 600–617.

Delille, Emmanuel. "L'organo-dynamisme d'Henri Ey: l'oubli d'une théorie de la conscience considéré dans ses relations avec l'analyse existentielle." *L'Homme et la Société* (2008): 167–169.

Evans, Philip. "Henri Ey's Concepts of the Organization of Consciousness and Its Disorganization: An Extension of Jacksonian Theory." *Brain* 95 (1972): 413–40.

Ey, Henri. "La conception de P. Janet sur les hallucinations et les délires." *L'Évolution psychiatrique: Hommage à Pierre Janet* 15 (1950): 437–449.

Ey, Henri. "La croyance de l'halluciné (À propos des études de M. Quercy sur les hallucinations)." *Annales médico-psychologiques* 11 (1932): 13–37.

Ey, Henri. *Hallucinations et délire: Les formes hallucinatoires de l'automatisme verbal*. Paris: Alcan, 1934.

Ey, Henri. "Hughlings Jackson's Principles and the Organo-Dynamic Concept of Psychiatry." *American Journal of Psychiatry* 118 (1962): 673–82.

Ey, Henri. "Paul Balvet, Le sentiment de dépersonnalisation dans les délires de structures paranoïdes (thèse de Lyon, 1936)." *L'encéphale: Journal de neurologie et de psychiatrie* 2 (1936): 226–228.

Ey, Henri. *Traité des hallucinations*. tome 1. Paris: Masson et Cⁱᵉ, 1973.

Ey, Henri, and Julien Rouart. "Essai d'application des principes de Jackson à une conception dynamique de la neuro-psychiatrie." *L'encéphale: Journal de neurologie et de psychiatrie* 1 (1936): 313–356.

Farrell, Patrick. "Mescaline Scribe." *Chacruna*. https://chacruna.net/mescaline-scribe-beauvoir-sartre/

Foucault, Michel. *Mental Illness and Psychology*, translated by Allan Sheridan with a foreword by Hubert Dreyfus. Berkeley-Los Angeles-London: University of California, 1987.

Gerassi, John. *Talking with Sartre: Conversations and Debates*. New Haven, CT, and London: Yale University Press, 2009.

Haziot, David. *Le roman des Rouart: Une famille de collectionneurs 1850–2000*. Paris: Fayard, 2012.

Janet, Pierre. "L'hallucination dans le délire de persécution." *Revue Philosophique de la France et de l'étranger* 113 (1932): 61–98.

Jaspers, Karl. *Psychopathologie générale, traduit d'après la 3e édition par A. Kastler et J. Mendousse, révisée par J.-P. Sartre et P. Nizan*. Paris: Alcan, Bibliothèque de philosophie contemporaine, 1928.

Jay, Mike. *Mescaline: A Global History of the First Psychedelic*. New Haven, CT: Yale University Press, 2019.

Lacan, Jacques. *De la psychose paranoïaque dans ses rapports à la personnalité*. Paris: Librairie E. Le François, 1932.

Lagache, Daniel *Les hallucinations verbales et la parole*. Paris: Alcan, 1934.

Lagache, Daniel. "Janet au Collège de France." *Évolution psychiatrique* 3 (1950): 417.

Lagache, Daniel, and Julien Rouart. "La psychopathologie générale de Karl Jaspers." *Journal de Psychologie Normale et Pathologique* 32 (1935): 776–797.

Merleau-Ponty, Maurice. *The Structure of Behavior*, translated by Alden L. Fischer with a foreword by John Wild. Boston: Beacon, 1963.

Mourgue, Raoul. "La méthode d'étude des affections du langage d'après Hughlings Jackson." *Journal de Psychologie Normale et Pathologique* 18 (1921): 752–764.

Patrouillard, Régis. "L'hallucination chez Henri Ey et sa signification aujourd'hui." *La Revue lacanienne* 1 (2007): 62–67.

Quercy, Pierre. *Études sur l'hallucination*, vol. 2. Paris: Alcan, 1930.

Rouart, Julien. "Du rôle de l'onirisme dans les psychoses de type paranoïaque et maniaque-dépressif." *L'Évolution psychiatrique* 4 (1936): 61–94.

Rouart, Julien. *Psychose maniaque dépressive et folie discordante: situation nosographique de quelques formes particulières par rapport à ces entités*. Paris: G. Doin, 1935.

Sartre, Jeabn-Paul. "L'image dans la vie psychologique: Rôle et nature." *Études sartriennes* 22 (2018): 246–243.

Sartre, Jean-Paul. *Les Mots et autres écrits autobiographiques*, vol. 560. Paris: Gallimard, 2010.

Šerko, Alfred. "Im Meskalinrausch." *Jahrbücher für Psychiatrie und Neurologie* 34 (1913): 355–366.

3 WOMEN, MENTAL ILLNESS, AND PSYCHEDELIC THERAPY IN POSTWAR FRANCE

Zoë Dubus

Set and setting are central concepts in today's models of psychedelic-assisted therapy. However, this has not always been the case: set and setting are theoretical constructs that emerged from fierce epistemological debate.[1] Schools of psychiatry in some parts of the world have relied on it more than others. Researchers in France who engaged in experiments with LSD between 1950 and 1970 distinguished themselves by not employing this new technique. They did not even consider it.[2] As a result, the therapeutic results by early French psychedelic researchers were generally inconclusive, and patients routinely reported unpleasant experiences, which made the clinical findings even more unreliable.

Understanding why French physicians ignored set and setting models requires appreciating the context of postwar psychiatry in France. Conventional approaches downplayed the importance of patients' feelings, while the long-established French institutional system viewed psychiatrists somewhat distinctly first and foremost as scientists, not therapists. Moreover, during a period when psychiatry was still dominated by men, female patients were cared for and evaluated through a patriarchal lens.[3] These contextual features help to explain how France developed its own psychedelic research culture, which ignored set and setting considerations in the psychedelic therapeutic context.

Two of the most influential French psychiatrists of the time studied the effects of LSD almost exclusively on women. By contrast, Erika Dyck and her colleagues gathered and transcribed over 1,000 patient observations at

Hollywood Hospital in British Columbia and in three other clinics elsewhere in Canada, and she reported that only 27 percent of all recipients of psychedelic therapy were women.[4] Consequently, it is crucial to examine how the experimental subjects' gender may have influenced the way that psychiatrists interpreted the phenomena caused by the psychoactive drug, as well as their disinclination to show care toward and support of their patients.

The first study of LSD in France began in 1951, when the psychiatrist Jean Thuillier at Sainte-Anne Hospital in Paris wrote to the Zurich-based Sandoz to request the drug "out of curiosity . . . to compare its effects to the delirium of certain types of psychosis."[5] At the time, Sainte-Anne was at the leading edge of psychedelic research; moreover, the hospital played an important role in training elite psychiatrists and broadly influenced French psychiatry as a result. This chapter is based on two archival documents resulting from research carried out by two "masters of French psychiatry":[6] Jean Delay (1907–1987) and Henri Ey (1900–1977). The first is a 1958 article published by the Sainte-Anne-based Delay and his intern Philippe Benda in the journal *Annales Médico-Psychologiques*,[7] in which the authors present seventy-five patients, including seventy-two women who recently had been admitted to the hospital. The paper reveals some particularly horrifying sessions, which Ey, who worked at the Bonneval Hospital, noted both at the time and years later, saying that "Delay and Benda's subjects were full of anxiety and said very little about states of euphoria."[8] As it happens, euphoric states were reported in the trials that used set and setting. To explore an early example of the clinical use of set and setting, therefore, it is useful to examine both Delay and Benda's paper and Ey and colleagues' unpublished report:[9] were Ey's nineteen female patients who were given LSD more inclined to report states of euphoria than those at Sainte-Anne?

THE THERAPEUTIC CONTEXT IN FRANCE

Between 1950 and 1970, at least eight research teams experimented with LSD on human subjects in France, but the drug never became part of a therapeutic process in any of these institutions. LSD remained an experimental substance, mainly used to induce temporary psychosis.[10] In postwar

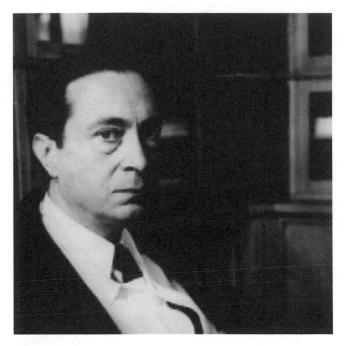

Figure 3.1
Jean Delay, ca. 1960, Sainte-Anne Hospital, reproduced with the permission of Florence Delay.

France, neuropsychiatry was taught by academics who were rarely psychiatrists themselves. This curriculum was "almost exclusively theoretical [and it] was influenced by the neuro-biological medical tradition." The careers were "quasi-dynastic,"[11] and knowledge and practices were passed from master to disciple. Delay was a member of this tradition of academic psychiatry and held the sole chair in mental illness in the entire country, at Sainte-Anne Hospital, the most prestigious institution of this time, from 1946 onward. He was part of what sociologist Robert Castel calls the "medical aristocracy," who had a "technicist [vision] of his vocation: it was all about 'treating cases' rather than taking care of human welfare."[12] Ey, on the other hand, was not working at Sainte-Anne: he chose to stay at the Bonneval public mental hospital south of Paris near Orléans (which now bears his name). However, from the 1930s onward, Ey traveled to Sainte-Anne's on a regular basis to give psychiatry lectures. The approach at the great Parisian research hospital at this time was informed by biological psychiatry, which disregarded the patients themselves in favor of concentrating on the scientific study of the physiological and neurological aspects of mental disorders.

This scientific and biological paradigm was dominant when these two authorities became interested in LSD in the early 1950s. As such, their first approach was to integrate LSD into the conceptual framework of the psychiatric treatment in France at the time: shock therapy. At a time when antipsychotic drugs were not yet available,[13] the medical interventions resorted to lobotomy, electroconvulsive therapy (ECT), insulin shock therapy, and amphetamine shock treatment in their attempts to treat mental illness. The idea was to trigger a "dissolution of the [ailing] spirit," which then could be reconstructed with the psychiatrist's help—in a way, it was hoped, that would eliminate the pathology. Delay was highly involved in the research into such treatments.[14] In fact, Thuillier described his approach as "too much science and not enough psychology; too much therapy and not enough analysis."[15] Hence, LSD arrived amid this therapeutic backdrop: the shock triggered by the experience must lead to the patient's improvement.

Some medical doctors, including British and American therapists, soon realized that LSD was even more beneficial when administered as part of a positive experience. They therefore discarded the notion of "shock" and began to develop the concept of "set and setting," a new approach that involved taking care to prepare the patient, creating a therapeutic alliance to give the subject a sense of trust and security in this relationship, and ensuring that the environment for the drug session was comfortable and cozy.[16] This new method called into question the psychiatric medical practices of the time.[17]

For Western medicine, attention to set and setting was novel and stood in stark contrast with the French model of psychiatry. The historian Aude Fauvel (2013) has explained the discrepancy between French and Anglo-American therapists and how they accounted for patients' feelings:

> Indeed, English law already offered the guarantee of always being able to summon *habeas corpus* and to demand to be heard by the courts. However, this procedure, which is typically initiated under exceptional circumstances, was diverted by mental patients to bypass the silence of the asylum. To prevent

this, there came a point in 1845 when the authorities even resorted to creating civil commissions to compile patients' complaints, without allowing doctors to oppose them. Because of this particular legislation, psychiatrists in Britain began to listen to the sick more than they did anywhere else.[18]

In contrast, consider the words of the French psychiatrist Paul Balvet, who said the following in 1950: "I admit it. I am my patient's enemy; in this way, I am the heir of the society that hates him."[19] For Balvet, a sadistic current was running through all forms of psychiatric intervention until the point where therapists abandoned their subjective attitude toward their patients and developed an empathic bond with them. However, it was difficult to be empathetic when asylums were overcrowded, often unsanitary, and violent places.[20] In 1952, another French psychiatrist, Henri Baruk, described the astonishment of therapists who adopted a caring approach and realized that "behind the apparently extinct or dead masks of the 'insane,' [is] an individual with a vibrant personality, with feelings."[21] He denounced the attitude of doctors who preferred to "take the easy way out" by avoiding "a daily effort of moral understanding," and instead were "destroying patients' reactions through trauma, shock, or brain destruction. The sick are thus transformed into apparently satisfied slaves, and all this is happening in a supposedly modern hospital."[22]

DESCRIPTION OF THE PATIENTS AND OF THE THERAPEUTIC METHOD

Nothing is known about Delay's patients other than that they were recently admitted to Sainte-Anne (which implies that the hospital staff did not really know them), suffering from neurosis or psychosis, had limited education, and came from relatively poor backgrounds. Information about their age (including average age) is not available, and neither is there any other biographical information. The reasons for their institutionalization and how often they were admitted are also unknown, beyond the general diagnosis of neurosis or psychosis. Since there were usually unhelpful treatments for mental illness, patients went in and out of institutions throughout the course of their lives. All the patients in Delay's study were institutionalized in compulsory care at Sainte-Anne (i.e., without their consent).

The article only presents an account of the sessions carried out with the patients, without individualizing them: the aim for the authors is not to present cases, and the transcription of the recordings is only partial. There is no indication that the treatment had been explained to the patients or that they were aware of what they were going to experience. These individuals received little attention during their LSD experiences. Rather, in his report on the treatments, Delay describes various types of reactions to the drug and concludes that he perceived LSD's possible clinical applications to be negligible. The seventy-two women in his study were perfectly interchangeable, and no details were provided about them as individuals. Moreover, the authors mentioned "minimal observer interference." The use of the word "observer" reveals the medical practitioners' attitude toward the experiment: they were not actively supporting the patients but rather taking a scientific approach, coldly observing phenomena. Furthermore, the various reactions to LSD were referred to as "arrays," which they used to capture the range of states that the patients were observed to have experienced. The duration of the sessions varied greatly, from as little as a few minutes to as many as two hours, at which time Delay would inject them with chlorpromazine to stop the psychedelic reaction; on the other hand, Ey's sessions lasted between one and seven-and-a-half hours.

Both Delay and Ey described their methods of applying the drug in a fairly comprehensive way (method of administration, dosage, duration of the session, and other details), but the actual therapeutic method was not specified. In some cases, there are hints about the attitude of the health-care team, but no specific information describing the therapeutic framework or approach. For example, in Ey's department, the notes reported "[s]creams when we try to hold her down."; doctors "force her to get up and look at herself in a mirror." This was a recurring issue in most LSD studies in France at that time: faced with an absence of established therapeutic techniques, each research team essentially had to start all over again and struggled to develop their protocols. As the historian Sarah Marks has noted, the methodologies used in psychedelic therapy were very rarely reported in the scientific literature of the time: it was in memoirs written decades later that psychiatrists like Stanislav Grof and Milan Hausner provided details of their anaclitic therapies, which integrated the concepts of set and setting. Indeed, set and setting are a variety of techniques developed from the mid-1950s onward to improve the management of patients under the influence of psychedelics in order to promote therapeutically beneficial experiences. Therapists considered the patients' state of mind, prepared them for the experience that they were about to have, organized the room so it was comfortable, and adopted a supportive, encouraging, and comforting attitude when necessary. At the time, the medical profession was very reluctant to adopt such practices: some doctors "even advised against shaking hands with patients, fearing interference with the transfer process."[23]

In Bonneval, Ey treated nineteen women with LSD, six of whom were institutionalized on a "voluntary basis," which in this case meant based on the opinions of the patient's relatives rather than what she herself wanted, and twelve were in an open ward attached to the mental hospital, which they entered of their own free will. Six of the women had received the most basic school education (*Certificat d'études primaire*), given between eleven and thirteen years of age, proving the student had acquired a basic level of knowledge. As with Delay's report, their intelligence was generally referred to as inferior. Table 3.1 summarizes both papers.

The observations of the LSD experiences recorded in the two reports are dominated by fear (mainly of going mad), shame (of not knowing how to answer the questions or being laughed at by observers), and silence (during the session or in the days afterward). Neither Delay or Ey mentions any approach to guiding or assisting the women during their experiences. Ey repeatedly refers to a "depressive tone" (*tonalité dépressive*) in the majority of the experiences, but not whether he had adopted a particular approach to help the women he treated navigate these difficult moments.

Childhood or adulthood trauma often lay behind the problems, ranging from depression to psychosis, that brought these women to the hospital. Early childhood abandonment, being an illegitimate child brought up by people other than her parents, the absence of affection during childhood, and physical violence were typical. During adulthood, heartbreak, domestic conflict, dread of the prospect of a new pregnancy, problems pertaining to

Table 3.1

Comparative descriptions of the LSD sessions carried out by Jean Delay and Henri Ey

	Delay and Benda (1958)	Ey and Colleagues (1959)
Gender	72 women—3 men	19 women
Age	Unknown	Average age: 30 years old Between 17 and 59 years old
Education level	Limited	6 with Certificat d'études primaire 1 with a more advanced diploma 4 without Certificat d'études primaire 8 with no curricula mentioned (education deemed as "bad")
Social background	Modest to poor	Modest to poor
Preparation	Unspecified	Very basic, not systematic
Number of sessions	Several sessions in a quarter of the cases Unspecified number	Sole session, save for one patient
Dosage	Between 1 and 2 μg per kilogram of body mass	Between 75 and 150 μg 10 = 100 μg / 8 = 150 μg / 1 = 75 μg
Administration	Mostly injection Oral = 10	Injection = 16 / Oral = 4 (one patient had two sessions)
Duration	1 to 2 hours	Between 1 and 7.30 hours
Chlorpromazine to end the session	Systematic	12 cases 8 unspecified cases

sexuality, and physical and sexual violence were also regularly mentioned. Hence, although in some cases the memories discussed under the influence of LSD were positive—"I saw the boarding school park; I saw flowers, I picked purple violets. A perfect life, these flowers that smelled good"[24]— their content much more often reflected pain, fear, and stress: "It seemed to me that he was there, I was overcome by fear"; "Her mother pushed her away when she wanted to comfort her"; "I saw my own rape and it was terrible"; "I thought about the sad child I was, with no mom." Several women shared the same symbolic experience about the meaning of colors: for instance, red symbolized "maternal hemorrhaging." In addition, the trauma of the war years was still firmly embedded in people's memories: the color green was reminiscent of the uniforms of German soldiers. Memories of the war surfaced on a regular basis in both Delay's and Ey's patients. Delay and Benda reported: "Corpses piling up like in 1940. I saw Daddy again with lots of little worms all over him."[25]

In 1950s France, psychiatrists were unconcerned about notions of patient consent regarding the treatments that they carried out. In Delay's and Ey's departments, preparation for the session was either nonexistent or extremely rudimentary. As far as follow-up after the sessions went, Delay reported that the patients talked to each other about the psychic phenomena they experienced and openly questioned the efficacy of their treatments, which strongly suggests that nobody had explained to them the purpose and potential value of their experiences. Ey's Bonneval report is unclear about whether each patient was forewarned of the effects of LSD, but it seems clear that she was often informed *after* the injection. The details were finally provided at the eighteenth observation: the patient was told that she was going to experience "feelings of cenesthesia, dry mouth, and blurred vision. In order to avoid the possibility of suggestion, no additional details were given."[26] This insufficient preparation partly explains the distressing tone recorded in the transcribed sessions, given that the patients had no idea what their experience of LSD would entail. In addition, several accounts in Ey's report mention doctors coercing patients into accepting the treatment, as in the observations of a twenty-seven-year-old nurse named Mireille F., who had been suffering from pangs of paroxysmal anxiety over the previous two months: "Anxious and recalcitrant. Only reluctantly accepts the injection." She received an injection of 100 μg.[27]

Regarding the issue of the presiding doctors and attendants and the patients establishing a therapeutic alliance, the Sainte-Anne patients were new to the institution, so they were likely unfamiliar with the ward staff or the doctors. Moreover, institutionalized mental patients at that time saw doctors only on rare occasions, which prevented them from establishing a genuine bond. The two reports indicate that the therapists placed a great deal of distance between themselves and the patients, and in some instances they displayed behavior designed to induce fear and anxiety in the patients during the session with LSD. In 1950, the journal *Esprit* published an issue devoted to the study of the ethics of psychiatric interventions. One paper called into question the notion of "personality rape," which patients undergoing narco-analysis[28] were subjected to in order to break their resistance and force them to tell their secrets against their will.[29] Yet from the 1940s to the end of 1960, Delay, Ey, and their French colleagues were particularly fond of this technique. They used LSD within a therapeutic model in which the patient's consent was deemed irrelevant. With LSD, Ey expresses his satisfaction at having been able to learn information that a patient "had never revealed" and other things that she had "concealed." In reaction, in the reports of both therapists, some patients refer to the substance as a "truth serum."

While their reports indicate that there was little emphasis on set, both Delay and Ey paid more attention to the setting. The room where Delay's experiments took place was filled with plants, with artwork displayed on the walls. The drawings and pictures were not just decorations; they were considered part of the experiment. Music was also occasionally played in Delay's sessions. In Ey's experiments at Bonneval, there was no music, but the room was painted sea green and decorated with a drawing and a plant. However, these tentative steps into issues of setting do not appear reflected in the way that the session was guided, which left much to be desired: in addition to the distant attitude and coldness of the observers, patients complained that they were often left alone, even when they were having a bad experience with LSD.

RESEARCH ANALYSIS

The first doctoral dissertation on the therapeutic use of LSD in France was carried out in 1957 by Daniel Widlöcher under Delay's supervision. Widlöcher was the first French psychiatrist to consider LSD as an adjunct to psychotherapy, and he used it with at least nine female patients in Sainte-Anne; he noted:

> In our observations, anxious and depressive reactions were more apparent among the patients who were hospitalized in open wards, where they could routinely criticize the appropriateness or the results of the treatment. On the other hand, among those who were institutionalized, for whom such problems were rather irrelevant compared to the issue of their institutionalization and of the duration of their stay, the experience was much easier to endure.[30]

Widlöcher tacitly admitted that institutionalized patients were less inclined to criticize and comment on the merits of their treatment, and more submissive and cooperative in order to be treated better and thus allowed to leave sooner. Because they were less inclined to rebel, the doctors did not give as much thought to how they were treated. The status of these women alone—that of patients often locked up against their will—does not explain their relative lack of resistance: gender played a key role in this instance. Discretion and submission were fundamental qualities for Frenchwomen in the postwar era.[31] From the perspective of institutional psychiatry, to go against this supposed "nature" was a transgression that could be interpreted as a worsening of the individual's mental state, and thus may lead to more stringent conditions of confinement. Within the asylum, women had more to lose than men if they resisted treatment: for the latter, unyielding and resistant behavior could be understood as a sign of recovery: the patient was beginning to recover his virile, "manly" qualities. In the words of the sociologist Joan Busfield (1989), "it would be impossible for any institution to escape the sexism that is endemic to society."[32]

GENDER, DISTANCE, AND A LACK OF EMPATHY

A wealth of scholarship now underscores a clear link between the oppression of women in society, particularly in connection with birth management and the onset of mental illness.[33] Several of Bonneval's patients were institutionalized for depression: most of them had suffered numerous and repeated pregnancies, late miscarriages, and difficult deliveries resulting in the death of the child. These tragic events were often what lay at the root of their mental distress. One of the women's valid fears was about getting pregnant again. In addition, the traumas that they experienced significantly affected their married lives and sexuality[34] and could lead to domestic violence. (It is important to note that in France, access to contraception was authorized only in 1969, via a law that did not enter into force until 1972.)

The way that the doctors judged these women is clear from their notes in Bonneval: thirty-six-year-old B., who had eight children in ten years, saw her third child die in childbirth, which triggered her first psychotic episode.

Her patient file reads "household neglect"—in other words, a pathological disorder linked to not keeping a tidy home. They noted her apathy, "with a general air of sadness"; her "impulsive runaways"; and her "oddities." B. no longer fully conformed to the female roles assigned to her by society. Her behavior was therefore interpreted in pathological terms according to a process that Phyllis Chesler analyzed in her 1972 book *Women and Madness*.[35] She described what a feminist way of caring for these women would look like: "A feminist therapist believes that a woman needs to be told that she is 'not crazy;' that it is normal to feel sad or angry about being overworked, undervalued and underpaid; that it is healthy to harbor fantasies of running away when the needs of others (aging parents, needy husbands, demanding children) threaten to overwhelm her."[36]

In French mental institutions, and in society more generally, gentleness, compassion, and empathy were attitudes typically ascribed to women. They were perceived as inherently "feminine," and therefore potentially pejorative. In a psychiatric context still dominated by men, these qualities were provided, in the best-case scenario, by female nurses.[37] Psychiatrists, for their part, needed to maintain a cold, stern manner when faced with suffering. For example, although the doctors realized that loneliness disturbed their patients, the latter were often left alone for the duration of the experiment. One of them "begged not to be left alone," while another called for help: "You have to help me, you can't leave me." According to the notes, thirty-six-year-old Ms. A "throws herself to the ground, tries to rip her clothes off and screams—it is impossible to get through to her." However, a few minutes later, Ms. A was left alone. The doctors noted that "her demeanor and her face show panic." In fact, Delay and Benda entitled one of their subsections "torture," in which seven of their subjects exhibited similar terrors. They transcribed a patient as saying: "Everything is hostile around me, nothing is familiar, stop torturing me," and "I don't understand how you can make people suffer like that." This transcript is not followed by any comment about advice aimed at helping the patients, who clearly begrudged the doctors for their cold manner: "an expressionless face. The closer I wanted to get to him, the more distant he seemed"; "You just stood there motionless, without a humane gesture. Instead of comforting me, you did nothing";

"You have a nasty look"; and so it goes on. As for the psychiatrists, they simply mention the "benevolent neutrality of the observers."

Both documents show a clear lack of empathy on the part of the therapists. Indeed, the Bonneval report reveals sessions dominated almost entirely by terror and suffering; yet it is clear that the physicians had their share of responsibility in leading the sessions in this direction, as the following example illustrates. Twenty-four-year-old Mrs. D. was given LSD orally five days after arriving at Bonneval. The session lasted seven hours and fifteen minutes: "Very strong levels of anxiety. We have to insist to make the patient agree to drink water containing 150 μg of LSD. Only *then*[38] do we warn her of the likely course of events." Two hours and forty minutes into the session, the doctors tried to make her believe that the water they had made her drink "contained no medication." It is hard to understand why doctors would suggest something so terrifying—namely, that the patient's disturbance was organic to her rather than drug induced. Moreover, the doctors later recorded that "the patient stubbornly and continuously refuses to admit the hypothesis put forth to her, she clings onto the conviction that she has been drugged, it is a link that connects her to reality. To deny the existence of this link is to admit her insanity!"

Another alarming session involved seventeen-year-old Simoneis, described as a "pervert" who had been prosecuted for a crime against decency. The doctors once again tried to upset their patient by making her believe something that they knew would disturb her: "The patient is very vigilant and she retains her self-control perfectly. However, she seems to panic when she is told of the prosecutor's (fictitious) visit." In addition to these attempts to destabilize the patients, members of Delay's team came in and out of the room, asking questions. In seven instances, the patient became aware that she was being laughed at and that the observers were laughing at the situation: "Please, Madam, this is not funny. I didn't think it, I can see it; they laughed, they laughed at me; it must be fun to watch the interrogation."[39]

Whether the doctors or the nursing staff were actually mocking her or not—though the quoted remarks by several patients suggest this possibility—is irrelevant: what I aim to demonstrate here is that there was a major difference between the emerging class of psychedelic therapists in other jurisdictions, who paid attention to the set and setting, and the French doctors, who did not. The former would have sought to avoid situations that could lead to patients having a bad impression of their experiences. In France, the classic shock therapeutic model created an environment of unease and paranoia in these early LSD treatments; the fact that these sessions were more experimental than therapeutic led the doctors to test their patients' reactions, with no regard for their feelings.

SYSTEMATIC EROTICIZATION

One of the reasons for doctors keeping their distance—beyond mere training, which recommended very minimal physical contact with patients—was in the systematic eroticization of the behavior of these vulnerable women. While scientists, especially Anglo-American researchers, very quickly noticed and recognized that individuals under the influence of LSD as part of a therapeutic process needed contact and had to be carefully looked after,[40] the patients' attempts to get close to the doctors in both Bonneval and Sainte-Anne were seen as "erotic pantomimes." For example, during sessions at Sainte-Anne, one patient attempted to lean on the doctor's shoulder and another tried to take his hand and apologized for the lack of respect. Delay and Benda, however, were aware of the need to establish physical contact with patients who were seeking support, given that they cited the psychiatrist Ronald Sandison's recommendation to that effect in their introduction. They also noted, "Various prompts from the observer interfere with the spontaneous behavior" of the patients, such as interjecting to encourage them to lie down. Instead, the doctors simply recorded observations about the patients' actions throughout the session be published in the reports. Indeed, one patient refused to lie down because she thought that her behavior was being interpreted as erotic: "I will not lie down, because they said that I was masturbating."

In Ey's ward, one patient was "forever holding the physician's hand. She strokes it in a manner which is unambiguous. . . . The patient can't stand it if the doctor moves away from her. It appears that this physical contact, in addition to its erotic nature, is also a way of 'orienting' herself." Another woman asks the doctor to "sleep" with her in order to "watch over [her] and keep [her] company." She adds: "I don't want to be alone" (this patient was in a terrified state throughout the entire session), which Ey understood to be a "furtively erotic demeanor" rather than a sign of fear. It should be noted that at that time, the word "sleep" was still commonly used to mean "lie down," and it did not suggest an obvious sexual connotation. Upon examining a third patient, who had been raped and was reliving the experience while on LSD, the doctors describe the young woman's actions using sensual words.

Colette is eighteen years old and was diagnosed as follows: "Severe neurosis with hysterical tendencies." She had recently been raped by a fifty-year-old man. The doctor observing her became the object of transference, a psychoanalytic term meaning the displacement of feelings, thoughts, and behavior onto someone other than the one from whom the original feelings, thoughts, and behavior had arisen. She mistook him for her rapist and tried to slap him. She shouted, "You have broken me" and lifted her skirt. The doctor commented, "Very erotic attitude—raises her skirt—rubs her thighs—violent gestures toward the doctors—repeats the words: bastard, disgusting . . . 'Doing that with men, it's too much'." Her attitude was repeatedly described as erotic and ambivalent. At the end of the session, the doctors nevertheless concluded that "the patient did not relive the traumatic rape experience. . . . The main thing which became apparent was a latent eroticism, combined with marked aggressiveness." The observations, which run over three pages, are quite explicit about her reliving the rape and make for particularly difficult reading. In addition, the aggressiveness that was mentioned earlier continued for several days, directed toward her presiding doctors, which they took to be proof of her transference, as well as her resentment toward them for making her relive her rape.

As mentioned here, many patients were afraid of being left alone and tried everything to convince the doctors to stay with them. Their pleas were often desperate, but the doctors tended to interpret them as erotic. For instance, thirty-two-year-old Jacqueline was prone to severe anxiety. She first called for her mother, then sobbed, and finally she thought she was going to die. The doctors noted that her anxiety was "extreme," and that she repeatedly made known that she did not want to be left alone. Then, they reported: "Erotic attitude, smiles, attempts to caress and grope, cuddly attitude. . . . Very rapid thymic oscillations ranging from the most intense anxiety to eroticism tinged with the fear of being abandoned."[41]

Physical contact between therapists and patients was indeed challenging in these institutions. As the historian Véronique Fau-Vincenti has shown, some female inmates were not shy about writing passionate letters to the interns they liked or walking around naked when there were men on the ward.[42] However, what is noteworthy here is that every attempt to make contact during both these LSD studies was systematically interpreted in erotic terms.

COMMUNICATION BREAKDOWN

At the end of the day, how could female patients properly share their life stories to facilitate therapy under such circumstances? Under the gaze of a male psychiatrist, some patients felt embarrassed and ashamed of their behavior and the image they presented. It should also be noted that one observer on Ey's team remarked that a patient who was "still young" had a "well-groomed" appearance. Because women were used to being assessed by what is now referred to as the "male gaze," patients were concerned about their appearance: "What a show I am giving you"; "I must look silly, unkempt. I feel belittled, ridiculous, I don't know what to do with myself"; "You are watching me, I don't like being watched"; "I must look like a dimwit."

The shame and embarrassment expressed by patients indicate that they did not feel safe; this was not an environment where they could be themselves. On the one hand, they were still weighed down by social conventions: for example, they had to try to look their best to maintain their femininity. If they did not, that would immediately be seen as a form of pathology, as previously shown. Yet the fact that they were being examined by men of higher social standing, who were better educated and had authority, who occupied the role of experts in relation to them, and who had control over their diagnosis and the duration of their institutionalization was particularly problematic. The doctor's power over these women was effectively almost absolute: he could decide to keep them in the asylum or allow them to be released, give permission for visits, or state that a particular kind of behavior deserved punishment. Thus, being worried about what the psychiatrist might find about you against your will (the idea behind the "truth serum" mentioned by Delay's and Ey's patients), as well as knowing that the scrutiny accompanying such discoveries could lead to an indefinite institutionalization due to your "madness" was not the ideal set and setting.

Nowadays, the inability to let go during the psychedelic experience is recognized as a major source of anxiety for subjects.[43] As early as 1959, the Canadian anthropologist Anthony Wallace had demonstrated the influence of certain parameters on the LSD experience. One of these factors was whether, from a cultural perspective, those experiencing a psychedelic session should fear being punished for their hallucinations.[44] In the Western world, this question was answered in the affirmative, and since the nineteenth century, it had been coupled with a pathological dimension. The female patients in question were aware of this fact and would sometimes strategically repress psychological symptoms for fear of an even more severe psychiatric diagnosis, or they would feel particularly helpless and terrified at the appearance of such symptoms which, for them, confirmed the diagnosis of madness. These women also assimilated the idea that if they expressed strong emotion, they would inevitably be seen as mad and as deviants from their femininity.

The treatment was aimed neither at psychotherapy nor specifically at reliving, processing, and accepting painful memories. The shock method was predominantly part of the context of biological psychiatry, using LSD as a form of shock therapy. After the chlorpromazine injection, which put an end to the session, the patients were once more left on their own. Yet it was sometimes precisely during this period, when the effects of LSD were waning and the patient was coming back to her senses, that she most needed to verbalize and analyze her experience. As one patient noted, "I would have liked to express my feelings." This reflection was noted in the paper but not commented upon.[45]

For Delay and Benda, it all just amounted to patients' complaints. The word "complaint" is used seventeen times in the first part of their paper; not only does this mean that the description of LSD's effects was expressed in purely negative terms, but also that these comments became tiresome for the doctors. It emphasizes the stereotype that women complain all the time. Yet the comments that are actually reported reveal that many statements alluded to a state of euphoria: one patient commented on the shape-shifting lines by saying, "It's funny"; another saw a plant and cried, "How pretty!" The way that these remarks were interpreted by supposedly neutral observers was in reality highly biased, even condescending.

Finally, these women found it impossible and frustrating to talk about their experiences when faced with psychiatrists who came from a very different social and cultural backgrounds. The patients at Sainte-Anne and Bonneval came from poor socioeconomic backgrounds, both economically and culturally. This created yet another barrier between the therapists and their patients, who were ashamed and conscious of the fact that they had difficulty expressing their feelings. They feared that words would fail them and they would be laughed at if they used expressions that were perceived as stupid. Many found solace in silence and refused to answer questions—in some cases, this lasted for several days after the experience, thus rendering any form of psychotherapy impossible. Their silence may indicate that some of these women attempted to resist treatment that they regarded as a form of brutality.[46]

CONCLUSION

Patriarchal and patronizing relationships between male psychiatrists and female patients is a key factor explaining the complex phenomenon of the systematic inattention to the notion of set and setting in early psychedelic therapeutic contexts in France. From a broader perspective, an intersectional frame of analysis could be used to focus on the impact of class on patients' lived experiences, and on the ways that therapists supervised—and neglected—those experiences. For example, in a fascinating book, the sociologists Claudine Herzlich and Janine Pierret demonstrate very clearly that people from lower social classes are considered tougher and better able to endure pain than those of higher social class. This implies that the medical profession is less interested in alleviating the suffering of the poor, whether physical or mental.[47] These women are therefore subjugated on three fronts: as patients facing doctors, as women facing men, and as proletarians facing a social and cultural elite.

Henri Ey and Jean Delay, as luminaries of the psychiatric profession of their time, had a decisive influence on steering subsequent French therapists interested in LSD away from considerations of set and setting. French researchers, particularly Delay, were pioneers in research into neuroleptics—drugs that lead the subject to experience indifference or ataraxia, reverse action mechanisms of LSD, which tends to evoke deep meaning and connection. With this drug model in mind, the psychiatrist's involvement was seen as unnecessary during such treatments—so much so that the French psychiatry professor Yves Pélicier explicitly referred to "the relational and psychological abandonment of the patient"[48] that resulted from this type of medication. It would seem that from their emergence in the 1950s, psychedelic theories were at odds with French psychiatry.

NOTES

1. Ido Hartogsohn, *American Trip: Set, Setting, and the Psychedelic Experience in the Twentieth Century* (Cambridge, MA: MIT Press, 2020).

2. Zoë Dubus, "Marginalisation, stigmatisation et abandon du LSD en médecine," *Histoire, médecine et santé*, no. 15 (2020): 87–105.

3. Phyllis Chesler, *Women and Madness* (New York: Doubleday, 1972); Elaine Showalter, *The Female Malady: Women, Madness, and English Culture, 1830–1980* (New York: Penguin Books, 1987); Lisa Appignanesi, *Mad, Bad and Sad: A History of Women and the Mind Doctors from 1800 to the Present* (London: Virago, 2009).

4. Erika Dyck, "What about Mrs Psychedelic? A Historical Look at Women and Psychedelics" (lecture, Breaking Convention, University of Greenwich, London, August 17, 2019): https://www.youtube.com/watch?v=T04atyEQqUk&t=112s.

5. Jean Thuillier, "Ma rencontre avec Albert Hoffman, l'inventeur du LSD," *Bulletin de L'Association des Amis du Musée et du Centre Historique de Sainte Anne* (October 2006): 1.

6. Alain Ehrenberg, *La fatigue d'être soi: Dépression et société* (Paris: Odile Jacob, 2008), 68.

7. Jean Delay and Philippe Benda, "L'expérience lysergique. LSD-25. A propos de 75 observations cliniques," *Encéphale*, no. 3/4 (1958): 169–209; 309–344.

8. Henri Ey, *Traité des hallucinations* (Paris: Masson et Cie, 1973), 568.

9. Henri Ey, Claude Igert, and Gabrielle Lairy, "Etat des recherches portant sur les hallucinogènes et les hallucinalytiques effectuées en 1958" (Avant rapport semestriel, Bonneval, mai 1959), no. 380 in Fonds Ey (7S), Archives municipales de Perpignan.

10. See, for instance, the research by Pinchas Borenstein, MD, in Villejuif, France: Pinchas Borenstein, Philippe Cujo, and Claude Olievenstein, "Epreuve à la iethylamide de l'acide

lysergique (LSD-25) et thérapeutiques psychotropes: étude électro-encéphalographique," *Annales Médico-Psychologiques* II, no. 2 (1965): 237–246.

11. Jean Garrabé, "Les chaires de clinique des maladies mentales et des maladies nerveuses à Paris," *L'information psychiatarique* 88, no. 7 (2012) : 551.

12. Robert Castel, "Genèse et ambiguïtés de la notion de secteur en psychiatrie," *Sociologie du Travail* 17, no. 1 (1975) : 57–77.

13. Anne Caldwell, *Origins of Psychopharmacology from CPZ to LSD* (Springfield: Thomas, 1970).

14. Edward Shorter and David Healy, *Shock Therapy: The History of Electroconvulsive Treatment in Mental Illness* (Toronto: University of Toronto Press, 2007).

15. Jean Thuillier, *Les dix ans qui ont changé la folie* (Paris : Robert Laffont, 1981), 25.

16. Maria Mangini, "Treatment of Alcoholism Using Psychedelic Drugs: A Review of the Program of Research," *Journal of Psychoactive Drugs* 30, no. 4 (1998): 381–418.

17. World Health Organization Study Group on Ataractic and Hallucinogenic Drugs, in *Study Group on Ataractic and Hallucinogenic Drugs in Psychiatry & World Health Organization*, vol. 152 (Geneva, Switzerland: World Health Organization, 1958)

18. Aude Fauvel, "Cerveaux fous et sexes faibles (France, 1860–1900)," *Clio Femmes, Genre, Histoir e* no. 37 (2013): 54.

19. "Médecine, qu atrième pouvoir? L'intervention psychologique et l'intégrité de la personne," *Esprit* 18, no. 165 (1950): 387.

20. Nicolas Henckes, *Le nouveau monde de la psychiatrie française. Les psychiatres, l'Etat et la réforme des hôpitaux psychiatriques de l'après-guerre aux ann ées 1970* (Paris: EHESS, 2007); Adeline Fride, *CHARENTON ou la chronique de la vie d'un asile de la naissance de la psychiatrie à la secto risation* (Paris: EHESS, 1983); André Roumieux, *Je travaille à l'asile d 'aliénés* (Paris: Champ libre, 1974).

21. Henri Baruk, "La Psychochirurgie frontale peut-el le se justifier?" *Revue PhiloFranceue de la France et de l'Étranger* 142 (1952): 393.

22. Baruk, "La Psychochirurgie frontale p eut-elle se justifier?" 420–421.

23. Sarah Marks, "From Experimental Psychosis to Resolving Traumatic Pasts: Psychedelic Research in Communist Czechoslovakia, 1954–1974," *Cahiers du Monde Russe* 56, no. 1 (2015): 70.

24. Delay and Benda, "L'expérience lysergique," 202.

25. Delay and Benda, "L'expérience lysergique," 208.

26. Ey et al., "Etat des recherches portant sur les hallucinogènes et les hallucinalytiques effectuées," 64.

27. Ey et al., "Etat des recherches portant sur les hallucinogènes et les hallucinalytiques effectuées," 30.

28. In this method, the patients were subjected to high doses of barbiturates, plunging them into a daze in which they unwittingly provided personal information. This in turn allowed the psychiatrist to undertake psychotherapy.

29. Juliette Boutonnier and Léon Michaux, "Le complexe de viol," *Esprit* 18, no. 165 (1950): 491–495.

30. Daniel Widlöcher, Le diéthylamide de l'acide lysergique: Étude de psycho-pathologie expérimentale (MD diss., Paris, 1957), 84.

31. To illustrate the way that sexism has permeated part of the French medical order, see André Soubiran, *Lettre ouverte à une femme d'aujourd'hui* (Paris: Albin Michel, 1967).

32. Joan Busfield, "Sexism and Psychiatry," *Sociology* 23, no. 3 (1989): 345.

33. See the literature review in Busfield, "Sexism and Psychiatry."

34. See this horrific account: R., "Moi, j'ai peur," *Les Temps Modern es* 12, no. 134 (1957): 1561–1567.

35. Phyllis Chesler, *Women and Madness* (New-York: Doubleday, 1972): 56.

36. Phyllis Chesler, "Twenty Years since 'Women and Madness,'" *Journal of Mind ¾ Behavior* 11, no. 3/4 (1990): 318.

37. See, for instance, R. Sandison, A. Spencer, and J. Whitelaw, "The Therapeutic Value of Lysergic Acid Diethylamide in Mental Illness," *Journal of Mental Science* 100, no. 419 (1954): 491–507. For an analysis of the gendered relations among health-care professionals in the time of shock therapy, see Coline Fournout, "L'imaginaire thérapeutique des chocs à l'insuline." *GLAD!. Revue sur le langage, le genre, les sexualités*, no. 12 (July 13, 2022): 1–16. https://doi.org/10.4000/glad.4437.

38. My emphasis.

39. Delay and Benda, 1958, 75 observations, 321.

40. See, for example, Joyce Martin, "L.S.D. Analysis," *International Journal of Social Psychiatry* 10 (1964): 165–69.

41. Ey et al., "Etat des recherches portant sur les hallucinogènes et les hallucinalytiques effectuées," 68–71.

42. Véronique Fau-Vincenti, "Des femmes difficiles en psychiatrie (1933–1960)," *Criminocorpus* (2019).

43. Max Wolff et al., "Learning to Let Go: A Cognitive-Behavioral Model of How Psychedelic Therapy Promotes Acceptance," *Frontiers in Psychiatry* 11 (2020): 1–13.

44. Anthony Wallace, "Cultural Determinants of Response to Hallucinatory Experience," *A.M.A. Archives of General Psychiatry* 1, no. 1 (1959).

45. Delay and Benda, "L'expérience lysergique," 327.

46. Erving Goffman, *Asiles* (Paris: Éditions de Minuit, 1968), 358.

47. Claudine Herzlich and Janine Pierret, *Malades d'hier, malades d'aujourd'hui* (Paris: Payot, 1984).

48. Yves Pélicier, "Neuroleptiques et modification des modes de prises en charge," *Tribune médicale* (1985): 414.

BIBLIOGRAPHY

Primary Sources

Dyck, Erika. "What about Mrs. Psychedelic? A Historical Look at Women and Psychedelics" (lecture, Breaking Convention, University of Greenwich, London, August 17, 2019), YouTube, https://www.youtube.com/watch?v=T04atyEQqUk.

Secondary Sources

Appignanesi, Lisa. *Mad, Bad and Sad: A History of Women and the Mind Doctors from 1800 to the Present*. London: Virago, 2009.

Baruk, Henri. "La Psychochirurgie frontale peut-elle se justifier?" *Revue Philosophique de la France et de l'Étranger* 142 (1952): 392–427.

Borenstein, Pinchas, Philippe Cujo, and Claude Olievenstein. "Epreuve à la diéthylamide de l'acide lysergique (LSD-25) et thérapeutiques psychotropes: étude électro-encéphalographique." *Annales Médico-Psychologiques* II, no. 2 (1965): 237–246.

Boutonnier, Juliette, and Léon Michaux. "Le complexe de viol." *Esprit* 18, no. 165 (1950): 491–495.

Busfield, Joan. "Sexism and Psychiatry." *Sociology* 23, no. 3 (1989): 343–364.

Caldwell, Anne. *Origins of Psychopharmacology from CPZ to LSD*. Springfield, Il: Thomas, 1970.

Castel, Robert. "Genèse et ambiguïtés de la notion de secteur en psychiatrie." *Sociologie du Travail* 17, no. 1 (1975): 57–77.

Chesler, Phyllis. "Twenty Years since 'Women and Madness.'" *Journal of Mind and Behavior* 11, no. 3/4 (1990): 318.

Chesler, Phyllis. *Women and Madness*. New-York: Doubleday, 1972.

Delay, Jean, and Philippe Benda. "L'expérience lysergique. LSD-25. A propos de 75 observations cliniques." *Encéphale*, no. 3/4 (1958): 169–209.

Dubus, Zoë. "Marginalisation, stigmatisation et abandon du LSD en médecine." *Histoire, médecine et santé*, no. 15 (2020): 87–105.

Ehrenberg, Alain. *La fatigue d'être soi: Dépression et société*. Paris: Odile Jacob, 2008.

Ey, Henri. *Traité des hallucinations*. Paris: Masson et Cie, 1973.

Ey, Henri, Claude Igert, and Gabrielle Lairy "Etat des recherches portant sur les hallucinogènes et les hallucinalytiques effectuées en 1958." (Avant rapport semestriel, Bonneval, mai 1959), no. 380 in Fonds Ey (7S), Archives municipales de Perpignan.

Fauvel, Aude. "Cerveaux fous et sexes faibles (Grande-Bretagne, 1860–1900)." *Clio. Femmes, Genre, Histoire*, no. 37 (2013): 41–64.

Fau-Vincenti, Véronique. "Des femmes difficiles en psychiatrie (1933–1960)." *Criminocorpus* (2019).

Fournout, Coline. "L'imaginaire thérapeutique des chocs à l'insuline." *GLAD!. Revue sur le langage, le genre, les sexualités*, no. 12 (July, 2022): 1–16.

Fride, Adeline. *CHARENTON ou la chronique de la vie d'un asile de la naissance de la psychiatrie à la sectorization*. Paris: EHESS, 1983.

Garrabé, Jean. "Les chaires de clinique des maladies mentales et des maladies nerveuses à Paris." *L'information psychiatarique* 88, no. 7 (2012): 549–57.

Goffman, Erving. *Asiles*. Paris: Éditions de Minuit, 1968.

Hartogsohn, Ido. *American Trip: Set, Setting, and the Psychedelic Experience in the Twentieth Century*. Cambridge, MA: MIT Press, 2020.

Henckes, Nicolas. *Le nouveau monde de la psychiatrie française. Les psychiatres, l'Etat et la réforme des hôpitaux psychiatriques de l'après-guerre aux années 1970*. Paris: EHESS, 2007.

Herzlich, Claudine, and Janine Pierret. *Malades d'hier, malades d'aujourd'hui*. Paris: Payot, 1984.

Mangini, Maria. "Treatment of Alcoholism Using Psychedelic Drugs: A Review of the Program of Research." *Journal of Psychoactive Drugs* 30, no. 4 (1998): 381–418.

Marks, Sarah. "From Experimental Psychosis to Resolving Traumatic Pasts: Psychedelic Research in Communist Czechoslovakia, 1954–1974." *Cahiers du Monde Russe* 56, no. 1 (2015): 53–70.

Martin, Joyce. "L.S.D. Analysis." *International Journal of Social Psychiatry* 10 (1964): 165–69.

"Médecine, quatrième pouvoir? L'intervention psychologique et l'intégrité de la personne," *Esprit* 18, no. 165 (1950): 387.

Pélicier, Yves. "Neuroleptiques et modification des modes de prises en charge." *Tribune médicale* (1985): 414.

R., "Moi, j'ai peur." *Les Temps Modernes* 12, no. 134 (1957): 1561–1567.

Roumieux, André. *Je travaille à l'asile d'aliénés*. Paris: Champ libre, 1974.

Sandison, Ronald A., A. M. Spencer, and J. D. A. Whitelaw. "The Therapeutic Value of Lysergic Acid Diethylamide in Mental Illness." *Journal of Mental Science* 100, no. 419 (1954): 491–507.

Shorter, Edward, and David Healy. *Shock Therapy: The History of Electroconvulsive Treatment in Mental Illness*. Toronto: University of Toronto Press, 2007.

Showalter, Elaine. *The Female Malady: Women, Madness, and English Culture, 1830–1980*. New York: Penguin Books, 1987.

Soubiran, André Lettre. *Ouverte à une femme d'aujourd'hui*. Paris: Albin Michel, 1967.

Thuillier, Jean. *Les dix ans qui ont changé la folie*. Paris: Robert Laffont, 1981.

Thuillier, Jean. "Ma rencontre avec Albert Hoffman, l'inventeur du LSD." *Bulletin de L'Association des Amis du Musée et du Centre Historique de Sainte Anne*, October, 2006.

Wallace, Anthony. "Cultural Determinants of Response to Hallucinatory Experience." *A.M.A. Archives of General Psychiatry* 1, no. 1 (1959): 58–69.

Widlöcher, Daniel. Le diéthylamide de l'acide lysergique: étude de psycho-pathologie expérimentale. MD diss., Faculty of Medicine, Paris, 1957.

Wolff, Max, Ricarda Evens, Lea J. Mertens, Michael Koslowski, Felix Betzler, Gerhard Gründer, and Henrik Jungaberle. "Learning to Let Go: A Cognitive-Behavioral Model of How Psychedelic Therapy Promotes Acceptance." *Frontiers in Psychiatry* 11 (February 2020): 1–13.

World Health Organization. "World Health Organization Study Group on Ataractic and Hallucinogenic Drugs." In *Study Group on Ataractic and Hallucinogenic Drugs in Psychiatry & World Health Organization*, 152. Geneva, Switzerland: World Health Organization, 1958.

4 MILAN HAUSNER, THE SADSKÁ CLINIC, AND THE FATE OF LSD PSYCHOTHERAPY IN COMMUNIST CZECHOSLOVAKIA

Ross Crockford

Hana K.'s third LSD experience was terrifying. Initially, the images that flashed before her eyes were beautiful: fountains of colors, fields of tulips, peacock feathers. Then they turned dark: monsters, claws, demonic eyes, vampires. She saw kings and beggars dead, buried, eaten by worms, providing food for animals and eventually for other people. "Imagine the countless atoms of our ancestors in this perpetual motion!" she cried aloud, describing everything she saw to another patient, sitting beside her bed.

Hana had a troubled life. Born in 1949, she grew up in a town south of Prague, in a family crushed by poverty. When Hana was a child, her father drank and her spiteful mother often hit her for wetting the bed. At school, classmates teased her for wearing secondhand clothes, which were often damp because she was too shy to ask permission to go to the bathroom. In her teens, she was lonely and angry, so tormented by vivid dreams of murdering her enemies that she asked to be hospitalized. At eighteen, she married a boy she barely knew, separated from him after four months, and then tried to kill herself by swallowing thirty sleeping pills.

After that, Hana's existence was a series of mind-numbing jobs, more suicide attempts, and stays in the massive, 2,000-patient Dobřany mental hospital, sixty miles southwest of Prague. Although intelligent, she was also considered hopelessly psychotic. But in 1969, when she faced another return to Dobřany, Hana told her family doctor she would rather kill herself—and this time the doctor referred her to the 112-bed clinic at Sadská, a facility east of Prague specializing in repeated sessions of LSD psychotherapy, directed by the psychiatrist Milan Hausner (1929–2000).

Hausner originally doubted that she could be helped. But as he listened to a recording of Hana's third LSD session, he saw some hope. "The most pronounced aspect of this session is her archetypal regression into the realm of antiquity and to the very beginnings of humanity," Hausner later wrote.[1] "Hana is beginning to formulate a new attitude toward death and eternity."

Over the next six months, Hana had twenty more sessions of LSD. Hausner told her that she might need sixty to be cured.

*   *   *

As Sarah Marks and others have detailed,[2] psychiatry in communist Europe was not merely an obedient lapdog to the Pavlovian conditioning promoted by the Soviet Union. It was far more varied and complex—and certainly one of its most unusual chapters concerns the use of LSD psychotherapy in 1960s Czechoslovakia, when that country's progression to a more humane government, its increasing openness to Western Europe, and its developments in psychiatry and pharmacology all coincided with a worldwide curiosity about psychedelic drugs.

Until recently, LSD therapy in Czechoslovakia was known mainly through the work of Stanislav Grof (1931–), who practiced at Prague's Psychiatric Research Institute, moved to the US in 1967, and is today celebrated as one of the founders of transpersonal psychology. But dozens of other Czech and Slovak psychiatrists also used LSD in psychotherapy, and the most dedicated and outspoken of them was Hausner, who supervised more than 3,000 LSD sessions, published research in more than 100 articles and books, and yet remains largely unknown, even in his homeland.

Hausner grew up in Prague, the only child of an insurance clerk and a pharmacist. He was drawn to the healing arts early: in May 1945, during the uprising against Nazi Germany's occupation of Czechoslovakia, he cared for fighters at Prague's barricades.[3] Germany had closed Czech universities during the six-year occupation, so after the war, the need for young doctors was acute, and in 1948—the same year the communists seized control of Czechoslovakia's government—Hausner enrolled in medicine at Prague's Charles University. After graduating in 1953, he practiced psychiatry in various places around the country, including a children's hospital. He married

Zdena Procházková, a medical statistician, completed his compulsory military service, and by 1958 was back in Prague, busily working on several psychiatric wards, often traveling from one hospital to another on the same day.

Hausner first experienced LSD in experiments conducted by Jiří Roubíček, likely in 1954. Roubíček, a neurologist, was interested in comparing the brain-wave patterns of schizophrenic patients with those of healthy subjects undergoing a "model psychosis" induced by LSD, which he obtained from Sandoz and started experimenting with in 1952.[4] Since LSD produces mind-altering effects in tiny amounts without inflicting physical harm, Roubíček's superiors considered it safe, and many young psychiatrists became his test subjects. (Czech doctors have a tradition of self-experimentation: the Czech medical society is named after Jan Evangelista Purkyně, a nineteenth-century physiologist who asserted that one learns best from direct experience and studied the effects that he underwent after ingesting such substances as digitalis and belladonna.) Unfortunately, it's not known what Hausner thought of his own LSD experiences, as he did not describe them in his writings.

In the late 1950s, Hausner started conducting his own medical research, publishing a study of his application of the new antipsychotic drug chlorpromazine combined with electroconvulsive therapy (ECT). Increasingly, however, he was interested less in biological psychiatry and more in psychotherapy—a controversial discipline, as it was often associated with Freudian psychoanalysis, which communists considered unscientific, individualistic, and likely to bankrupt national health-insurance programs. In 1959, Czech ideologues denounced Ferdinand Knobloch (1916–2018), the head of psychiatry at Charles University's medical-faculty polyclinic, for advocating the use of psychotherapy to treat neuroses, and Hausner came to his defense. In the journal *Czechoslovak psychiatry*, Knobloch assured his readers that he was developing a "materialistic" psychotherapy, with measurable results,[5] and Hausner provided a survey of recent Soviet medical literature showing that Russian doctors already were practicing psychotherapy in various forms, using suggestion (often with hypnosis) and persuasion, in an effort to fully understand "the personality of socialist man in unity with the socialist environment."[6] (Hausner read and spoke Russian, along with English and German.) Czechoslovakia held an international congress on treating neuroses later that year, so a wider acceptance of psychotherapy was already underway. But Knobloch likely appreciated Hausner's support, because he soon hired Hausner to work at the university polyclinic.

Between seeing patients, Hausner wrote his first book, *The Mentally Ill among Us* (1961), a guide to the mental-health system for patients and their families that told the story of a young man's psychotic break, his treatment through medication and psychotherapy, and his return to work. In the preface, Hausner noted that Czechoslovakia's third Five-Year Plan (1961–1965) called for wider treatment of "nervous diseases," and he hoped that his readers would learn that "mental illness does not equal disgrace, but can be successfully treated like any other physical illness."[7] (Hausner's compassionate book was so popular that it was republished in 1969, 1978, and 1981.) During this time, he also began paying privately to undergo psychoanalysis, perhaps with Knobloch, as part of his training to become a psychoanalyst himself. Most fatefully, though, he became interested in treating patients with LSD, newly available from Czechoslovakia's government laboratories.

In 1956, chemists at the Research Institute for Pharmacy and Biochemistry in Prague filed a patent for a new process for making LSD,[8] and in 1959, the ministry of health gave the institute permission to begin producing the drug, trademarked Lysergamid, "primarily for experimental purposes."[9] So Hausner devised an experiment. In 1954, R. A. Sandison and other British doctors had reported benefits in neurotic patients who received small-to-substantial doses of LSD (25–400 μg) in conjunction with individual psychotherapy, applied repeatedly over several months[10]—a method that Sandison later called "psycholytic" therapy. Hausner wondered if this would work in groups. Through the university, he knew Vladimír Doležal, a medical doctor and chemist specializing in toxicology, and they proposed using LSD in a therapeutic community established by Hausner's boss.

At the polyclinic, Knobloch had become intrigued by the self-defeating behavior of his neurotic patients, so he'd developed a retreat for them on a state farm in Lobeč (thirty-five miles north of Prague), modeled on the therapeutic community for traumatized soldiers that Maxwell Jones had established near London in 1947. Even under communism, Czechs with "bad nerves" were typically treated with baths at the country's opulent nineteenth-century spa resorts, and Knobloch wanted to prove that he could help more people at less cost. At Lobeč, fifteen men and fifteen women spent several hours every day working on the farm, and several additional hours with a rehabilitation aide engaged in group discussions or various types of therapy, producing art or music or acting out events from their lives via psychodrama or "psychogymnastics," a nonverbal exercise incorporating movement and mime.[11] A psychiatrist from Prague visited to direct individual and group psychotherapy only once or twice a week, so the patients effectively became cotherapists, a design that Hausner tried to duplicate at Sadská.

In their experiment, Hausner and Doležal gave eleven neurotic patients 100 μg of LSD in conjunction with six hours of individual psychotherapy; seven got 50 μg and group therapy, and seven got saline as a control. After several weeks, the patients who'd received LSD and individual therapy showed the most improvement, displaying new insights and changed attitudes in their relationships with staff and other patients. Those who received LSD in the group had the worst results: "Patients were more concerned about their unusual experiences than to expose them to the therapeutic effect of the collective." It was a modest study,[12] but the first on LSD psychotherapy to appear in the Czech medical literature.

Other Czech doctors were starting to use the drug. Stanislav Grof began psycholytic therapy with neurotic patients at the Psychiatric Research Institute in 1961, and that year the authorities approved Lysergamid for outpatient psychiatry, encouraging other doctors around Czechoslovakia to test it in their own practices. Individual psychotherapy expanded, and soon it was possible to discuss concepts that were essentially Freudian: in 1963, Hausner and Doležal published a remarkable how-to guide for hallucinogens in the journal *Czechoslovak psychiatry*,[13] citing the West German psychiatrist Hanscarl Leuner's contention that such drugs "reawakened psychic dynamics" by evoking "age regression going to the first years of life," "re-living of forgotten traumatic events," and providing "abreactive emotional release with subsequent insight." They outlined radical techniques, some borrowed from Leuner and other Western LSD doctors, that they used at Lobeč: getting patients to write out their autobiographies, using family photos to encourage associations, having the doctor play characters perceived in patients' hallucinations, and even recruiting other patients to assist with the sessions. Hausner and Doležal quoted their patients endorsing LSD therapy, included samples of patients' artwork, and claimed that after a year, 75 percent of their patients receiving LSD and individual therapy had improved, although the best results were in those who'd combined such therapy with a stay at Lobeč, where they could practice insights acquired from their LSD experience.

Through such research, Hausner established contact with Leuner, who became the principal advocate for psycholytic therapy after Sandison moved on from LSD in 1964. Hausner started getting published in international journals, Czechoslovakia began permitting academics to travel to capitalist countries, and in August 1964, Hausner summarized his Lobeč work at the Sixth International Congress of Psychotherapy in London. By 1965, Czechoslovakia's authorities had approved commercial production of its LSD,[14] and Hausner wrote a paper—published in English—for the state pharmaceutical export firm, noting that Lysergamid was indistinguishable from Sandoz's product and describing its effectiveness in outpatient psychiatry. He would run 104 sessions with sixty-five patients, using doses of 50 to 300 μg, and found LSD was "a valuable means for deepening and accelerating the psychotherapy."[15] (Perhaps reluctant to limit foreign interest in Lysergamid to therapeutic communities, Hausner downplayed his Lobeč research, writing that he'd seen "no impressive differences" in results with outpatients.)

Hausner had credentials, contacts, and a steady supply of LSD. He was ready to apply everything that he'd learned at a clinic of his own.

*　*　*

The psychiatric clinic at Sadská, a town of 3,000 residents forty miles east of Prague, consisted of a pair of two-floor pavilions originally constructed in the 1920s as a retreat for postal employees to enjoy a nearby lake and mineral spa, or walk along the Elbe River and through the Kersko forests. To meet the growing demand for psychiatric care, the ministry of health acquired the facility and began admitting patients in 1962. But by the autumn of 1965, Sadská's chief physician was losing his eyesight. The clinic was affiliated with Charles University's faculty of medicine, so Hausner, then thirty-six, got the job, and he quickly made changes.

Pavilion A remained devoted to standard psychiatry for inpatients suffering issues from hysteria to psychosis. But Hausner had Pavilion B remodeled as an open ward to suit a therapeutic community. He selected some fifty inpatients for it, to stay six to eight weeks, and from them, he chose one or two groups of twelve to fourteen patients who he thought were most likely to benefit from LSD, to stay six months. As at Lobeč, the patients spent mornings laboring in the forest or in the clinic's garden and workshop, afternoons in group discussions, and evenings hearing lectures, creating dances or plays, or watching films. But with his own facility, Hausner could fully implement psycholytic therapy, and every day several patients underwent LSD.

The drug was usually delivered by injection to control the dosage, and before breakfast so the patients wouldn't be hungry in the middle of their trip. Sessions were conducted in the patients' rooms—LSD groups were on the ground floor—and the patients were accompanied by a sitter. Outpatients also came to Sadská for "weekend therapy," undergoing LSD and individual or group analysis and returning to work on Monday.[16] Like the inpatients, these visitors underwent dozens of treatments: one forty-two-year-old male received 300 μg thirty-seven times in eighteen months.

Hausner wrote up a guide for patients, introducing them to psycholytic therapy. Many instructions were typical of clinics elsewhere—he advised patients to keep their eyes closed while on LSD and to accept unpleasant or frightening episodes, as they might reveal the sources of their psychological difficulties—but others seemed worded to reassure patients who had lived under totalitarianism. "Talk openly about everything that comes to mind while using the substance," Hausner advised. "The purpose of sitting is not to 'extract' experiences that you would not discuss in a completely awake state."[17]

He also wrote detailed instructions for the staff. Nurses were to supervise patients filling out the numerous questionnaires, to conduct art and occupational therapy, and to sit with patients during LSD sessions. Some patients might undergo psychotic episodes, he warned: "Remember that kindness, an effort to understand seemingly bizarre behavior, and minimal restraints can usually eliminate even the most violent manifestations." Any doctor or therapist working with LSD was required to have at least three experiences with the drug themselves so that they could better understand their patients, and nurses had the option to undergo LSD as well. "When work started at Sadská, the personnel took a very sceptical attitude to the whole undertaking," Hausner told a reporter, but most employees came around. "Their first eye-opener is that as 'normal' people they are not so very different from the patients under LSD intoxication. This discovery breaks down the barrier of prejudice in them."[18]

The LSD therapy at Sadská was also greatly influenced by Zbyněk Havlíček (1922–1969), a psychologist and surrealist poet who had worked at

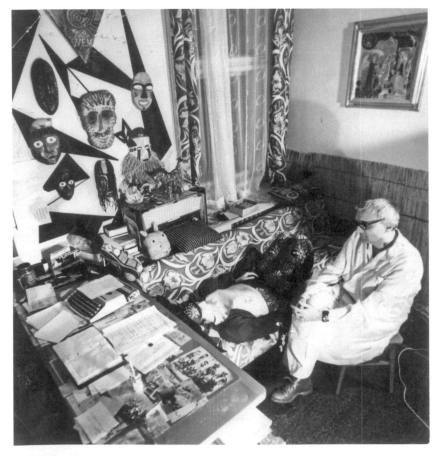

Figure 4.1
Milan Hausner counsels a patient in his office at the Sadská clinic in 1974. A color photo of the same scene in a popular magazine contributed to the end of LSD psychotherapy in Czechoslovakia. Reproduced courtesy of Vladimír Lammer.

the Dobřany mental hospital in the 1950s and was at Sadská when Hausner arrived. Fascinated by psychoanalysis, Havlíček considered LSD a "miracle" compared to the mind-numbing drugs issued by most psychiatrists, and he ran many of the early psycholytic groups at Sadská, interviewing patients while they were hallucinating.

In letters to his girlfriend, Havlíček described his method in detail, playing with patients' symptoms "like a bullfighter, waving a red cloth to their statements,"[19] probing their visions and memories and finding connections in their biographies and patterns of behavior. This LSD analysis apparently worked: Hausner reported that eighty hospitalized patients underwent psycholytic therapy at Sadská in 1966, mainly suffering from neuroses, sexual disorders, and psychosomatic syndromes that hadn't responded to other treatments for years, and forty-seven of them improved enough to be discharged. "The more sessions, the better the results," Hausner said: patients who improved significantly had an average of twelve sessions (average dose 250 μg), while those showing no improvement had an average of six.[20]

This was good news at a time when moral panic about LSD was cresting elsewhere. In April 1966, a few days after the *New York Times* reported that a man claiming to be "flying" on LSD had stabbed his mother-in-law to death, Sandoz announced that it was stopping all distribution of its product, and therapists from the US, the UK, Italy, and other countries started visiting the Sadská clinic, hoping to buy Lysergamid. Stanislav Grof knew many prominent LSD doctors after presenting his own psycholytic research at a conference in New York, and he brought several of them to Sadská, including Harvard's Walter Pahnke. But the panic elsewhere reached Czechoslovakia, too: the communist daily *Rudé Právo* ran an article denouncing LSD as a "new god" that had unleashed madness in the West,[21] and Hausner had to respond. No misuse of Lysergamid had occurred in Czechoslovakia, he assured readers; only trained psychiatrists could request the drug after approval by a special committee of the ministry of health. (Hausner was the committee secretary, and he directed foreigners' inquiries to the state export company.) Besides, LSD was too valuable a tool to be outlawed. The drug was a "probe into the subconscious," Hausner wrote—and "the probe goes very deep, often into the first days of life, if not further."[22]

This was an extraordinary claim, especially for the pages of the official Communist Party newspaper, but it did reflect what the doctors were seeing. Hausner reported elsewhere that two-thirds of his LSD patients "relived phantasies concerning their birth, intrauterine life, 'birth trauma,' [or] first events of the sucking age."[23] At an October 1966 conference in Amsterdam, Grof theorized that LSD brought forth constellations of emotionally charged, condensed experiences (COEX), individual to each patient's life, and these earliest memories or fantasies lay at the core of each COEX system, providing a key to understanding the patient's problems. Havlíček, the Freudian, disagreed, arguing that such experiences were merely "a retroprojection of later conflicts" onto the richly symbolic moment of birth.[24] To Hausner, these were theoretical differences; he was focused on managing his clinic, and he instructed Sadská's nurses to comfort patients in a "pediatric regression" by "stroking, taking a hand, etc."—which required "a certain skill" in distinguishing regression from "adult manifestation on an erotic level."[25]

The most fundamental dispute between the doctors, however, occurred over how LSD therapy should be conducted. In 1967, Grof got a fellowship to work at Baltimore's Spring Grove State Hospital, which used "psychedelic" therapy, giving alcoholics one huge dose of LSD (400 μg or more) to induce a life-changing spiritual experience.[26] Grof started thinking that Europe's psycholytic advocates were on the wrong track: repeated sessions of psychoanalysis were time-consuming and couldn't grasp the profound sensations of ego death, rebirth, or cosmic unity that LSD patients often experienced at higher doses, which he saw could be beneficial. Havlíček had none of it: he argued that the psychedelic experience was essentially narcissistic and typically American—a retreat into a "luxurious uterus," providing feelings of divine exaltation but socially worthless, separating the patient from the real world where their problems began, and where they had to learn to survive.[27] Hausner, who'd been elected vice president of the European Association for Psycholytic Therapy, agreed: "In my experience," he later wrote, "achieving true transcendental insight is rare unless the subject succeeds in discarding the negative aspects of his unconscious and erases the faulty programming that is causing the problem."[28] (To avoid confusion with psychedelic therapy,

Hausner usually referred to the drugs as "psychodysleptics," meaning that they induced a dreamlike state.)

Grof prepared a response,[29] proposing a way to integrate psycholytic and psychedelic techniques at an international LSD congress to be held in Prague in September 1968, but the paper was never heard. On August 20, Soviet troops invaded Czechoslovakia to crush the democratic progress emerging during the Prague Spring. Then, on January 7, 1969, Havlíček died of leukemia. Sadská's fortunes were destined to change after that.

* * *

When Hana K. arrived at Sadská in 1970, she spent four months in group therapy while Hausner assessed her. She answered questionnaires and wrote her autobiography, read books by Freud and Erich Fromm, and sat in on discussions about relationships—many of the patients were young and had family conflicts because the state wouldn't assign them apartments of their own unless they were married. Then Hana started the LSD treatments, and by sharing work and experiences with other patients, for the first time in her life she made some friends.

After twenty-two sessions, Hausner decided that Hana had improved enough to join a group psycholytic session. Although his early research suggested that group LSD sessions had little value, Hausner found that low doses of the drug helped some patients see their own "faulty, unbalanced behavior" when interacting with others.[30] Hana received 100 μg with half the patients in her group. At first, the experience was unpleasant, like she was being watched on a stage. But soon members of the community started violently arguing with each other—and Hana was flooded with empathy.

"I am actually beginning to understand and to relate to people," Hana wrote in her diary. "I can see and understand the reason for the things they do, and I don't hate them anymore! Poor doctor. He's got so many children. How can he cope with it all?"[31]

After the 1968 invasion, it took Czechoslovakia's new Soviet-backed government several years to replace key officials with hardline communists, and during that time Hausner was able to continue LSD therapy. Newcomers joined Sadská, including a psychoanalyst from Poland and a group therapist from Barcelona, and foreigners continued to tour the clinic—R. A. Sandison visited in 1970—but increasingly from the Soviet bloc, curious about methods unavailable in their own countries. "We have found your system of contacting LSD group's therapy very fascinating," two Polish psychologists wrote in Sadská's guestbook after staying several weeks in the summer of 1969. "We have seen wonderful results. We have taken LSD ourselves and experienced that it helps very much in speeding up psychotherapy. We would like to arrange LSD group's psychotherapy in Poland."[32]

To hear the people who worked there describe it, Sadská was more like an offbeat arts college than a Soviet medical facility. Hausner brought his three children to the clinic, and sculptors and dream interpreters came from Prague to give classes to the patients. Some evenings, they held masquerades or parties; the doctors and nurses and patients would dance together, and the next day, they would discuss in group how they had interacted. There were a few suicide attempts, but there were also romances: one older LSD patient, who had spent his youth in a Nazi concentration camp and suffered from depression, was so impressed by Sadská that after his discharge, he became a therapist at the clinic and married one of the psychiatrists. As one patient later wrote, "At Sadská, it was Freud and love."[33]

Sadly, that love wasn't felt in the Czech capital. Communists feared that the Western scourge of narcotics addiction was leaking into Czechoslovakia, and in December 1969, the popular magazine *Květy* ran an article about drug abuse by Prague youths, opening with a rumor that LSD could be bought in front of a downtown cinema from a car with Austrian license plates.[34] Hausner increasingly had to defend the psychiatric use of LSD and the distribution scheme that he helped administer. At the prestigious Collegium Internationale Neuropsychopharmacologicum, held in Prague in 1970, he spoke on the "therapeutic and illegal use of Lysergamide": after some 3,000 sessions with 300 patients at Sadská, he reported, general health improved for 60 percent of them, and life satisfaction increased for 70 percent. "Nobody of these 300 patients became habituated to LSD," he asserted; distribution of the drug was under "rigorous governmental control," and "no misuse has been observed."[35] But he was swimming against the tide. In February 1971, thirty-four countries adopted the UN

Convention on Psychotropic Substances, classifying LSD as a drug of abuse with no therapeutic value. Czechoslovakia was only an observer of the proceedings, but the Soviet Union soon signed on, and Sadská came under scrutiny.

In May of that year, a panel of doctors conducted a comprehensive audit of the clinic "due to frequent negative comments" from the regional health authority. Hausner prepared a table showing that LSD patients were a small percentage of Sadská's admissions, and the time they spent there was decreasing (see table 4.1).

The panel commended Hausner for fulfilling the planned number of treatments, his focus on "modern currents" in psychiatry, such as "group psychotherapy and active pursuit of cooperation of the patient," and his "progressive efforts" to reduce hospitalization via his "weekend" LSD therapy. But, "[a]s far as LSD treatment is concerned, we reiterate the fact that this method is not generally accepted. The number of patients treated in this way needs to be limited as much as possible, or to stay with LSD for a few cases that would only go to outpatient treatment."[36]

Hausner complied, increasingly putting new LSD patients on weekend therapy. Every third or fourth weekend, about forty patients would endure a "psycholytic marathon," taking turns sitting for each other and heading back to work on Monday. Each of them would have been hospitalized an average of sixty-four days without the program, Hausner calculated, so it saved the state 1.34 million Crowns per year.[37] (At the time, the average salary in Czechoslovakia was 26,844 Crowns per year.) To save more money, Hausner

Table 4.1 Changes to LSD Therapy at Sadská, 1967–1970				
	1967	**1968**	**1969**	**1970**
LSD patients	82	49	57	84
Percentage of admitted patients	8.6	6.5	6.0	11.8
LSD intoxications	587	313	405	416
LSD used (μg)	160,100	93,500	121,000	157,500
Days off work by LSD patients	5,832	3,841	4,369	2,625

recruited psychology students to assist on weekends, and many underwent a "training intoxication" with LSD for university credit.

Hausner continued to publish articles internationally, including one comparing the symbology of dreams to LSD hallucinations that was subsequently reprinted in a Czech journal for general practitioners.[38] In March 1973, he chaired a conference on psychotherapy in socialist countries that was attended by experts from across the Soviet bloc—although he was careful to mention psycholytic therapy only once in his own paper, surveying the range of techniques used in Czechoslovakia at the time. (For example, Hausner, then president of the psychotherapeutic section of Czech Psychiatric Society, noted that 250 of its 300 members used hypnosis.) In June, he traveled to Oslo for the 9th International Congress of Psychotherapy, where he identified his practice as "dynamic confrontation therapy," in which a patient faces the problems of past, present, and future (!) in a controlled environment, with psychodysleptic drugs targeting the "neurochemical, intrapsychic, interpersonal, psychosomatic and the valuation system area[s]," and ultimately providing a corrective emotional experience.[39]

But officials back in Prague were likely suspicious of the relative freedom that Hausner enjoyed without a Communist Party membership. Drug abuse was becoming a problem in Czechoslovakia, and though nearly all the cases involved prescription medicines, often containing ephedrine or codeine, the bureaucrats feared that LSD was next. In October 1973, they inspected the Sadská clinic, and in its safe, they found 619 ampoules of LSD that had expired in 1969. In January 1974, they consulted the pharmacy that distributed the drug and learned it had another 2,400 ampoules that Hausner had ordered in 1971 and were about to expire. In a series of letters, Hausner apologized. Supplies from the factory had been unpredictable, he said, and LSD remained stable in glass ampoules for many years. Besides, the drug hadn't been stolen or turned up on the black market, so what was the harm?[40]

Hausner needed some good press, so he invited journalists from *Květy* to visit Sadská. The resulting article[41] described a traumatized eighteen-year-old girl arriving at the clinic, and Hausner's plans to treat her with LSD, accompanied by a full-page color photo of Hausner ministering to a female patient lying on a wildly patterned couch in his office under a wall of primitive masks. The deputy director of the regional health authority demanded that LSD therapy be stopped. Hausner apologized again, admitting the photo was "too provocative," and he got letters from other doctors supporting the continued use of LSD. But the health authority ordered Hausner to send reports on every patient receiving the drug, and it started conducting spot checks of the clinic's supply.

In the late summer of 1974, Hausner's father died, and Hausner had a nervous breakdown. "He had the worst fears for the future, he was anxious about his family, and concerned about material security," one of his colleagues later said.[42] Hausner admitted that he'd considered suicide and was hospitalized in Prague for several months. The regional pharmacist came to Sadská, collected all the ampoules of LSD, and stomped on them in Hausner's office.

"They took away all his appetite for work," a nurse said years after this incident. Hausner suffered another breakdown and received treatments from his Prague colleagues that he'd tried to avoid in his own practice, including ECT, antidepressants, and lithium. When he finally returned to Sadská in 1975, he was emotionally flattened, a changed man. A nearby hospital took over administration of the Sadská clinic and converted the psychotherapeutic pavilion into a ward for chronic psychiatric patients. LSD was still theoretically available with permission from the health ministry, but nobody risked ordering it.

Hausner left Sadská in 1981, after he and Zdena divorced. Czechoslovakia drifted into a stultifying political "normalization," and Hausner ended up in the industrial north, providing psychiatry to the employees of a uranium mine. When he died in 2000, Czech medical journals did not mention his passing.

*   *   *

For many decades, even after the communist regime fell in 1989, Czech medical authorities resisted any talk of reviving LSD therapy, and the few doctors interested in the drug were limited to conducting animal studies. But possibilities are beginning to reopen. Prague psychiatrists are studying the neurobiological effects of psilocybin—in a suite designed to resemble Hausner's office as it appeared in *Květy*—and have established a private clinic offering ketamine-assisted psychotherapy, the first in central Europe, although such treatments are not yet covered by Czech medical insurance.

Hausner's correspondence, patient files, and hundreds of pieces of artwork reside in the Czech Academy of Sciences archive, but they are currently inaccessible to the public. Thanks to the growing interest in psychedelics, a book that Hausner wrote in 1997 about psycholytic therapy at Sadská has finally been published,[43] but to get a more complete picture of what happened at the clinic, the author also sought out people who were there. Some thirty psychiatrists and psychologists worked or trained at the clinic; the author and his colleagues interviewed nine of them, and while many said that Hausner was a superb administrator and psychiatrist, they also said that LSD didn't "accelerate" psychotherapy because so much time was spent in sessions and analyzing the patients' experiences. Several said that therapists were overwhelmed by the volume of material that LSD evoked and Hausner tried to do too much: many of the LSD patients had neuroses or depression, but the conditions of others ranged from alcoholism to schizophrenia to psychopathy. The author also interviewed five Sadská nurses, all of whom said that it was the most interesting period of their careers, and the clinic was "like a big family." But did LSD therapy help the patients? "Well, they did not come back," one nurse said. "They went back to life and everything was OK," said another. "It is true that it was a half-year-long treatment. But it was successful, at least according to me."[44]

The author also interviewed fifteen former Sadská patients. Three said that psycholytic therapy hadn't substantially changed their condition, and four said that it made their condition worse. One woman said that she felt "broken" after every session and experienced unnerving flashbacks years later. A man who suffered sexual neuroses said that he didn't consider LSD useful because "it opened everything in allegorical terms" and confused the therapeutic relationship: in one session, he tried to rest his head in his doctor's lap, and she rejected him, which took him a long time to overcome. But eight thought that Sadská's therapy had helped. A woman who suffered from posttraumatic stress disorder (PTSD) and sexual dysfunction said that she was "newly born" after her third session; she had been raised Catholic, and she said that LSD showed her "what belief really is." A male alcoholic said that "LSD made the first step" to his sobriety and inspired him to become a therapist for other alcoholics.

Hana K. was discharged not long after her group LSD session. In 1972, she married a fellow Sadská patient, and eventually they had two sons. Today, she says that she's become happier as she gets older, and the worst time of her life was just before she went to Sadská.

"A home, and kind people around me, that is something I never had before," she said of the clinic nearly fifty years later. "And with LSD they taught me things I never came across anywhere else. But whether the treatment would be equally as successful without LSD I cannot say."[45]

NOTES

1. Milan Hausner and Erna Segal, *LSD: The Highway to Mental Health* (Malibu, CA: ASC Books, 2009), 248.

2. *Psychiatry in Communist Europe*, ed. Mat Savelli and Sarah Marks (Hampshire, UK: Palgrave Macmillan, 2015); Sarah Marks, "From Experimental Psychosis to Resolving Traumatic Pasts: Psychedelic Research in Communist Czechoslovakia, 1954–1974," *Cahiers du monde russe* 56, no. 1 (2015): 53–76.

3. Hausner autobiographical summary, January 14, 1982, typescript, author's files.

4. Jiří Roubíček and Jan Srnec, "Experimentální psychosa vyvolaná LSD," *Časopis lékařů českých* 94, no. 8 (February 18, 1955): 189–195.

5. F. Knobloch, "Ideologický boj a formy kritiky," *Československá psychiatrie* 55, no. 5 (1959): 337–339.

6. Milan Hausner, "Pohledy na Sovětskou psychoterapii," *Československá psychiatrie* 55, no. 5 (1959): 339–349.

7. *Duševně nemocný mezi námi* (Prague: Státní zdravotnické nakladatelství, 1961), 8.

8. Republika Československá statni uřád pro vynalezy a normalisaci, Patentní spis č. 86727.

9. Memo from MUDr. Jan Stříteský on behalf of the Scientific Council of the Ministry of Health, October 3, 1959. Author's copy.

10. R. A. Sandison, et al., "The Therapeutic Value of Lysergic Acid Diethylamide in Mental Illness," *Journal of Mental Science* 100. no. 419 (1954): 491–507.

11. F. Knobloch, "The Diagnostic and Therapeutic Community as Part of a Psychotherapeutic System," *Acta Psychotherapeutica, Psychosomatica et Orthopaedagogica* 7 supplementum (1959): 195–204.

12. V. Doležal and M. Hausner, "Naše zkušenosti s individuální a kolektivní psychoterapií za pomoci LSD," *Activitas Nervosa Superior* 4, no. 2 (1962): 241–242.

13. M. Hausner and V. Doležal, "Praktické zkušenosti s halucinogeny v psychoterapii," *Československá psychiatrie*, 59, no. 5 (1963): 328–335.

14. *Seznam československých farmaceutických přípravků 1965–1967*, SPOFA, 302–304.

15. M. Hausner and V. Doležal, "The Experience with Psychedelics in Outpatient Psychotherapy," *Medical Information Service of SPOFA-Chemapol* 3, no. 4 (1966): 79–83.

16. Hausner repeatedly used the phrase "weekend therapy" to describe his two-day LSD outpatient therapy, which was likely unique to Sadská. See note 37 that specifically deals with this weekend therapy.

17. "Rules for patients of the psycholytic department," February 15, 1966, in *Terapeutická komunita POS: Ruzně materialy*, Milan Hausner fonds, Masaryk Institute and Archives of the Czech Academy of Sciences. Author's translation.

18. Lieko Zachovalová, "Why Does Czechoslovakia Still Make LSD?" *Czechoslovak Life* 22, no. 3 (1967): 9.

19. Zbyněk Havlíček and Eva Prusíková, *Dopisy Evě / Dopisy Zbyňkovi* (Prague: Torst, 2003), 515.

20. "Psycholytická psychoterapie," *Activitas Nervosa Superior* 10, no.1 (1968): 50.

21. "Nový bůh povstal na západě: jmenuje se LSD," *Rudé Právo*, May 22, 1966, příloha 3.

22. "LSD-25: skalpel, nebo dýka?" *Rudé Právo*, June 25, 1966, příloha 2, author's translation.

23. Hausner and Doležal, "Psychedelics in Outpatient Psychotherapy," 81.

24. Milan Hausner and Zbyněk Havlíček, "Catarctic and Interpretive Attitude to Regressive Events in Psychodysleptic Psychotherapy," Fourth Psychotherapeutic Congress, Wiesbaden, Germany, August 1967.

25. "Instructions for staff of the psycholytic department," February 15, 1966, in *Terapeutická komunita*, Hausner fonds, author's translation.

26. Matthew Oram describes the work at Spring Grove in *The Trials of Psychedelic Therapy: LSD Psychotherapy in America* (Baltimore: Johns Hopkins University Press, 2018).

27. Z. Havlíček, "Autenticita a význam regresívních prožitků v průběhu analytické LSD-psychoterapie," *Československá psychiatrie* 64, no. 4 (1968): 236–240.

28. Hausner and Segal, *Highway*, 16.

29. Stanislav Grof, "Psycholytic and Psychedelic Therapy with LSD: Toward an Integration of Approaches," typescript prepared for the IV Congress of the European Medical Association for Psycholysis, 1968.

30. Hausner and Segal, *Highway*, 39.

31. Hausner and Segal, *Highway*, 249.

32. *Navštěvní kniha POS*, Hausner fonds.

33. Karel Šebek, "Doktor Zbyněk Kaligari," in *Skutečnost snu*, ed. Stanislav Dvorský (Prague: Torst, 2003), 446.

34. "Mezi pražskými narkomany," *Květy* 19, no. 48 (1969): 4–9.

35. "Therapeutic and Illegal Use of Lysergamide," typescript, Hausner fonds.

36. "Review of the psychiatric ward at the University Hospital at Sadská," a report by MUDr. Josef Šulc, dated May 6, 1971, in *Terapeutická komunita*, Hausner fonds, author's translation.

37. M. Hausner, "Frakcionovaná víkendová psychoterapie chronických psychogenních, charakterogenních a sociogenních poruch," *Československá psychiatrie* 70, no. 3 (1974): 195–99.

38. M. Hausner, "LSD a sen," *Praktické lékař* 53, no. 15–16 (1973): 576–79.

39. M. Hausner, "The Dynamic Confrontation Model as an Integration of Psychotherapy," *Psychotherapy and Psychosomatics* 24 (1974): 497–99.

40. *Lysergamid POS Hospodaření*, Hausner fonds.

41. "Šifry z Mozku," *Květy* 24, no. 9 (March 2, 1974): 18–20.

42. Discussion between Miloš Vojtěchovský, Vladimír Hort, and Hana Junová, 2004, author's files.

43. Hausner and Segal, *Highway*, published in Czech as *LSD: Výzkum a klinická praxe za železnou oponou* (Prague: Triton, 2016).

44. Author's interview, April 2008.

45. Interview conducted by Michal Vančura, presented at *75. narozeniny LSD*, Prague, April 19, 2018.

BIBLIOGRAPHY

Primary Sources

Discussion between Miloš Vojtěchovský, Vladimír Hort and Hana Junová, 2004, author's files.

Grof, Stanislav, "Psycholytic and Psychedelic Therapy with LSD: Toward an Integration of Approaches," typescript, prepared for the IV Congress of the European Medical Association for Psycholysis, 1968.

Hausner autobiographical summary, January 14, 1982, typescript, author's files.

Hausner, Milan. *Duševně nemocný mezi námi* (Prague: Státní zdravotnické nakladatelství, 1961).

Hausner, Milan. "LSD-25: skalpel, nebo dýka?" *Rudé Právo*, June 25, 1966, příloha 2.

Hausner, Milan. "Psycholytická psychoterapie," *Activitas Nervosa Superior* 10, no. 1 (1968): 50.

Hausner, Milan, and Erna Segal. *LSD: The Highway to Mental Health*. Malibu, CA: ASC Books, 2009.

Havlíček, Zbyněk, and Eva Prusíková. *Dopisy Evě / Dopisy Zbyňkovi* (Prague: Torst, 2003).

"Instructions for staff of the psycholytic department," February 15, 1966; "Rules for patients of the psycholytic department," February 15, 1966; "Review of the psychiatric ward at the University Hospital at Sadská," a report by MUDr. Josef Šulc, May 6, 1971; *Terapeutická komunita POS: Ruzně materialy*, Milan Hausner fonds, Masaryk Institute and Archives of the Czech Academy of Sciences.

Interview conducted by Michal Vančura, presented at a one-day conference, held in Czech; "75th Birthday of LSD", Prague, April 19, 2018.

Lysergamid POS Hospodaření, Hausner fonds.

Memo from MUDr (a one-day conference, held in Czech; "75th Birthday of LSD"). Jan Stříteský on behalf of the Scientific Council of the Ministry of Health, October 3, 1959. Author's copy.

Navštěvní kniha POS, Hausner fonds.

Republika Československá statni uřád pro vynalezy a normalisaci, Patentní spis č. 86727.

Seznam československých farmaceutických přípravků 1965–1967, SPOFA, 302–304.

"Šifry z Mozku," *Květy* 24, no. 9 (March 2, 1974), 18–20.

"Therapeutic and Illegal Use of Lysergamide," typescript, M.H. *Anglické listy duplikaty*, Hausner fonds.

Secondary Sources

Doležal, V. and M. Hausner. "Naše zkušenosti s individuální a kolektivní psychoterapií za pomoci LSD." *Activitas Nervosa Superior* 4, no. 2 (1962): 241–242.

Hausner, M. "LSD a sen," *Praktické lékař* 53, no. 15–16 (1973): 576–579.

Hausner, M. "The Dynamic Confrontation Model as an Integration of Psychotherapy." *Psychotherapy and Psychosomatics* 24 (1974): 497–499.

Hausner, M. "Frakcionovaná víkendová psychoterapie chronických psychogenních, charaktero-genních a sociogenních poruch." *Československá psychiatrie* 70, no. 3 (1974): 195–199.

Hausner, Milan. "Pohledy na Sovětskou psychoterapii." *Československá psychiatrie* 55, no. 5 (1959): 339–149.

Hausner, M., and V. Doležal. "Praktické zkušenosti s halucinogeny v psychoterapii." *Československá psychiatrie* 59, no. 5 (1963): 328–335.

Hausner, M., and V. Doležal. "The Experience with Psychedelics in Outpatient Psychotherapy." *Medical Information Service of SPOFA-Chemapol* 3, no. 4 (1966): 79–83.

Hausner, Milan, and Zbyněk Havlíček. "Catarctic and interpretive attitude to regressive events in psychodysleptic psychotherapy." Fourth Psychotherapeutic Congress, Wiesbaden, Germany, August 1967.

Havlíček, Z. "Autenticita a význam regresívních prožitků v průběhu analytické LSD-psychoterapie." *Československá psychiatrie* 64, no. 4 (1968): 236–240.

Knobloch, F. "The Diagnostic and Therapeutic Community as Part of a Psychotherapeutic System." *Acta Psychotherapeutica, Psychosomatica et Orthopaedagogica* 7 supplementum (1959): 195–204.

Knobloch, F. "Ideologický boj a formy kritiky." *Československá psychiatrie* 55, no. 5 (1959): 337–339.

Marks, Sarah. "From Experimental Psychosis to Resolving Traumatic Pasts: Psychedelic Research in Communist Czechoslovakia, 1954–1974." *Cahiers du monde russe* 56, no. 1 (2015): 53–76. https://journals.openedition.org/monderusse/8165.

Marks, Sarah, and Mat Savelli, eds. *Psychiatry in Communist Europe*. London: Palgrave Macmillan, 2015.

"Mezi pražskými narkomany," *Květy* 19, no. 48 (1969): 4–9.

"Nový bůh povstal na západě: jmenuje se LSD," *Rudé Právo*, May 22, 1966, příloha 3.

Oram, Matthew. *The Trials of Psychedelic Therapy: LSD Psychotherapy in America*. Baltimore: Johns Hopkins University Press, 2018.

Roubíček, Jiří, and Jan Srnec. "Experimentální psychosa vyvolaná LSD." *Časopis lékařů českých* 94, no. 8 (1955): 189–195.

Sandison, Ronald A., A. M. Spencer, and J. D. A. Whitelaw. "The Therapeutic Value of Lysergic Acid Diethylamide in Mental Illness." *Journal of Mental Science* 100, no. 419 (1954): 491–507.

Šebek, Karel. "Doktor Zbyněk Kaligari." In *Skutečnost snu*, edited by Stanislav Dvorský. Prague: Torst, 2003.

Zachovalová, Lieko. "Why Does Czechoslovakia Still Make LSD?" *Czechoslovak Life* 22, no. 3 (1967): 8–11.

5 REMEMBERING TO FORGET: HOW THE UK DISAPPEARED FROM THE PSYCHEDELIC MAP

Wendy Kline

Whenever young Frank Crompton accompanied his grandmother on the bus through Worcester, England, in the 1950s, she made him put a bag over his head as the bus drove by Powick Psychiatric Hospital. "Don't look that way or you'll get damaged by it," she would say.[1] The stigma of Powick was widespread in the local community. Beryl Kendall, whose mother was institutionalized at Powick, remembers an old saying that if you were naughty, you would be sent there. "Horrific, that was," she remembered of the rumors, which added to her stress when she got off the bus in front of the hospital. "I never knew what I was going to find."[2]

The looming presence of the asylum was enough to give just about anyone pause. When W. V. Caldwell first laid eyes on Powick in the 1960s, he understood why passersby might look the other way. He described the hospital as "gray and dismal, its stones piled upon one another in monumental unimaginative weariness." This American observer interpreted the view as characteristically British: "Tall curtainless windows stared blankly at us through the first spatter of cold rain. Here were all the schools, orphanages, and prisons of Charlotte Bronte and Dickens wrapped into one. Here was the English 'institutions,' bleak and somber."[3] Two local high school students visited in the summer of 1962, noting that the hospital "presents rather a grim sight when viewed from Hospital Lane, with its high walls and rectangular windows." No wonder, they wrote, "that those who judge the hospital on this appearance imagine it to be a place of straight-jackets and padded cells."[4]

But what about the inside? Over 26,000 people passed through Powick's doors between 1852 and 1989 for treatment.[5] What was the experience like for them? "I could see the lights all along the Malvern Hills and bank of hills near which I know must be very near home," wrote one patient as she looked out from inside the institution's walls just after being admitted. "I thought of the prospect of about a month in this place and wept."[6] The medical superintendent Ronald Sandison saved her undated account of her first thirty hours at Powick, noting that her unhappy experience served as a "reminder of the immenseness of the task of turning Powick Hospital into a therapeutic unit."[7]

This chapter addresses Ronald Sandison's role in temporarily putting Powick on the psychiatric map through his introduction of LSD-assisted therapy. From 1952 until 1964, Sandison treated over 500 patients with LSD, published a series of papers in psychiatric journals, presented his work at conferences in the UK, Europe, and the US, and in 1961 organized a historic three-day conference in London on the therapeutic use of LSD. His findings were received "almost with hysteria," he reflected later. "You see psychiatrists at that time were under such pressure . . . people were hungry for anything they could get their hands on." As a result, the practices implemented at Powick "very quickly spread to most countries."[8] Despite these successes, however, Sandison ultimately remained skeptical about a future psychedelic renaissance. In the 1950s, LSD was "a highly regarded and precious substance, used with care and some reverence by a small group of physicians," he wrote. "Sadly, it became in the next decade the playthings of millions, thus devaluing its significance as a therapeutic tool almost to nil."[9] As a result, he wrote later, the therapeutic use of LSD "has gone forever."[10] But Sandison's skepticism came at a price: UK's founder of psychedelic treatment found his contributions, with few exceptions, essentially erased from the historical record by the 1990s.[11]

BECOMING A PSYCHIATRIST

As a child, Sandison was passionate about astronomy and the weather. He recalled his father taking him to Greenwich Observatory, where he studied the stars, as well as eyeing minute objects under his uncle's microscope. "I was always observing and measuring things," he wrote.[12] "There was something in me from a very early age which gave me an intense curiosity about things, both living and non-living."[13] He would later apply this fascination to the human psyche. "Psychotherapy is a process of exploration and detection as surely as the unravelling of the mystery of the galaxies had been to astronomers," he reflected. He went on to study medicine at King's College in London, where he originally intended to study surgery. But his experiences gave him pause. "The study of medicine did not encourage any great sensitivity toward the human condition," he wrote. Most of his time studying medicine was spent dissecting a cadaver, but "dead bodies cannot speak or protest," a problem that did not seem to bother his classmates. Sandison bought his own skeleton, named her Henrietta, and reflected on what her life might have been like. Henrietta, along with the decision to take elective courses in theology and psychology, marked the beginnings of his "study of the mind and of mental and unconscious processes."[14]

Other forces that undoubtedly propelled Sandison into psychiatry were his mother's struggle with depression and then the impact of World War II. During the long, bitterly cold winter of 1929, Sandison's family life "suddenly collapsed" as his mother moved out of the home, suffering from a breakdown. Sandison, an only child, was thirteen at the time, and he was told very little about what was happening to his mother, or even where she was. Although she returned the following summer, she continued to struggle with depression until he was sixteen. Sandison barely discusses his childhood in his lengthy (unpublished) memoir, but in other writings, he reflects on the impact of her breakdown and recovery. His mother later explained that on Sandison's sixteenth birthday, he asked her when she was going to get better. The mere question prompted her recovery. "I have gradually come to understand more about the dynamic causes of this breakdown," he wrote, though how she recovered remained a mystery.[15] "I can see why you are a therapist," she told him. "It wasn't just the words you used, it was the implication that I had to get better for a reason."[16] His later determination to make sense of mental illness, and to help his patients improve in any way possible, undoubtedly started with his mother.

But it was World War II that drew Sandison, as well as many others, into the field of psychiatry, "partly arising from their [personal] experiences of that war."[17] In 1940, Sandison began his first medical appointment as house physician to the Emergency Medical Service at Warlingham Park Hospital, in Surrey south of London. He spent six months there, during the "most dangerous and precarious stage of the war."[18] Every single day, he witnessed an air raid, including one direct hit on his ward, which killed a patient. "The war and its consequences were always with us," he wrote.[19] Many of his patients were air raid victims, and most needing care were "psychological casualties of war."[20] For the remainder of the war, he abandoned medicine, serving in the Royal Air Force as head of the Physiological Development Panel at Central Fighter Establishment. It was not an easy position; Sandison noted that his wartime experience had left him "drained, depressed, and lacking a sense of direction."[21]

After the war, Sandison returned to Warlingham Park Hospital as a trainee psychiatrist, now convinced that his future lay in mental health. It was a transitional period for psychiatry, he later reflected, which made it an exciting time to enter the field.[22] Both Sigmund Freud and Carl Jung had started to influence the British medical establishment in the early twentieth century, and psychoanalysis gained significant followers after World War I. Indeed, Britain witnessed a "sudden 'craze' for psychoanalysis after 1918," as Freud's theories helped many come to terms with the psychological devastation brought on by the war.[23] "There was something very British about the early excitement aroused by Freud's work," noted Sandison in an address to the Wessex Psychotherapy Society in 2003. British psychotherapists drew on the discoveries of Freud and Jung rather eclectically, often with "little popular differentiation between those terms and concepts originating in Freud's own work" and those introduced by his others such as Alfred Adler and Jung.[24] But by midcentury, a revolution in drug therapy dramatically changed the nature of the field,[25] and "almost all traces of the doctor, nurse, or other vanished from the therapeutic equation."[26]

Sandison remained at Warlingham Park from 1946 until 1951, just as the hospital was "juggling with this transition."[27] This institution, under the direction of the superintendent, T. P. Rees, offered him considerable training opportunities in the use of the new physical treatments of the day, including electroconvulsive therapy (ECT), deep insulin coma therapy, and leucotomy. One of the hardest things about training during these years, Sandison stressed, was "to avoid being seduced by the physical treatments," which focused on dramatic results and (supposedly) rapid recovery. Physical and drug innovations represented "a huge challenge to psychotherapy."[28] But Rees also believed in the therapeutic benefits of psychotherapy, maintaining three analysts on the staff, two Freudian and one Jungian, and thus "every shade of current psychiatric practice was present."[29] Rees—and eventually Sandison—also believed in the idea that mental hospitals should be managed as "therapeutic communities," in which the gates were left unlocked and patients were encouraged to actively participate in their own treatment, as well as group activities.[30] While at Warlingham, Sandison engaged in therapy with a Jungian therapist, which helped crystalize his belief that the best way to treat the mentally ill was through talk therapy: "I was far more interested in what patients had to say, and in their actions, than in classifying their 'symptoms.'"[31]

TRANSFORMING POWICK

Sandison knew little about Powick's history when he arrived there in 1951 as the deputy medical superintendent and consultant psychiatrist. Perhaps that was for the best; he quickly discovered that it was a "deeply dismal and anti-therapeutic place."[32] Compared to Warlingham, he found "an air of poverty about the place." Both the grounds and the interior appeared "gloomy." Conditions there were atrocious; originally built for 200 patients in 1847, it housed nearly 1,000 by 1951. Therapy was virtually nonexistent; "no doctor had had an interview alone with a female patient for many years, and this had also become the norm on the male side of the hospital."[33] But the position provided him with an opportunity to explore his therapeutic goals. "I think that I wanted to do my own thing," he explained about why he chose to go there. "I had a lot of ideas of my own and wanted to develop them." His goal was to create a hospital modeled on Warlingham Park, and to "get a therapeutic community going."[34]

At the end of his first year, Sandison was invited with about ten other psychiatrists to a study tour of Swiss mental hospitals. Included on this trip was a visit to Sandoz pharmaceutical laboratories in Basel, where he first witnessed the work being done on LSD. "In an instant I knew that my destiny lay with this substance," he later wrote, "and that it would unlock secrets and enable healing if only I could learn to master its mysteries."[35] In 1952, he returned to Powick with 100 ampoules of LSD from Sandoz, where "the serious application of the use of LSD as a therapeutic tool undisputedly began" under his design and direction.[36]

Sandison was one of many psychiatrists who saw LSD as an opportunity to transform the field in the midst of transition and to replace what he called the "therapeutic vacuum in psychiatry."[37] He agreed with Stanislav Grof, a psychiatrist in Prague also enthusiastic about the therapeutic potential of LSD, that psychoanalytic theory was highly valuable, but also "long and costly."[38] Grof decided to study medicine after reading Freud's *Introductory Lectures to Psychoanalysis* (1917), which made a "deep impression" on him. But he was frustrated by the disconnect between theory and practice. "I had great difficulty coming to terms with this situation," Grof reflected. "To become a psychoanalyst, one had to study medicine. And in medicine, if we really understand a problem, we are usually able to do something pretty dramatic about it."[39] This was not the case in psychiatry. As a past president of the American Psychiatric Association, Jeffrey Lieberman (2016) claims that while "oncologists can touch rubbery tumors [and] pulmonologists can peer through a microscope at strings of pneumonia bacteria," psychiatry "has struggled harder than any other medical specialty to provide tangible evidence that the maladies under its charge even exist."[40]

LSD appeared to offer an answer. "It is almost impossible to describe in a connected manner the sequence of this remarkable emotional experience," declared Sandison after first taking LSD.[41] The first time Grof tried it, the results were about as dramatic as could be: "I was hit by a radiance that seemed comparable to the epicenter of a nuclear explosion," he recalled. "At an inconceivable speed my consciousness expanded to cosmic dimensions."[42] Their experiences convinced them that Freud's study of human personality was only the tip of the iceberg. The drug appeared to be "bringing into consciousness the contents from the depth of the unconscious."[43] Sandison described in his memoir "an orgasm of excitement" upon learning about LSD's potential; Grof described it as important a tool for psychiatry as "that of the microscope for medicine or the telescope for astronomy."[44] LSD could help psychiatrists "understand the nature of the bridge between the conscious and the unconscious," in Sandison's words, thereby dramatically transforming our understanding of the mind.[45]

Two years after Sandison obtained LSD, he and his colleagues published the results of their first study of its use with patients at Powick. "It marked the end of an era," he later claimed of the paper's publication. "This paper generated both national and international interest in the possibilities of the use of LSD in psychiatry."[46] Actually, Sandison published two separate articles in the April 1954 volume of the *Journal of Mental Science*. The first, "The Therapeutic Value of Lysergic Acid Diethylamide in Mental Illness," which he coauthored, described the results of his study of thirty-six "psycho-neurotic" patients who had received the LSD treatment. "The significance of this paper," he reflected later, is that it "helped to give me the courage to start thinking about LSD as an adjunct to psychotherapy."[47] Fourteen of the cases had recovered, and another twenty had demonstrated improvement in their conditions; only two had not shown improvement by the time of publication.[48] And unlike other drug treatments, it appeared to enhance talk therapy rather than silence it. "It really looked as if my dream could come true," Sandison recalled, "that of joining physical methods of treatment and psychotherapy."[49]

Why treatment proved so effective was another matter, and the authors were cautiously speculative. A patient's reaction to the drug could vary dramatically on different days, even with the same dosage, making it difficult to determine exactly what the drug was doing. The key, which had been overlooked by other LSD researchers, was that "objective findings and subjective experiences are not to be regarded separately."[50] Sandison believed that these subjective experiences were "manifestations of the patient's unconscious" as experienced through the "reliving of repressed personal memories."[51] Indeed, it was the "surging up of repressed experiences" that appeared to cause "some of the most intense abreactions we have ever seen."[52] The LSD sessions needed to take place in a "carefully prepared environment" and "should be used only by experienced psychotherapists and their assistants" as "an adjunct to skilled psychotherapy."[53] The patient should "lie or sit on a bed" in a private, "tastefully furnished" room until the "more disturbing psychic effects have subsided," at which point he or she could join a larger group in the ward also undergoing LSD treatment.[54] After the effects wore off, patients were asked to write a full account of the experience, as well as expressing it in artwork.[55] Treatment should take place weekly in a hospital setting for "at least six weeks" (and in some cases, up to a year). Sandison administered very small doses (starting at 25 μg), gradually increasing the amount "until an adequate reaction is obtained."[56] He would later coin the term "psycholytic," meaning "mind loosening," as a counter to the North American term "psychedelic," which required much higher doses of LSD.[57]

Sandison was the sole author of "Psychological Aspects of the LSD Treatment of the Neuroses," the second article to appear in the April 1954 volume, which delved more deeply into how and why LSD seemed to be such an effective therapeutic tool. Psychoneurotic patients, the focus of the Powick study, suffered from "a faulty relationship between the conscious and the unconscious," Sandison explained, "leading to a one-sided or prejudiced conscious point of view."[58] LSD appeared to enable these patients to begin to assimilate their unconscious, effectively doing the work of a psychotherapist in a more timely manner. "It is for at least some of these patients that LSD treatment may offer a new hope," he explained. He provided two examples "for whom little could have been done" from his Powick study to illustrate how LSD psychotherapy enabled them to recover.[59]

The two publications, and their positive reception, enabled Sandison to make a case to the regional hospital board to build a separate facility for his "LSD family,"[60] which became known as the "LSD block." It contained five patient rooms (each complete with a couch, a chair, and a blackboard), a meeting room, and two rooms for the nurses. "Roughly the therapeutic arrangement ran like this," wrote W. V. Caldwell during his 1963 visit. "The ward was an extremely long narrow room running north and south." Private rooms lined the east wall and were filled with patients who on occasion would "come out to socialize or have tea." Nurses would visit periodically, and they appeared warm and friendly. They dealt directly with the patients, "supporting them in time of trouble, easing their fears, good-humoredly tolerating emotional outbursts," he observed. Sandison's assistant, Dr. Grenville Davies, was "friendly, loquacious, and dynamic," and she interacted "informally with both patients and nurses." Caldwell was struck by how different the LSD block felt from the rest of the institution—"different not so much in equipment or furnishing as the psychological ambience which had been provided."[61]

Visitors came anywhere from down the road to the US and Australia to observe Sandison's treatment. "With the growth of interest in LSD," he wrote, "I found myself much in demand from those hungry to learn about this new approach to psychiatric treatment."[62] The two local high school students who visited in 1962 found the tour of the LSD block "the most fascinating episode of our whole stay." After lunch, they entered one of the private rooms of a patient about to receive LSD. "He had no objection to our witnessing the whole operation," they wrote, "and so we settled down for the afternoon." After the patient was injected intravenously with LSD, they stayed with the nurse, who explained that "she was the mother-figure" to help him through his session. He was "troubled by impotence and generally distressed by life." Under LSD, the nurse explained to the students, "he had learned to face an underlying fear of his mother and went through many experiences mostly unpleasant . . . that had affected his mental outlook." The patient began to shake violently, then began to suck the nurse's hands. "At one time he went through the motions of sexual intercourse, or motions very similar, but at no time did he use any part of the nurse's body except her arms and hands, to express his feelings." Surely, this was an experience like no other for these high school students. They stayed with the patient for a few hours after he came out of his "stupor," and listened as he described what he had just experienced. He "talked about his problems which obviously must remain private in detail, although I have outlined some of them," one of them wrote. "We were very glad when he said that we had helped him a great deal that afternoon with his terrible problems."[63]

To the twenty-first century observer, allowing high school students into Sandison's "carefully prepared environment" to be used "only by experienced psychotherapists and their assistants" (in Sandison's words) appears problematic. Perhaps descriptions such as these prompted Sandison to be a bit more exclusive in whom he allowed into the room. Certainly, the staff was highly restricted; only designated nurses and doctors entered the ward. "To get inside the LSD unit was impossible," remembered Ken Crump, who worked as a nurse at Powick from 1963 to 1989. "Worse than getting in the Vatican. Everybody who worked there was sworn to secrecy," he declared. "You would never get anything out of anybody who had anything to do with the LSD treatment at Powick."[64]

NETWORKS AND ALLIES

But researchers were another matter. Sandison welcomed, even encouraged, colleagues to witness firsthand what was happening in his LSD block. He also welcomed invitations to present his findings at international conferences, as another way to publicize his methods and further influence psychiatric practice. In 1955, he was invited to speak at the annual meeting of the American Psychiatric Association in Atlantic City. This was his first invited talk at a scientific conference, and it was the first time that they included a roundtable on "LSD and Mescalin in Experimental Psychiatry."[65] Although Sandison did not think that his paper was particularly well received, he himself was greeted "as a sort of saviour or guru. . . . It was an expression of the vast hunger felt in the USA, and indeed in most of the rest of the world, for healing and enlightenment."[66] He also received media attention back in the UK: the national newspaper *News Chronicle* not only wrote a flashy article about the "[a]mazing new drug [that] recalls every childhood memory," which was the subject of Sandison's talk; they also funded his travel to the US, suggesting their belief that his research was media worthy.[67]

Sandison suddenly found himself in the midst of an international network of LSD researchers who saw him as a leader in the field. Dr. Herman Denber, the director of psychiatric research at Manhattan State Hospital, visited Powick in 1954. Interested in transforming his hospital into a therapeutic community, he was impressed with the amount of freedom that Sandison granted patients at Powick (including their freedom to roam about the property), as well as his LSD treatment. When Sandison returned the visit in 1957, he was "delighted" with the changes that Denber had made.[68] Hanscarl Leuner was a professor and director of the department of psychotherapy and the *Nervenklinik* (psychiatric clinic) at Germany's University of Goettingen when he read Sandison's Powick studies.[69] "In our method of treatment we followed the experiences gained by Dr. Sandison . . . in 1954," he explained in his paper on "Psychotherapy with Hallucinogens," presented at Sandison's 1961 "Hallucinogenic Drugs and Their Psychotherapeutic Use" conference held in London.[70]

Perhaps Sandison's biggest fan was Betty Eisner, a clinical psychologist and LSD researcher from Los Angeles. "This letter should have been written some time ago," she wrote in 1958, introducing herself. "The more work that I have done therapeutically with LSD, the more I have appreciated your inspiring and provocative pioneering with it," she explained. "I think that you will be interested to see how closely our work parallels yours," she continued, in the first of over sixty letters she would write to Sandison between 1958 and 1997. At the time, she was working with Sidney Cohen at the Neuropsychiatric Hospital of the Veterans Administration Center in Los Angeles. She had just completed a draft of an article describing their study of twenty-two patients treated with LSD, and she was hoping for Sandison's feedback. "There are so many aspects of this remarkable drug which I feel you understand better, perhaps, than anyone." She wanted, therefore, to "check my observations against yours." She was extremely excited that she was getting "the same sort of material that you do" regarding the reliving of past memories. She noted, however, that her study incorporated props into the treatment, something that Sandison had not done: "We found that music, originally used for relaxation, so facilitated drug action that it was incorporated as part of the treatment." She was eager to get any feedback he might have about the results of her study.[71]

Sandison responded with equal enthusiasm. "It is very encouraging to me to find that other people are obtaining much the same results as we are here with treatment," he wrote. The matter that interested him the most in her letter was "the use of music to stimulate the response to LSD"—this had never occurred to him. "We should very much like to make use of this suggestion of yours and will be glad to let you know what results are obtained."[72] From this initial exchange, a friendship grew, as Eisner and Sandison bounced ideas back and forth, compared results, shared connections, and even patients. For example, when Cary Grant, who had done several LSD sessions with Eisner in Los Angeles, was traveling through the UK, he sought treatment from Sandison at Powick. "You are the only one I would really trust him to because of his unresolved relationship with his mother and the circumstances of her illness and that of her brothers and sisters," Eisner explained to Sandison.[73]

At Sandison's suggestion, Eisner presented her research findings at the first international conference of the Collegium Internationale Neuropsychopharmacologicum in Rome in 1958, where they first met face to face. From there, she came to the UK to visit Powick and meet Sandison's colleagues, and she returned a few years later as the only American LSD researcher to present at Sandison's 1961 London conference. Even after they were both forced to stop working with LSD as it became criminalized beginning in the mid-1960s, they continued to visit each other and correspond about their divorces, remarriages, research, and writing. As a reserved, "very quiet Scotsman,"[74] he often chafed at her blunt mannerisms, but Sandison viewed Eisner as "a charismatic and able therapist whose friendship I owe much." She was also his "principal connection with many American workers," introducing him to influential researchers and encouraging him to consider moving to the US.[75]

Although his work as superintendent at Powick Hospital lasted only thirteen years, it still assumed a major presence in his eighteen-chapter autobiography. His decision to leave his post in 1964 was more personal than professional, involving an affair and a divorce. Sandison later wrote that "leaving Powick was more traumatic than I had expected."[76] After its closure in 1992, he reflected that Powick stood as a "scene of decades of the human struggle to come to terms with its own insanity." He did not believe, in the end, that LSD had solved the problems of mental illness, which had become "even more frightening and inexplicable to people." As he stood across the road from the deserted building, he "felt the ghosts of the tortured minds of those who had been put away, hovering strongly on the wind."[77]

Perhaps Sandison's 1992 visit to Powick was intended to provide him with some closure and long-needed reflection. But that year also led to a reevaluation of LSD's past. The growing interest in neuroscience helped to relegitimate research interest in hallucinogens, "not as symbols of social dissent or as magic drugs, but as tools to study different neurotransmitter systems."[78] Research scientists who had long given up hope that psychedelics would ever again be deemed therapeutic or medicinal eagerly embraced what came to be called a "psychedelic renaissance" beginning in the 1990s.

Sandison and Eisner agreed. Perhaps their efforts had not been in vain. "I have been going over old letters and meetings from way back when we were doing LSD work, and I must say that those were very exciting times!" Eisner wrote Sandison in June 1992. "I remember coming to Powick on my way to Rome in 1958 and being amazed and delighted at all the wonderful work that you were doing there." She had begun to dig into her old files, noting that her memories were "assuming the proportions of a book."[79]

Eisner's memories triggered similar reflections in Sandison. "Yes, the LSD days were massive landmarks in both our lives and no doubt in the lives of many others, not forgetting our patients," he wrote. "You and I have a long history, which is also part of what I am now. I look back on the heady days of the fifties and early sixties with some awe, but also with much pleasure."[80] He, too, was determined to tell his story, and when he finally did write it, he explained why: "I feel there is a place for me to write the story from the inside. One cannot do this adequately in scientific papers, so I take the opportunity here."[81]

The real reason why he set out to "write the story from the inside," however, grew out of frustration. If there was to be a renaissance, he believed that his contributions should be part of it. But events commemorating the fiftieth anniversary of Albert Hofmann's discovery of LSD and its transformative properties in 1993 suggested to Sandison that his contributions had been forgotten. The Swiss Academy of Medical Sciences hosted a two-day symposium in Lugano, Switzerland, funded by Sandoz pharmaceuticals. "50 Years of LSD: State of the Art and Perspectives on Hallucinogens" was an invitation-only affair that featured lectures on the psychopathology and clinical aspects of LSD given by European and American scientific experts. Eisner was invited, but Sandison was not.

Sandison's omission from the conference, as well as a lack of media coverage about his contributions to LSD research, gave him pause. It was time to reach out to Hofmann himself. "I believe I am almost the only British survivor of those days in the 1950s when there were at least 16 clinics using LSD therapeutically in the UK. . . . Now, almost two generations later, I find that people have forgotten about the early use of LSD." Perhaps it was his own fault, as his own interest in the therapeutic use of LSD also declined after his research shut down in the mid-1960s. "I can understand that people outside the UK may have forgotten the work we did in those far-off days," he concluded.[82]

It was not only Sandison who had been forgotten. Powick Hospital, which had formally closed its doors in 1989, was torn down and redeveloped as a housing estate. "Powick's been—for thirty years—was forgotten about [sic]. It's thirty years since it closed," states Crump, who worked as a charge nurse at Powick from 1964 until its closure. "There's nothing left of the hospital, just the medical superintendent's house. Most people who live there, it's all houses, haven't got a clue what was there before." Crump is part of a team that wants to keep Powick's history alive, through history exhibits, oral history interviews, and presentations. He regularly gives a talk entitled "Remembering Powick Hospital," most recently for the Malvern Civic Society in 2019, about fifteen minutes down the road from where Powick had been. Normally about eighty people turn up to society talks, but two hundred attended Ken's talk that night. "And it went down well," he says. "Got phone calls, and people, 'Can you come and talk to us?'" He appears teary-eyed as he speaks. "I'm getting a bit emotional, talking about this," he admits. He remembers his early years at Powick as positive ones. "When I started there, [Sandison and Superintendent Arthur Spencer] had been working hard to restore respectability in the mental hospital. They removed the walls, they'd unlocked the wards, they'd allowed the patients to have their own clothes, they had their own allowances." He remembered Sandison as a "very good bloke—you'd feel confident when you're talking to him."[83]

But most people want to forget. Those who have bought property on which Powick used to stand certainly don't want the word to spread that their houses were constructed on asylum grounds. When a plaque was placed on the wall of the local pub commemorating the institution, many wrote letters of complaint. Crump ponders this: "Should we remember it? Or should we forget it?" He believes strongly that it should be remembered. Powick was home to over 26,000 people between 1852 and 1989. "That's a lot of people. How can you forget that that place ever existed?"[84]

Ronald Sandison passed away in 2010, at the age of ninety-four. He left behind hundreds of pages of unpublished material, as he spent the last decade or so of his life writing letters, poems, short stories, and a lengthy memoir, determined that his contributions would not be forgotten. Although psychedelic research had regained a great deal of ground beginning in the 1990s, he ultimately remained skeptical of its use, believing that too much time had transpired since the heady days of the 1950s. Perhaps this skepticism makes him an unlikely candidate as a psychedelic pioneer, but his initial passion for LSD's potential therapeutic use in the 1950s and early 1960s is certainly worthy of reflection and recognition.

NOTES

1. Frank Crompton, interview with author, November 26, 2019.

2. "Beryl," an interview with Beryl, whose mother was put into Powick Mental Hospital, describing her mother's mental illness and the impact it had on her as a child, March 30, 2010, video, 4:21:00, https://www.youtube.com/watch?v=dDTji3cpqgU.

3. W. V. Caldwell, *LSD Psychotherapy: An Exploration of Psychedelic and Psycholytic Therapy* (New York: Grover Press, 1968), 92.

4. J. E. Stredder and S. J. S. W. Curry, "A Three-Day Study of Powick Hospital," 1, Dr. Ronald A. Sandison Papers, Wellcome Library Archives and Manuscripts (hereafter "Sandison Papers").

5. Ken Crump, interview with author, November 26, 2019.

6. "Thirty Hours at Powick," p. 1, PP/SAN/B/2, file 1 of 2, Sandison Papers.

7. "Thirty Hours at Powick," Sandison's handwritten note attached to the document.

8. David Healy, interview with Ronald Sandison, 2002, PP/SAN/B1/2, Sandison Papers.

9. Sandison, *In-Tide Out*, ch. 6, 1, PP/SAN/A/1, Sandison Papers.

10. Sandison, *In-Tide Out*, ch. 6, 20.

11. His work is cited briefly in histories such as Martin A. Lee and Bruce Schlain's *Acid Dreams* (1985), but the primary focus on psychedelic pioneers remains on figures from the US and Europe.

12. Sandison, "Who Become Psychotherapists, and Why?" n.d., D6, Sandison Papers.

13. Sandison, *In-Tide Out*, ch. 4, 18.

14. Sandison, "Who Become Psychotherapists, and Why?" n.d., D6, Sandison Papers, 7–8.

15. Sandison, "Who Become Psychotherapists, and Why?"

16. Sandison, "Who Become Psychotherapists, and Why?"

17. Sandison, *In-Tide Out*, ch. 1, 26.

18. Sandison, *In-Tide Out*, ch. 1, 5.

19. Sandison, *In-Tide Out*, ch. 1, 7.

20. Sandison, *In-Tide Out*, ch. 1, 6–7.

21. Sandison, *In-Tide Out*, ch. 4, 11.

22. Sandison, *In-Tide Out*, ch. 6, 20.

23. Graham Richards, "Britain on the Couch: The Popularization of Psychoanalysis in Britain 1918–1940," *Science in Context* 13, no. 2 (2000): 183–230.

24. Richards, "Britain on the Couch," 185.

25. Edward Shorter, *A History of Psychiatry* (New York: Wiley, 1997), 190.

26. Sandison, "The Changing Face of Psychotherapy: A Retrospect over the Past Century," Sandison Papers.

27. Sandison, "The Changing Face of Psychotherapy."

28. Sandison, "The Changing Face of Psychotherapy."

29. Sandison, *In-Tide Out*, ch. 2, 9–10.

30. Healy interview.

31. Sandison, *In-Tide Out*, ch. 3, 1.

32. Sandison, *In-Tide Out*, ch. 5, 1.

33. Sandison, *In-Tide Out*, ch. 5, 5.

34. Healey interview.

35. Sandison, *In-Tide Out*, ch. 5, 25.

36. Sandison, *In-Tide Out*, ch. 6, 1.

37. Sandison, *In-Tide Out*, ch. 2, 4.

38. Sandison, "Consciousness in the Twentieth Century: The Role of the Group," n.d., D6, Sandison Papers.

39. Stanislav Grof, "The Great Awakening: Psychology, Philosophy, and Spirituality in LSD Psychotherapy," in *Higher Wisdom: Eminent Elders Explore the Continuing Impact of Psychedelics*, ed. Roger Walsh and Charles Grob (Albany: SUNY Press, 2005), 120–121.

40. Jeffrey A. Lieberman, *Shrinks: The Untold Story of Psychiatry* (Boston: Back Bay Books, 2016), 106.

41. Sandison, "Personal Experiences with LSD, Transcript of a Tape," n.d., folder B.1, Sandison Papers.

42. Stanislav Grof, "Search for the Self," interviewed by Keith Thompson, *Yoga Journal*, July/August 1990, 57.

43. Grof, "The Great Awakening," 125.

44. Stanislav Grof, "Implications of Psychedelic Research for Anthropology: Observations from LSD Psychotherapy," at the "Ritual: Reconciliation in Change" conference, July 21–29, 1973; Paper prepared in advance for participants in Burg Wartenstein Symposium No. 59, p. 8, Box 1, Folder 3, MSP 1, Stanislav Grof Papers, Karnes Archives and Special Collections, Purdue University Libraries, West Lafayette, Indiana.

45. Sandison, *In-Tide Out,* ch. 14, 6.

46. Sandison, *A Century of Psychiatry*, 46.

47. Sandison, *In-Tide Out,* ch. 6, 12.

48. R. Sandison, A. Spencer, and J. Whitelaw, "The Therapeutic Value of Lysergic Acid Diethylamide in Mental Illness," *Journal of Mental Science*, April, 1954, 502.

49. Sandison, "The Changing Face of Psychotherapy: A Retrospect over the Past Century," Sandison Papers.

50. Sandison, Spencer, and Whitelaw, "The Therapeutic Value of Lysergic Acid Diethylamide in Mental Illness," 492.

51. Sandison, Spencer, and Whitelaw, "The Therapeutic Value of Lysergic Acid Diethylamide in Mental Illness," 494.

52. Sandison, Spencer, and Whitelaw, "The Therapeutic Value of Lysergic Acid Diethylamide in Mental Illness," 497.

53. Sandison, Spencer, and Whitelaw, "The Therapeutic Value of Lysergic Acid Diethylamide in Mental Illness," 503–504.

54. Sandison, Spencer, and Whitelaw, "The Therapeutic Value of Lysergic Acid Diethylamide in Mental Illness," 505.

55. Sandison, Spencer, and Whitelaw, "The Therapeutic Value of Lysergic Acid Diethylamide in Mental Illness," 506.

56. Sandison, Spencer, and Whitelaw, "The Therapeutic Value of Lysergic Acid Diethylamide in Mental Illness," 504.

57. Ben Sessa, "Ronald Sandison," *The Psychiatrist* 34, no. 11 (2010): 503; On Betty Eisner's use of psycholytic therapy, see https://chacruna.net/women-and-history-of-set-and-setting/.

58. Sandison, "Psychological Aspects of the LSD Treatment," *Journal of Mental Science*, April, 1954, 508.

59. Sandison, "Psychological Aspects of the LSD Treatment," 509.

60. Sandison, Spencer, and Whitelaw, "The Therapeutic Value of Lysergic Acid Diethylamide in Mental Illness," 506.

61. Caldwell, *LSD Psychotherapy*, 93.

62. Sandison *A Century of Psychiatry, Psychotherapy and Group Analysis* (London: Jessica Kingsley Publishers, 2001), 50.

63. Stredder and Curry, "A Three-Day Study of Powick Hospital," 7–8.

64. Ken Crump, interview with author, November 26, 2019.

65. Sandison, notes on his copy of the American Psychiatric Association program, Sandison Papers.

66. Sandison, *In-Tide Out*, ch. 5, 25.

67. Sandison, *In-Tide Out*, ch 6, 21.

68. Sandison, *In-Tide Out*, ch 6, 5.

69. Caldwell, *LSD Psychotherapy*, 104.

70. Hanscarl Leuner, "Psychotherapy with Hallucinogens," in *Hallucinogenic Drugs and Their Psychotherapeutic Use*, ed. Richard Crocket, Ronald Sandison, and Alexander Walk (London: H K Lewis, 1963), 67.

71. Eisner to Sandison, January 25, 1958, box 8, folder 11, SC 924, Betty Eisner Papers, Stanford University Special Collections.

72. Sandison to Eisner, February 13, 1958, Betty Eisner Papers.

73. Eisner to Sandison, June 21, 1960, Betty Eisner Papers.

74. Crump, interview with author, November 26, 2019.

75. Sandison, *In-Tide Out*, ch. 6, 28. For more on Betty Eisner, see Tal Davidson, *The Past Lives of Betty Eisner,* (master's thesis, York University, 2017), https://yorkspace.library.yorku.ca/xmlui/handle/10315/34493.

76. Sandison *In-Tide Out*, p. 37.

77. Sandison *In-Tide Out*, ch. 15, 16–17.

78. Nicolas Langlitz, *Neuropsychedelia: The Revival of Hallucinogen Research since the Decade of the Brain* (Berkeley: University of California Press, 2013), 1.

79. Eisner to Sandison, June 17, 1992, Betty Eisner Papers.

80. Sandison to Eisner, December 15, 1992, Betty Eisner Papers.

81. Sandison, *In-Tide Out*, ch. 6, 2.

82. Sandison to Hofmann, July 19, 1993, B1.2, Sandison Papers.

83. Crump, interview with author, November 26, 2019.

84. Crump, interview with author, November 26, 2019.

BIBLIOGRAPHY

Primary Sources

Beryl, interview by Ken Crump. 4:21, George Marshall Medical, March 30, 2010. https://www.youtube.com/watch?v=dDTji3cpqgU.

David Healy, interview with Ronald Sandison, 2002, PP/SAN/B1/2, Sandison Papers.

Eisner to Sandison, June 17, 1992, Betty Eisner Papers.

Eisner to Sandison, June 21, 1960, Betty Eisner Papers.

Eisner to Sandison, January 25, 1958, box 8, folder 11, SC 924, Betty Eisner Papers, Stanford University Special Collections.

Grof, Stanislav. "Implications of Psychedelic Research for Anthropology: Observations from LSD Psychotherapy." at the "Ritual: Reconciliation in Change" conference, July 21–29, 1973; paper prepared in advance for participants in Burg Wartenstein Symposium No. 59, p. 8, Box 1, Folder 3, MSP 1, Stanislav Grof Papers, Karnes Archives and Special Collections, Purdue University Libraries, West Lafayette, Indiana.

Sandison, "The Changing Face of Psychotherapy: A Retrospect over the Past Century," Sandison Papers.

Sandison to Eisner, February 13, 1958, Betty Eisner Papers.

Sandison to Eisner, December 15, 1992, Betty Eisner Papers.

Sandison to Hofmann, July 19, 1993, B1.2, Sandison Papers.

Sandison, "Consciousness in the Twentieth Century: The Role of the Group," n.d., D6, Sandison Papers.

Sandison, "Personal Experiences with LSD, Transcript of a Tape," n.d., folder B1, Sandison Papers.

Sandison, "The Changing Face of Psychotherapy: A Retrospect over the Past Century," Sandison Papers.

Sandison, "Who Become Psychotherapists, and Why?" n.d., D6, Sandison Papers.

Sandison, *In-Tide Out,* ch. 6, 1, PP/SAN/A/1, Sandison Papers.

Stredder, J. E. and S. J. S. W. Curry, "A Three-Day Study of Powick Hospital." Dr. Ronald A. Sandison Papers, Wellcome Library Archives and Manuscripts.

"Thirty Hours at Powick," p. 1, PP/SAN/B/2, file 1 of 2, Sandison Papers.

Secondary Sources

Caldwell, W. V. *LSD Psychotherapy: An Exploration of Psychedelic and Psycholytic Therapy*. New York: Grover Press, 1968.

Davidson, Tal. "The Past Lives of Betty Eisner." Master's thesis. York University, 2017.

Dubus, Zoë. "Women's Historical Influence on 'Set and Setting.'" Translated by Robert Savery. Women in the History of Psychedelic Plant Medicine Series. Accessed November 26, 2019. https://chacruna.net/women-and-history-of-set-and-setting/.

Grof, Stanislav. "The Great Awakening: Psychology, Philosophy, and Spirituality in LSD Psychotherapy." In *Higher Wisdom: Eminent Elders Explore the Continuing Impact of Psychedelics*, edited by Roger Walsh and Charles Grob. Albany, NY: SUNY Press, 2005.

Grof, Stanislav. "Search for the Self." Interviewed by Keith Thompson. *Yoga Journal*, July/August 1990, 57.

Langlitz, Nicolas. *Neuropsychedelia: The Revival of Hallucinogen Research since the Decade of the Brain*. Berkeley: University of California Press, 2013.

Leuner, Hanscarl. "Psychotherapy with Hallucinogens." In *Hallucinogenic Drugs and Their Psychotherapeutic Use*, edited by Richard Crocket, Ronald Sandison, and Alexander Walk, 67–73. London: H. K. Lewis, 1963.

Lieberman, Jeffrey A. *Shrinks: The Untold Story of Psychiatry*. Boston: Back Bay Books, 2016.

Richards, Graham. "Britain on the Couch: The Popularization of Psychoanalysis in Britain 1918–1940." *Science in Context* 13, no. 2 (2000): 183–230.

Sandison, R. *A Century of Psychiatry, Psychotherapy and Group Analysis*. London: Jessica Kingsley Publishers, 2001.

Sandison, R. "Psychological Aspects of the LSD Treatment." *Journal of Mental Science* (April 1954): 508–515.

Sandison, R. A. Spencer, and J. Whitelaw. "The Therapeutic Value of Lysergic Acid Diethylamide in Mental Illness." *Journal of Mental Science* (April 1954): 491–507.

Sessa, Ben. "Ronald Sandison." *The Psychiatrist* 34, no. 11 (2010): 503.

Shorter, Edward. *A History of Psychiatry*. New York: Wiley, 1997.

6 EARLY EXPERIMENTAL LSD CULTURES IN THE CLINIC

Magaly Tornay

From its very beginning, when a drop of LSD-25 permeated the skin of Albert Hofmann's fingertips in Sandoz laboratories in 1943, the substance has been a negotiator of boundaries. Symbolized by Hofmann's bicycle ride, the first intentional trip with the mysterious drug, it has since stood for journeys into unknown realms, expanding limits, and subverting authority. In its early history, however, it initially reinforced a demarcation that is central to modern societies: the one between normal and pathological.[1] It was not until the 1960s that LSD became a political substance filled with subversive potential. In the two decades prior, it had been used to study differences between healthy and ill, body and mind, and subjective and objective.[2]

This chapter analyzes early practices of meaning-making around LSD in the clinic, a crucial site for negotiating the normal and the pathological. During the second half of the twentieth century, these categories became increasingly flexible and disputed in psychiatry, culminating in the anti-psychiatry movement of the late 1960s. Psychiatric clinics are closely intertwined with the history of hallucinogens, and not just in terms of clinical trials on patients. In Switzerland, some institutions were also involved in several stages of the production process, such as harvesting rye and sorting ergot for Sandoz.[3]

It was also in these psychiatric settings that most early experiments with LSD and psilocybin were conducted on healthy subjects, such as chemists, laboratory personnel, students, artists, musicians, and writers, temporarily expanding their subjects beyond the usual nurses, patients, and physicians.

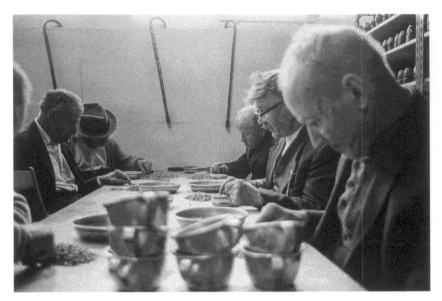

Figure 6.1
Patients sorting ergot from rye. Retirement and nursing home, Bärau, Switzerland (1971/1972).
© Werner Haug

Unlike private self-experimentation, the psychiatric setting provided credibility, appropriate methods, and access to tools such as Rorschach tests and audiovisual recordings.

It seems necessary, then, to rethink the concept of the clinic as a closed or remote entity for it to emerge as a site of everyday life, in line with a practical turn in the historiography of psychotropic drugs and the clinic.[4] The site of analysis is hence the clinic in a broader sense, reimagined as a crucial node of an intense but unequal exchange of material, knowledge, and meanings. The case of Switzerland is particular since it was here that LSD first found its way into psychiatry through personal connections. The links between the Swiss pharmaceutical companies and many of the larger clinics, notably in Basel and Zurich, were exceptionally close. When Sandoz began testing new ergot drugs for possible therapeutic use in the 1930s, a system was set up whereby the company temporarily paid the salary of an assistant doctor. Thus, psychiatric clinics became laboratories of sorts, springing into action shortly after a new compound left the firm. From these close interactions

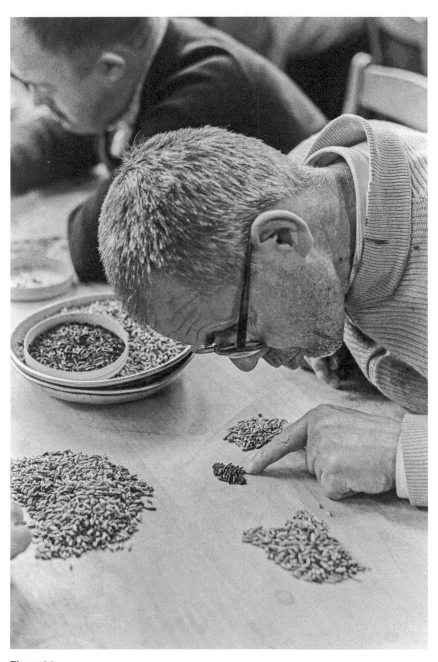

Figure 6.2
Patients sorting ergot from rye. Retirement and nursing home, Bärau, Switzerland (1971/1972).
© Werner Haug

between the clinic and the industry, an experimental culture emerged that eventually transcended its boundaries.

The early history of hallucinogens in Swiss clinics shaped narratives that proved influential: the analogy of LSD intoxication with psychosis, the biochemical basis of the psyche, and the first conceptualization of LSD as a subjective substance. But to enter the clinic, LSD had to transcend it. It was framed not only as a possible drug for patients by Sandoz, but also as a substance with the potential to turn the clinical order on its head—a drug for the doctors themselves.

ENTERING THE CLINIC

Before LSD became an imagination-sparking *"Phantastikum,"*[5] it had to be introduced into the clinic and reinterpreted accordingly. Albert Hofmann had first compared its effects with Pervitin, a methamphetamine, which as a stimulant provided him with a contemporary interpretative foil (see chapter 9). The transcendental aspects (namely, the demons that took hold of him) actually emerged only in his later retellings of his first intentional self-experiment on bicycle day.[6] The clinic added new registers to these interpretations.

LSD entered the clinical scene through a personal connection at Zurich's prestigious Psychiatric University Clinic, Burghölzli. The first LSD experiments were conducted by Werner A. Stoll (1915–1995), a young psychiatrist in training, and the son of Hofmann's boss, Sandoz director Arthur Stoll (1887–1971).[7] The company had been trying to find a way to test the new substance on "the only suitable organism, the human" for a while.[8] They had already been testing another ergot substance used to ameliorate against migraine headaches at the clinic, and in December 1945, they started paying Werner a monthly salary of 625 Swiss francs to test LSD.[9]

In February 1947, he sent a letter from his vacation in the Swiss mountains to the director of the Burghölzli, Manfred Bleuler (1903–1994), announcing he was ready to "finally send [his] LSD-work."[10] In his resulting article, he reclassified the substance as belonging to the "*Magika*" or "*Phantastika*," stressing its imagination-sparking, even transcendental properties: "It transports the subject into a magical world" and "gifts him supernatural powers and overwhelming experiences inaccessible to his mundane surroundings."[11] What later became one of the main strands of LSD interpretation—its revelatory, spiritual, and transcendental aspects— appeared in these notes for the first time.

More important, however, were observations by the younger Stoll that effectively anchored the new substance in psychiatry. He interpreted the experiences through his own professional lens and described them in psychopathological language: the subjects who took LSD fundamentally experienced a psychosis triggered by a substance he classified as "toxic" and called a "trace substance."[12] The observation that LSD led to temporary schizophrenic states in effect renewed interest in investigating the core of mental illnesses using hallucinogens—model psychosis research. Although this had already been pursued with mescaline, it gained new momentum precisely because LSD was a trace substance and very potent in small doses, which made it a "precision tool," unlike earlier substances that were thought to flood the system.[13]

Stoll also found that LSD had only very weak effects in psychotic patients, while "profoundly transforming the normal psyche with a few hundred thousandth of a gram."[14] This finding introduced an essential distinction between healthy and ill, and LSD promised to be a tool to make that demarcation firmly. An initial series of pretrials had been conducted by Sandoz staff and unspecified doctors, presumably at Sandoz and Burghölzli. Stoll then began his actual trial with sixteen supposedly "normal" subjects and six schizophrenic patients. Psychological tests, such as the Rorschach, were performed only on the healthy subjects. The so-called normal cohort consisted of chemists, doctors, laboratory workers, technical staff, and clerks, "all well versed with scientific observation," numbering eleven males and five females. Since Stoll thanked the members of the pharmaceutical division at Sandoz for their "daringness towards this little-known substance," it likely consisted of Sandoz employees and Burghölzli doctors again.[15]

Besides general difficulties to find words for what they experienced, three lines of interpretations were salient: a suspicion of technology, a scientific outlook, and an aesthetic sensibility. Hofmann, for one, experienced an estrangement from the laboratory and saw the "ugliness of the technical world" and the "useless activities" of his colleagues "in white coats."[16] The setting itself became overly characterized as ugly or distracting; some subjects also experienced the psychological tests as meaningless. A senior chemist reported seeing apparatuses and "Benzene rings everywhere!" without any estrangement. A third subject introduced literary and artistic references and felt "at one with all romantics and fantasists; I thought of E. T. A. Hoffmann, saw Poe's maelstrom . . . reveled in the colors of the Isenheim Altarpiece, felt the exhilaration and sublimity of an art show. . . . I seemed to grasp [abstract painting] for the first time."[17]

The trials with patients were "sparser and less colorful," in Stoll's view. They were evenly split in terms of gender and consisted of a pupil, a housewife, an au pair, a farmer, a student, and a debt collector; in all cases, previous therapies had shown no success. Since these subjects were not "scientifically literate," Stoll explained the disappointing results by their suspected lack of interest and the symptoms of psychosis, which may have prevented a clear recounting of the drug effects.[18]

However, the debt collector clearly distinguished anything he saw with LSD—"beautiful colorful rainbow pictures"—from his tormenting nocturnal visions, undermining the soon-to-be-prevalent analogy of psychosis and LSD intoxication.[19] Although Stoll acknowledged this, it did not challenge his hypothesis linking LSD and psychosis. The setting of this first trial—with one cohort described as scientifically literate and "normal," the other as illiterate and pathological—left the door wide open for confirmation bias. The differences in methods, including psychological testing and self-reports for the healthy cohort, as well as physical measurements and observation for the patients, reinforced these other differences.

Stoll nevertheless argued that his findings directly "led to central problems in psychiatry," notably the difference between the normal and the pathological psyche, highlighted by LSD.[20] Thus, he not only opened the way for LSD to become a Phantastikum (i.e., a transcendental, supernatural magic drug), he also brought into play a contrary line of thinking that cemented distinctions between normal and pathological and introduced a psychopathological language to describe the LSD experience, laying the groundwork for further research at Burghölzli.

DOCTORS TRIPPING THROUGH THE CLINIC

Manfred Bleuler, whose father Eugen (1857–1939) had been director of the Burghölzli, where he famously coined the term "schizophrenia," reacted with enthusiasm to Werner Stoll's report.[21] He immediately asked Sandoz to continue these "interesting experiments," particularly to find out "whether the metabolism of psychotic and non-psychotic people is different after ingesting LSD."[22] Picking up on Stoll's description of LSD as a trace substance, Bleuler brought the body into play. Since the reactions of patients and "normal" subjects were so different, he reasoned, it might well be that mental disorders have a physical cause.[23] A possible key seemed to lie in LSD, which was surprisingly associated with the body more than the mental sphere at that time.

He wanted to pursue two aspects in his clinic: use LSD to explore the differences between psychotic and healthy people, and examine its use as a "shock treatment" for patients, inducing "hallucinosis" and "euphoria," with the shock potentially changing the course of the illness.[24] Bleuler's own euphoria about the substance's potential for research persisted even after Stoll was no longer available for further trials, and he became personally involved in LSD experiments more intensely than previously suspected. In the spring of 1947, Bleuler tested LSD on three cases of severe hallucinosis, suspecting a sedative effect if given in smaller doses. "The experiment was entirely negative," he reported to Sandoz, abandoning this low-dose approach for further embracing trials with higher doses "in the sense of a shock therapy."[25]

Stoll was replaced by Gion Condrau (1919–2006), an assistant doctor, despite concerns about his tendency to be "done with his scientific tasks a bit too quickly."[26] His project was to determine any differences between healthy and psychotic subjects and to test LSD as a "psychic retuning" similar to insulin shock treatments.[27] However, he experienced difficulties gaining consent for this "unconventional therapy"; the negotiations with patients or their relatives proved to be "very time-consuming, tedious and lengthy."[28] Sandoz reassured him that "nothing unpleasant was to be feared" from this substance, possibly marking a departure from Stoll's first trials, which, as

Bächi notes, were likely conducted without proper consent, "disguised" as an unspecific new form of shock treatment.[29]

Sandoz continued to pay 550 Swiss francs monthly for the trials until mid-November 1947, when Condrau's work was done, seamlessly transitioning to paying Werner Stoll for an article that he was planning on the Rorschach tests.[30] Ernst Rothlin (1888–1972), the head of Sandoz's pharmaceutical division objected to Condrau's description of the substance as "unspecific"; to him as a pharmacologist, it was really anything but. He also expressed bewilderment at the use of the term *vergiftung* ("intoxication"), pointing to differences in the approaches of psychiatrists and pharmacologists around the category of the toxic.[31]

Especially striking were Condrau's findings with respect to subjects who received LSD without "appropriate preparation" (i.e., without their knowledge).[32] Some of the "normal" subjects (of a total of seven, including one self-experiment), mainly consisting of assistant doctors, were given the substance "blind," in their morning coffee or tea. All healthy subjects followed their normal routine and reported increasing difficulty fulfilling their normal tasks—"unable to find two telephone numbers in the directory," they lost interest in office work and any motivation at all, "walking around the office without doing anything" without even being bothered by it. A doctor reported, after unwittingly having drunk LSD-spiked coffee, feeling as if under a "glass bell jar" (an apparatus used in laboratory experiments) and thinking "quite indifferently that I might have gone mad."[33]

The results with the patients were again rather disappointing. Even though Condrau used relatively high dosages (up to 280 μg), he could not observe any new mental states. Their hallucinations, he said, were embedded in their usual hallucinations and could not be distinguished as a specific LSD effect. This finding led him to theorize that patients—in his case, no specific diagnosis was selected—had some kind of resistance to LSD because they already had a similar substance present in their body, again paving the way for a potential metabolic basis of psychosis.[34]

However, the difference between normal and pathological was inscribed in this setting from the very beginning. While the healthy subjects wrote their own protocols, patients were denied the opportunity to provide a first-person report, not least because they were presumed to have reduced language capacities. The self-reports of medical personnel were evaluated in detail, but with the patients, Condrau recorded mainly vegetative reactions and neurological symptoms using clinical observation and measurements. Reliable witnesses for these LSD sessions were only the dosed medical staff themselves, wandering around their work environments and observing themselves, and Condrau himself, trying to detect the effects of the drug on the patients' bodies, but not how the patients were experiencing the effects themselves.

The scene at Burghölzli in the late 1940s had in a sense become quite paradoxical: doctors walking around tripping, unable to perform their duties, perceiving their colleagues' heads as small as a pea or huge as a melon, indifferently thinking that they might have gone mad—from the outside, they may well have. The patients, on the other hand, behaved as they usually did and were the only ones able to clearly distinguish between what they experienced on LSD and their normal hallucinations. In retrospect, they somehow seem abler—and more literate—when making sense of this new substance.

VARIATION AND PERSONALITY

This closely interwoven group of actors from Sandoz and Burghölzli successfully introduced LSD to the human, leading to its reinterpretation as a phantastikum and a tool for delineating the boundaries between the normal and the pathological—even if, in the process, the psychiatrists themselves felt temporarily mad. Sandoz then introduced another aspect by asking the Burghölzli to investigate LSD by using it as a "personality test," since those who have experienced it themselves "are likely to attach particular importance to this aspect."[35] Personality tests of various types had long been used in psychiatric settings, and LSD appeared to bring to light even more aspects of a person than the psychotic or nonpsychotic state.

This line of research revealed new methodological challenges. The main method used to investigate LSD as a personality test was the Rorschach test—itself a personality test. This projective test had already gained traction for its perceived ability to render an objective image of the self through associations on a series of inkblots.[36] Projective techniques such as the Rorschach test have been described as "X-ray-like tools" of postwar technicism, designed to capture, measure, and ultimately make machine-readable the elusive parts of the human condition: dreams, hallucinations, fears, or altered internal states.[37] These instruments of a science of subjectivity generate evaluable information about inner states, with the advantage of focusing neither on behavior alone nor self-reports.[38]

With hallucinogens, the experimental setting became strangely doubled, with LSD and the inkblots both potentially providing a window into a subject's personality. But what was actually shown in the results? Was it the effect of the drug under investigation or the personality of the test subject? Or even traces of a disorder that had not yet broken out? And was LSD able to reveal the true nature of a personality under exceptional circumstances, hidden in everyday life?

Bleuler, who along with a colleague had already used mescaline in this way, noted similar difficulties in determining what was actually shown: Was the true self the one with or without drugs? "Which of the two formulations of the personality corresponds to reality?"—the one shown in the Rorschach before or during a trip? To the researchers' surprise, a Rorschach test taken without drugs gave a less truthful picture of the personality than the mescaline one: sober, only the subject's "distrust of his own originality," "exaggerated self-critique," and "extremely severe self-control" were displayed; inhibition fell with mescaline to give a "truer," less veiled image of the self. Personality, they concluded, must thus be a more flexible, multilayered category than previously thought.[39]

Condrau, describing LSD as a similarly revelatory tool, theorized that the substance provided a "caricature" of personality by exaggerating existing traits. In psychotic patients, for example, it seemed to intensify their specific form of schizophrenia.[40] The characterization of LSD as an amplifier of what is lingering or hidden brought a diagnostic use into view. It could potentially confirm diagnoses, predict future illnesses, or merely paint a portrait of someone with strokes that are slightly too thick.

Werner Stoll, in contrast, was opposed to drawing conclusions "from exceptional circumstances." He gave an example of a craftsman who, in alcoholic stupor, demolished his apartment and consequently behaved in a manner contrary to his authentic nature. This made LSD unsuitable as a personality test because it turned normal behavior into its opposite. In his view, intoxications were, after all, exceptional, even pathological states contrary to the true nature of most people.[41] In his 1952 article on Rorschach tests, Stoll emphasized individual differences and fluctuations; in his view, clearly defined personality traits ("abstractions") were not obtainable by observing someone on LSD. It was precisely each individual's subjective differences that became salient with this substance—the "variability" in humans. He conceded that the substance might serve to unveil a hidden potential in a person by loosening repression. But to Stoll, it still seemed wrong to believe that LSD would reveal one's true personality—in his eyes, normal was only ever a sober state.[42]

The underlying idea of normalcy was still strongly tied to a concept of everyday life, with pathologies as preformed, normative, and stable entities that could be clearly distinguished from normal. This categorization began to change in the 1960s when psychiatry was challenged politically and normal and pathological became increasingly seen as continuous and flexible categories.[43]

Not long after, a new psychodynamic interpretation came to the fore in Zurich: Gaetano Benedetti (1920–2013), then a doctoral student under Bleuler and later a psychoanalyst at Burghölzli, made a singular LSD case study with a patient diagnosed with alcohol hallucinosis (i.e., hallucinations caused by alcohol) in the early 1950s. The Rorschach protocols before, during, and after administering LSD showed, according to Benedetti, an astonishing change: "A 'new' man meets us here." The patient had a profound experience under LSD and reached a turning point in his life: "The die is cast and a new life has begun." Here, LSD was interpreted as a cathartic agent: during his intoxication, the patient had gone through his entire biography again and in "triple repetition."[44] Benedetti drew an analogy between the LSD trip and his patient's life story, which had a healing effect by intensifying the same themes. He reimagined LSD as a door opener to the unconscious not only of patients, but of everyone—after all, in contrast to psychiatry, psychoanalysis considered all people in need of therapy.

SCHIZO-URINE BETWEEN THE CLINIC
AND THE LABORATORY

While the Burghölzli psychiatrists began to acknowledge the immense variability of the LSD experience, questions concerning the normal and the pathological remained unsolved. Another path toward it had already been laid out: the idea that the psyche might be biochemically steered. This idea opened up another field for LSD to perform its boundary work and brought into play another pair of opposites: the age-old mind-body problem, contrasting the two fundamental constituents of mind and matter.

Albert Hofmann framed the problem as material versus spiritual when he referred to his later problem child as almost-non-matter. He described LSD as a go-between from the material to the spiritual world and vice versa. As he wrote to the German philosopher Ernst Jünger, "the effect of magic drugs happens at the borderline where mind and matter merge . . . these substances are themselves cracks in the infinite realm of matter, in which the depth of matter, its relationship with the mind, becomes particularly obvious."[45] It was precisely its extraordinary potency in extremely small doses that led Hofmann to conceive of it as almost immaterial substance: LSD's effects on "purely spiritual or psychological regions," he wrote, may also explain why "almost no matter is needed, that is, why LSD is effective in such incredibly small doses."[46]

Hofmann had opened a space of ambivalence between the material and the immaterial. His research partners in Zurich and Basel, on the other hand, set out to investigate it in a more robust and materialistic way. In the process, they set in motion a wholly different flow of matter, which further expanded the clinical world toward the animal kingdom.

In 1953, as Hofmann was working on the full synthesis of LSD, researchers from the Psychiatric University Clinic of Basel (then called Friedmatt) shipped over 50 liters of patients' urine to the Sandoz laboratory. More would arrive, not only from Basel, but also from Burghölzli and several smaller asylums.[47] LSD was not entirely new to the Basel clinic since its director, John Staehelin (1891–1969), a member of the editorial board of the *Swiss Archives of Neurology, Psychiatry and Psychotherapy*, first read a draft of Werner Stoll's 1947 article and wanted to test it as well.[48] In close collaboration with the Zurich clinic, the Basel group had started investigating the biochemical basis of schizophrenia mediated by LSD in 1948. They were looking for an LSD-like substance, organically occurring in the body, which might be triggering psychosis, unknown but equally potent and almost undetectable. Hofmann's task was to help the team by distilling and fermenting the urine of schizophrenic patients to detect traces of this anticipated unknown substance. Even though urine has a long history as a research material and medical resource, such as a healing fluid or an indicator of human health, it had so far been considered mainly a "window into the body," not into the mind or psyche.[49]

On the one hand, the different reactions to LSD from healthy and ill subjects seemed to support the idea that a similar substance already existed in the bodies of psychotic patients, continuously causing "bad trips" and explaining their weak reaction to the drug itself. On the other hand, and in contrast to earlier hallucinogens, the high potency of LSD gave hope that an equally invisible, odorless, and barely traceable substance exists but had just not yet been found. Although not new, this autotoxin hypothesis gained traction precisely because LSD was considered a trace substance.[50] Furthermore, LSD found an important ally in chlorpromazine, the first antipsychotic introduced into psychiatry in the early 1950s.[51] It seemed not only to "heal" psychoses, but also to interrupt LSD trips, and it was later described as LSD's "counterpoison," (i.e., antidote).[52] This alliance led to further experimentation since for the first time, there seemed to be a stable, controlled setting—the psychiatric hospital, which increased the importance of clinics as laboratories.

In this vein, the team in Basel set out to find a mysterious substance in the urine of patients. Rolf Weber, a researcher, even made a vast series of self-experiments drinking thirty-one "normal" urine samples and thirty-one samples of "schizo-urine," distilled and fermented by Hofmann at Sandoz. While the normal samples had no effect, the schizo-urine had, according to Weber, effects similar to autism: "pensiveness, flight of thought, difficulty to focus." Despite again noting a difference between the bodily fluids of patients and healthy subjects, he deemed his trial too small to be conclusive. He nonetheless saw indications that there might be a "principle" in schizophrenic patients that triggered reactions similar to those with "smaller doses of LSD."[53]

Together with Peter Witt, who later became famous for his spider tests with various psychotropic drugs, Weber fed the schizo-urine to spiders. The method had already been applied to study various drugs to see if they affected how spiders wove their webs (i.e., their symmetry, precision, and rich detail), but also the willingness of the spiders to weave. It promised, in a sense, a quite literal trace substance underlying schizophrenia by way of spiders. However, the webs woven under the influence of schizo-urine were not particularly accurate, chaotic, or close to the webs spun while under LSD or other hallucinogenic substances. The authors speculated that their method might not be sensitive enough, ending their paper with a programmatic quote by an American neurophysiologist: "There can be no twisted thought without a twisted molecule."[54]

Far from a fringe trend, similar research was conducted in the US and Canada, leading some historians to point out the obsession in the 1950s with the search for a "schizophrenic serum" in the blood, urine, or spinal fluid of psychotic patients.[55] Psychiatry had become biochemical, and the widely accepted idea that mental processes were biochemically steered eventually paved the way for neurotransmitter research.[56] A schizophrenic serum, however, was never found.

As the decade obsessed with the schizophrenic serum ended, new ways were found in the 1960s to investigate the mind-body problem with hallucinogens. The body still played an important role, but now as a surface. Hans Heimann (1922–2006), a psychiatrist in Berne, turned his attention to the phenomenology of expressions of subjects on LSD and psilocybin (i.e., their posture, voice, gestures, or sighs), while the content of an experience did not matter to him. He intended to cancel the "dualism of the mind-body-problem," as expressions were a link between the inside and outside: they lie "transversal to all opposites of conscious-unconscious, of inside and outside."[57] His research had received a boost from technology, since recording devices were more easily available. A camera hidden behind darkened glass was crucial to his setting, with the observer operating it by remote control. Technology served as a means to blur subjective aspects and to carve out a general typology through the objectifying camera lens. While the mind-body dichotomy dissolved in Heimann's concept of the significance of expression, materiality had found a way back in through the back door of technology.

EPILOGUE: AND WHAT ABOUT THE PATIENTS?

While the experimental culture that emerged between Sandoz and the psychiatric clinics expanded to encompass more actors, border crossings, and boundary shifting toward wider social and global circulation, little is graspable about the patients themselves. Apart from case reports in published articles, sources remain scarce to this day. Looking at the flow of knowledge and material in and out of the clinics, it is clear that patients played a role on multiple levels in this uneven setting: As late as the 1970s, patients in Swiss asylums were in contact with ergot, once the basic source for LSD and now for other Sandoz drugs, as a form of therapy (see chapter 9). Pictures taken by a young photographer inspired by anti-psychiatry, who visited several institutions around Berne around that time, showed patients sorting through rye to collect ergot for Sandoz as a form of work therapy.[58] Since the end of the 1930s, patients had been crucial in cultivating and especially harvesting and collecting rye and ergot, with their integration in this production process being a part of work therapy.[59] It may well be that some of the patients occupied with ergot production were the same people on whom LSD or psilocybin was tested (e.g., in the Basel area), adding a curious twist to this story.

Notwithstanding the narratives that emerged from the early hallucinogenic setting in Switzerland—such as its use conceptualized as shock therapy, personality test, the chemical basis of the psyche, and model psychosis—patients contributed to the production of stable knowledge and material and were important actors in involuntarily shaping what later circulated around the globe. Among the flow of material coming in and out of the clinics was not least their valuable waste—urine—which was seen as a possible key to the biochemistry of psychosis.

While LSD had initially served to reinforce the normal and the pathological as preformed, normative, and stable entities, it also produced paradoxical effects: the Burghölzli medical staff tripped around the clinic and the Basel team went so far as to drink urine in an effort to finally solve the puzzle of the mind. Researchers and psychiatrists, in a sense, had become closer to their patients and seemed, at times, in need of medication too. It is only fitting, then, that Sandoz, when preparing the launch of LSD as a medicine under the brand name Delysid, framed it not only as a drug for patients, but for doctors as well: "By taking Delysid himself, the psychiatrist is able to gain an insight into the world of ideas and sensations of mental patients," the leaflet read.[60]

In psychiatry, the late 1960s saw a shift toward a more "flexible normal-ism,"[61] which was no longer so strongly characterized by stable, preconceived norms, but rather gave way to a view of illness and health as a continuum in which potentially everyone may need therapy. LSD in this setting was a tool to do boundary work, but not a subversive substance in itself. It became a negotiator of boundaries that remained connected to professional and social practices of meaning-making.

In the process, the question of the normal and the pathological was reframed by some as one of elites and masses. Albert Hofmann, for one, opposed the idea of LSD for the masses of the late 1960s, considering it essentially a bourgeois drug. It is noteworthy in this context that he took LSD with Ernst Jünger in an utterly nonclinical setting, featuring red-violet roses and a Mozart concerto.[62] Interpretations of LSD are ultimately perhaps inseparable from the question of who takes it.[63] Throughout its history, it has mattered whether the LSD takers were college students, European artist bohemians, or psychiatric patients sorting through ergot.

NOTES

1. See Georges Canguilhem, *Le normal et le pathologique* (Paris: Presses Universitaires de France, 1966); Jürgen Link, *Versuch über den Normalismus. Wie Normalität produziert wird* (Göttingen, Germany: Vandenhoeck & Ruprecht, 2006).

2. For a discussion of these dichotomies, see also Sarah Shortall, "Psychedelic Drugs and the Problem of Experience." Supplement 9, *Past and Present* (2014), 187–206.

3. On ergot production, see Beat Bächi, *LSD auf dem Land. Produktion und kollektive Wirkung psychotroper Stoffe* (Konstanz, Germany: Konstanz University Press, 2020).

4. See, for example, Monika Ankele and Benoît Majerus, eds., *Material Cultures of Psychiatry* (Bielefeld, Germany: Transkript, 2020); Kijan Espahangizi and Barbara Orland, ed., *Stoffe in*

Bewegung. Beiträge zu einer Wissensgeschichte der materiellen Welt (Zürich: Diaphanes, 2014); on the practical turn in the history of science, see Hans-Jörg Rheinberger, Historische Epistemologie zur Einführung (Hamburg: Junius, 2007), 119–121; Andrew Pickering, The Mangle of Practice: Time, Agency, and Science (Chicago: University of Chicago Press, 1995); for a critique, see Philipp Felsch, "Die Arbeit der Intellektuellen. Zur Vorgeschichte des 'Practical Turn'." Nach Feierabend, Wissen, ca. 1980 (2016): 255–262.

5. Werner A. Stoll, "Lysergsäure-diäthylamid, ein Phantastikum aus der Mutterkorngruppe." Schweizer Archiv für Neurologie und Psychologie 60 (1947): 279–323. The term Phantastikum is originally from Louis Lewin.

6. A. Hofmann to A. Stoll, April 22, 1943, Novartis Archive, Sandoz, H 105.022. See also Bächi, LSD, 80.

7. See chapter 9 in this volume.

8. A. Stoll and E. Rothlin to M. Bleuler, February 13, 1947, State Archive of Zurich, PUK, Z 99.4379. (All source translations by the author.)

9. A. Stoll and E. Rothlin to M. Bleuler, February 13, 1947, monthly pay slips from December 1945 to July 1946. It is striking that despite these regular contributions, trials were conducted in a researcher's spare time, which explains a general lack of sources on experiments in Swiss archives, as many records were considered private property. W. Stoll to M. Bleuler, February 8, 1947; M. Bleuler to E. Rothlin, April 29, 1947. For another example of troves of patient files in a private estate, see Marietta Meier, Mario König, Magaly Tornay, Testfall Münsterlingen: Klinische Versuche in der Psychiatrie, 1940–1980 (Zürich: Chronos, 2019).

10. W. Stoll to M. Bleuler, February 8, 1947, State Archive of Zurich, PUK, Z 99.4379.

11. Stoll, Phantastikum, 317. On imaginary and transcendental dimensions, see Jakob Tanner, "'Doors of Perception' Versus 'Mind Control'. Experimente mit Drogen zwischen kaltem Krieg und 1968," in Kulturgeschichte des Menschenversuchs im 20. Jahrhundert, ed. Birgit Griesecke et al. (Frankfurt am Main: Suhrkamp, 2009), 340–72; Nicolas Langlitz, "Political Neurotheology: Emergence and Revival of a Psychedelic Alternative to Cosmetic Psychopharmacology," in Neurocultures. Glimpses into an Expanding Universe, ed. Francisco Ortega and Fernando Vidal (Frankfurt am Main: Peter Lang, 2011), 141–165. For a more detailed analysis of these early trials, see Magaly Tornay, Zugriffe auf das Ich. Psychoaktive Stoffe und Personenkonzepte in der Schweiz, 1940–1980 (Tübingen, Germany: Mohr Siebeck, 2016).

12. Stoll, Phantastikum, 315.

13. Mike Jay, Mescaline: A Global History of the First Psychedelic (New Haven, CT: Yale University Press, 2019), 192. See also Nicolas Langlitz, Neuropsychedelia: The Revival of Hallucinogen Research since the Decade of the Brain (Berkeley: University of California Press, 2013).

14. Werner A. Stoll, "Ein neues, in sehr kleinen Mengen wirksames Phantastikum." Schweizer Archiv für Neurologie und Psychiatrie 64 (1949): 483–484.

15. Stoll, Phantastikum, 283.

16. For these quotes, see Bächi, *LSD*, 89.

17. Stoll, *Phantastikum*, 302.

18. Stoll, *Phantastikum*, 305; 310.

19. Stoll, *Phantastikum*, 309.

20. Stoll, "Mengen", 484.

21. See also Brigitta Bernet, *Schizophrenie: Entstehung und Entwicklung eines psychiatrischen Krankheitsbildes um 1900* (Zürich: Chronos, 2013).

22. M. Bleuler to A. Stoll, February 11, 1947, State Archive of Zurich, PUK, Z 99.4379.

23. See also Nikolas Rose, "Neurochemical Selves." *Society* 41, no. 1 (2003): 46–59; Jeannie Moser, "'The Cure Is Biochemical'. Drogen und die Arbeit am Selbst in den sozialutopischen 1950er- und 1960er-Jahren," in *Handbuch Drogen in sozial- und kulturwissenschaftlicher Perspektive*, ed. Robert Feustel, Henning Schmidt-Semisch, and Ulrich Bröckling (Wiesbaden, Germany: VS Verlag für Sozialwissenschaften, 2019), 81–92.

24. M. Bleuler to E. Rothlin and A. Stoll, February 18, 1947, State Archive of Zurich, PUK, Z 99.4379.

25. Bleuler to Rothlin, May 29, 1947, State Archive of Zurich, PUK, Z 99.4379.

26. Bleuler to Rothlin, July 9, 1947, ibid.

27. Rothlin to Bleuler, August 9, 1947, ibid.

28. Bleuler to Rothlin, August 16, 1947, ibid.

29. Bächi, *LSD*, 86 f.; Rothlin to Bleuler, August 26, 1947, State Archive of Zurich, PUK, Z 99.4379.

30. Bleuler to Rothlin, November 15, 1947, State Archive of Zurich, PUK, Z 99.4379; Rothlin to Bleuler, November 17, 1947, State Archive of Zurich, PUK, Z 99.4379. It would take until 1952 for Stoll to publish these results. Werner A. Stoll. "Rorschach-Versuche unter Lysergsäure-Diäthylamid-Wirkung." *Rorschachiana* 1, no. 3 (1952): 249–270.

31. Rothlin to Bleuler, August 9, 1947, State Archive of Zurich, PUK, Z 99.4379; Rothlin to Bleuler, April 9, 1948, State Archive of Zurich, PUK, Z 99.4379.

32. Rothlin to Bleuler, 22 December 1947, State Archive of Zurich, PUK, Z 99.4379.

33. Gion Condrau, "Klinische Erfahrungen an Geisteskranken mit Lysergsäure-Diäthylamid." *Acta Psychiatrica et Neurologica* 24 (1949): 9–32, 16 f.; Edwin Blickenstorfer, "Zum ätiologischen Problem der Psychosen vom akuten exogenen Reaktionstypus. Lysergsäurediäthylamid, ein psychisch wirksamer toxischer Spurenstoff," *Archiv für Psychiatrie und Nervenkrankheiten* 188, no. 3 (1952): 226–236, 229.

34. Condrau, *Erfahrungen*, 22, 26. In Canada, Abram Hoffer and Humphry Osmond picked up on precisely this point. See Erika Dyck, *Psychedelic Psychiatry: LSD from Clinic to Campus* (Baltimore: Johns Hopkins University Press, 2008), 31–38, 44–49.

35. Rothlin to Bleuler, August 9, 1947, State Archive of Zurich, PUK, Z 99.4379.

36. See Damion Searls, *The Inkblots. Hermann Rorschach, His Iconic Test, and The Power of Seeing* (New York: Crown Publishing, 2017); Naamah Akavia, *Subjectivity in Motion. Life, Art, and Movement in the Work of Hermann Rorschach* (New York: Routledge, 2013); Rebecca Lemov, *Database of Dreams. The Lost Quest to Catalog Humanity* (New Haven, CT: Yale University Press, 2015).

37. Rebecca Lemov. "X-Rays of Inner Worlds, The Mid-Twentieth-Century American Projective Test Movement." *Journal of the History of Behavioral Sciences* 47, no. 3 (2011): 251–254.

38. Peter Galison, "Image of Self," in *Things That Talk: Object Lessons from Art and Science*, ed. Lorraine Daston (Cambridge, MA: MIT Press, 2004), 257–296.

39. Frederic Wertham and Manfred Bleuler, "Inconstancy of the Formal Structure of the Personality: Experimental Study of the Influence of Mescaline on the Rorschach Test." *Archives of Neurology and Psychiatry* 28, no. 1 (1932): 52–70, 67. On the history of mescaline, see Jay, *Mescaline*.

40. Condrau, *Erfahrungen*, 31.

41. Stoll, *Phantastikum*, 319.

42. Stoll, *Rorschach-Versuche*, 264, 268.

43. See Link, *Normalismus*; on antipsychiatry, see Benoît Majerus, "Mapping antipsychiatry: Elemente für die Geschichte einer transnationalen Bewegung." *Themenportal Europäische Geschichte* (2010), http://www.europa.clio-online.de/2010/Article=440; Duncan D. Double, ed., *Critical Psychiatry. The Limits of Madness* (Basingstoke, UK: Palgrave Macmillan 2006); Nick Crossley, *Contesting Psychiatry: Social Movements in Mental Health* (Abingdon, UK: Routledge, 2006).

44. Gaetano Benedetti, "Beispiel einer strukturanalytischen und pharmakodynamischen Untersuchung an einem Fall von Alkoholhalluzinose, Charakterneurose und psychoreaktiver Halluzinose." *Zeitschrift für Psychotherapie und medizinische Psychologie* 1 (1951): 177–192, 183, 188 f.

45. Albert Hofmann, *LSD—mein Sorgenkind* (Stuttgart: Fischer, 1979), 163.

46. A. Hofmann to A. Stoll, June 2, 1947, Novartis Archive, Sandoz, H 105.022.

47. F. Georgi to A. Hofmann, July 8, 1953, Novartis Archive, Sandoz, H 105.022; R. Weber to A. Hofmann, March 26, 1953, Novartis Archive, Sandoz, H 105.022.

48. M. Bleuler to A. Stoll, May 13, 1947, State Archive of Zurich, PUK, Z 99.4379.

49. See Tamar Novick, "Die Entdeckung des Urins." *Nach Feierabend. Materialgeschichten* (2018): 139–150, 143.

50. On the autotoxin hypothesis and mescaline, see Jay, *Mescaline*, ch. 8.

51. See David Healy, *The Creation of Psychopharmacology* (Cambridge, MA: Harvard University Press, 2002).

52. Hofmann, *Sorgenkind*, 55.

53. Typescript by R. Weber, December 16, 1952, Novartis Archive, Sandoz, H 105.002.

54. P. Witt and R. Weber, "Biologische Prüfung des Urins von drei Kranken mit akut psychotischen Zustandsbildern auf pathogene Substanzen mit dem Spinnentest." *Monatsschrift für Psychiatrie und Neurologie* 132 (1956): 193–207; Weber, *Urin*, 205.

55. Humphry Osmond coined this term; see Jay, *Mescaline*, ch. 8; Erika Dyck, "Flashback: Psychiatric Experimentation with LSD in Historical Perspective." *Canadian Journal of Psychiatry* 50, no. 7 (2005): 381–387. See also Jeannie Moser, *Psychotropen. Eine LSD-Biographie* (Konstanz, Germany: Konstanz University Press, 2013), 190; Healy, *Psychopharmacology*, 186–192.

56. Healy, *Psychopharmacology*, 186–192.

57. Hans Heimann, "Ausdrucksphänomenologie der Modellpsychosen (Psilocybin). Vergleich mit Selbstschilderung und psychischem Leistungsausfall." *Psychiatria et Neurologia* 141 (1961): 69–100, 70 f.

58. Werner Haug, *Gesichter einer anderen Schweiz* (unpublished manuscript, 2021).

59. On ergot cultivation, see Bächi, *LSD*.

60. Hofmann, *Sorgenkind*, 55.

61. See Jürgen Link and Mirko M. Hall, "On the Contribution of Normalism to Modernity and Postmodernity." *Cultural Critique* 57 (2004): 33–46.

62. For this episode, see Jay, *Mescaline*, 189.

63. For a similar argument in the US context, see David Herzberg, *Happy Pills in America: From Miltown to Prozac* (Baltimore: Johns Hopkins University Press, 2009), 3–5.

BIBLIOGRAPHY

Primary Sources

M. Bleuler to A. Stoll, February 11, 1947, State Archive of Zurich, PUK, Z 99.4379.

M. Bleuler to E. Rothlin and A. Stoll, February 18, 1947, State Archive of Zurich, PUK, Z 99.4379.

M. Bleuler to E. Rothlin, April 29, 1947, State Archive of Zurich, PUK, Z 99.4379.

M. Bleuler to A. Stoll, May 13, 1947, State Archive of Zurich, PUK, Z 99.4379.

F. Georgi to A. Hofmann, July 8, 1953, State Archive of Zurich, PUK, Z 99.4379.

A. Hofmann to A. Stoll, April 22, 1943, Novartis Archive, Sandoz, H 105.022.

A. Hofmann to A. Stoll, June 2, 1947, Novartis Archive, Sandoz, H 105.022.

E. Rothlin to M. Bleuler, August 9, 1947, State Archive of Zurich, PUK, Z 99.4379

E. Rothlin to M. Bleuler, August 26, 1947, State Archive of Zurich, PUK, Z 99.4379.

E. Rothlin to M. Bleuler, April 9, 1948, State Archive of Zurich, PUK, Z 99.4379.

W. Stoll to M. Bleuler, February 8, 1947, State Archive of Zurich, PUK, Z 99.4379.

A. Stoll and E. Rothlin to M. Bleuler, February 13, 1947, State Archive of Zurich, PUK, Z 99.4379.

Werner Haug. *Gesichter einer anderen Schweiz*. Unpublished manuscript, 2021.

Secondary Sources

Ankele, Monika, and Benoît Majerus, eds. *Material Cultures of Psychiatry*. Bielefeld, Germany: Transkript, 2020.

Bächi, Beat. *LSD auf dem Land. Produktion und kollektive Wirkung psychotroper Stoffe*. Konstanz, Germany: Konstanz University Press, 2020.

Benedetti, Gaetano. "Beispiel einer strukturanalytischen und pharmakodynamischen Untersuchung an einem Fall von Alkoholhalluzinose, Charakterneurose und psychoreaktiver Halluzinose." *Zeitschrift für Psychotherapie und medizinische Psychologie* 1 (1951): 177–192.

Bernet, Brigitta. *Schizophrenie: Entstehung und Entwicklung eines psychiatrischen Krankheitsbildes um 1900*. Zürich: Chronos, 2013.

Blickenstorfer, Edwin. "Zum ätiologischen Problem der Psychosen vom akuten exogenen Reaktionstypus. Lysergsäurediäthylamid, ein psychisch wirksamer toxischer Spurenstoff." *Archiv für Psychiatrie und Nervenkrankheiten* 188, no. 3 (1952): 226–236.

Canguilhem, Georges. *Le normal et le pathologique*. Paris: Presses Universitaires de France, 1966.

Condrau, Gion. "Klinische Erfahrungen an Geisteskranken mit Lysergsäure-Diäthylamid." *Acta Psychiatrica et Neurologica* 24 (1949): 9–32.

Crossley, Nick. *Contesting Psychiatry: Social Movements in Mental Health*. Abingdon, UK: Routledge, 2006.

Double, Duncan D., ed. *Critical Psychiatry. The Limits of Madness*. Basingstoke, UK: Palgrave Macmillan 2006.

Dyck, Erika. "Flashback: Psychiatric Experimentation with LSD in Historical Perspective." *Canadian Journal of Psychiatry* 50, no. 7 (2005): 381–387.

Dyck, Erika. *Psychedelic Psychiatry: LSD from Clinic to Campus*. Baltimore: Johns Hopkins University Press, 2008.

Espahangizi, Kijan, and Barbara Orland, eds. *Stoffe in Bewegung. Beiträge zu einer Wissensgeschichte der materiellen Welt*. Zürich: Diaphanes, 2014.

Felsch, Philipp. "Die Arbeit der Intellektuellen. Zur Vorgeschichte des 'Practical Turn'." *Nach Feierabend, Wissen, ca. 1980* (2016): 255–262.

Galison, Peter. "Image of Self." In *Things That Talk: Object Lessons from Art and Science,* edited by Lorraine Daston, 251–278. Cambridge, MA: MIT Press, 2004.

Healy, David. *The Creation of Psychopharmacology*. Cambridge, MA: Harvard University Press, 2002.

Heimann, Hans. "Ausdrucksphänomenologie der Modellpsychosen (Psilocybin). Vergleich mit Selbstschilderung und psychischem Leistungsausfall." *Psychiatria et Neurologia* 141 (1961): 69–100.

Herzberg, David. *Happy Pills in America: From Miltown to Prozac.* Baltimore: Johns Hopkins University Press, 2009.

Hofmann, Albert. *LSD—Mein Sorgenkind.* Stuttgart: Fischer, 1979.

Langlitz, Nicolas. *Neuropsychedelia: The Revival of Hallucinogen Research since the Decade of the Brain.* Berkeley: University of California Press, 2013.

Langlitz, Nicolas. "Political Neurotheology: Emergence and Revival of a Psychedelic Alternative to Cosmetic Psychopharmacology." In *Neurocultures. Glimpses into an Expanding Universe,* edited by Francisco Ortega and Fernando Vidal, 141–165. Frankfurt am Main: Peter Lang, 2011.

Lemov, Rebecca. "X-Rays of Inner Worlds: The Mid-Twentieth-Century American Projective Test Movement." *Journal of the History of Behavioral Sciences* 47, no. 3 (2011): 251–278.

Link, Jürgen. *Versuch über den Normalismus. Wie Normalität produziert wird.* Göttingen, Germany: Vandenhoeck & Ruprecht, 2006.

Link, Jürgen, and Mirko M. Hall. "On the Contribution of Normalism to Modernity and Post-modernity." *Cultural Critique* 57 (2004): 33–46.

Majerus, Benoît "Mapping antipsychiatry: Elemente für die Geschichte einer transnationalen Bewegung." *Themenportal Europäische Geschichte* (2010): 440. http://www.europa.clio-online.de /2010/Article.

Meier, Marietta, Mario König, Magaly Tornay. *Testfall Münsterlingen: Klinische Versuche in der Psychiatrie, 1940–1980.* Zürich: Chronos, 2019.

Mescaline, Mike Jay. *A Global History of the First Psychedelic.* New Haven, CT: Yale University Press, 2019.

Moser, Jeannie. "'The Cure Is Biochemical'. Drogen und die Arbeit am Selbst in den sozialuto-pischen 1950er- und 1960er-Jahren." In *Handbuch Drogen in sozial- und kulturwissenschaftlicher Perspektive,* edited by Robert Feustel, Henning Schmidt-Semisch, and Ulrich Bröckling, 81–92. Wiesbaden, Germany: VS Verlag für Sozialwissenschaften, 2019.

Moser, Jeannie. *Psychotropen. Eine LSD-Biographie.* Konstanz, Germany: Konstanz University Press, 2013.

Novick, Tamar. "Die Entdeckung des Urins." *Nach Feierabend. Materialgeschichten* 2018: 139–150.

Pickering, Andrew. *The Mangle of Practice: Time, Agency, and Science.* Chicago: University of Chicago Press, 1995.

Rheinberger, Hans-Jörg. *Historische Epistemologie zur Einführung.* Hamburg: Junius, 2007.

Rose, Nikolas. "Neurochemical Selves." *Society* 41, no. 1 (2003): 46–59.

Shortall, Sarah. "Psychedelic Drugs and the Problem of Experience." *Past and Present* Supplement 9 (2014): 187–206.

Stoll, Werner A. "Lysergsäure-diäthylamid, ein Phantastikum aus der Mutterkorngruppe." *Schweizer Archiv für Neurologie und Psychologie* 60 (1947): 279–323.

Stoll, Werner A. "Ein neues, in sehr kleinen Mengen wirksames Phantastikum." *Schweizer Archiv für Neurologie und Psychiatrie* 64 (1949): 483–484.

Stoll, Werner A. "Rorschach-Versuche unter Lysergsäure-Diäthylamid-Wirkung." *Rorschachiana* 1, no. 3 (1952): 249–270.

Tanner, Jakob. "'Doors of Perception' Versus 'Mind Control'. Experimente mit Drogen zwischen kaltem Krieg und 1968." In *Kulturgeschichte des Menschenversuchs im 20. Jahrhundert*, edited by Birgit Griesecke et al., 340–372. Frankfurt am Main: Suhrkamp, 2009.

Tornay, Magaly. *Zugriffe auf das Ich: Psychoaktive Stoffe und Personenkonzepte in der Schweiz, 1940–1980*. Tübingen, Germany: Mohr Siebeck, 2016.

Wertham, Frederic, and Manfred Bleuler. "Inconstancy of the Formal Structure of the Personality: Experimental Study of the Influence of Mescaline on the Rorschach Test." *Archives of Neurology and Psychiatry* 28, no. 1 (1932): 52–70.

Witt, P., and R. Weber. "Biologische Prüfung des Urins von drei Kranken mit akut psychotischen Zustandsbildern auf pathogene Substanzen mit dem Spinnentest." *Monatsschrift für Psychiatrie und Neurologie* 132 (1956): 193–207.

II GLOBAL NETWORKS OF PSYCHEDELIC KNOWLEDGE

In this part, the authors of the various chapters highlight some of the ways that psychedelic knowledge networks remained rooted in place, regardless of their expansive potential. While people and substances traversed the globe, the specific contexts of knowledge production still mattered. Here, we see examples of psychedelic histories where locations, context, or setting are paramount in the way that knowledge is generated. These chapters help us to better understand the subtle tension between globalizing trends that conflict with cultural influences.

We witness evidence of the transnational circulation of plants, substances, and ideas, but we also discover that universalizing trends could be met with resistance and cultural contexts continued to shape psychedelic knowledge. The authors here tackle big themes related to transnational history. To various extents, industrialization, tourism, agriculture, food production, Christianity, and Cold War political radicalism all have connections with psychedelic history. These themes circumnavigated the globe and indeed were often used to symbolize large-scale, extranational challenges requiring multilateral investments.

Yet, despite the large global trends, these chapters also drill down into some of the on-the-ground realities that challenge sweeping generalizations about how psychedelics fit into a Western, Christian, and capitalist framework of permanent modernization and progress. Empire-building and colonialism, for instance, went hand-in-hand with commodifying plants for industrial and commercial production. Psychedelic plants became part of a larger global commercializing trend, but they did not entirely get consumed by it either. African flora and fauna, for example, fueled industrial imaginations that projected a kind of cultural ignorance of science on the part of Indigenous populations, whether that applied to medical understandings of mental illness or rubber production. Viewed through a colonial lens, Indigenous landscapes represented opportunities for modernization, and with modernization came commodification and medicalization. Neo-Malthusian concerns about food production also traveled around the globe, reinforcing another set of tensions between international trends and local conditions. We are reminded here that these trends are deeply imbricated with the history of medicine, especially pharmaceutical production and its corollary, psychiatric categorization. In response to some of the erasures of national boundaries that made way for commercial ones, local political movements fought back using do-it-yourself ideologies to address their own experience of the problems of the modern condition, crystalizing most notably in a Cold War conflict, but also inspiring a number of localized experiments in political radicalism.

Psychedelics course through these topics in ways that remind us of their pervasiveness in shaping this modern period, while also demonstrating how plant- and laboratory-based psychedelics tethered these trends to particular settings. In some cases, this meant coveting and preserving plant-based knowledge to escape the colonizer's gaze and grip; in others, it meant ramping up the production of psychedelic-based pharmaceuticals to gain a competitive advantage in a global marketplace. and elsewhere still, merging psychedelics into modern medical practices offered a testament to the virtues of open-minded progress and proof of distinct participation in cutting-edge psychiatric practices.

And still, psychedelics lubricated radical political movements that attempted to poke holes in a Cold War logic that pitted capitalism against communism, as if this binary set of options provided those frameworks to organize modern civilization. Fusing psychedelics with politics, we see another set of transnational themes that permeate the zeitgeist of this period; again, psychedelics become part of—and at times, arguably integral to—stimulating local responses to the modern human condition.

7 FROM RUBBER ADULTERANT TO CEREMONIAL PSYCHEDELIC: *VOACANGA AFRICANA* IN THE TRANSNATIONAL IMAGINATION, 1894–2018

Timothy Vilgiate

Online ethnobotanical retailers in the Netherlands, the US, and elsewhere have sold *Voacanga africana* seeds and root bark since the late 1990s as a "legal high." Copying and pasting slightly adjusted descriptions of the plant from other websites and reference books, most sellers describe the plant in some form as a "poison, stimulant, aphrodisiac, and ceremonial psychedelic" used in Ghana, rarely providing citations. Supporting this idea, their product descriptions conjure up murky images of a distant African landscape, claiming that "sorcerers in West Africa use the seeds to induce visions," or describing "arduous hunting expeditions" and "tribal celebrations." While little evidence exists to support these claims, the lack of clarity only reinforces the allure of what sellers describe as a "closely guarded secret of the African magic healers."[1] This language appeals to a stereotyped idea of Africa as a primitive and distant place, which resurfaces intermittently in the language of trip reports, as in the case of one individual who described feeling "like the only desirous situation would be loud chanting and banging on drums, or perhaps stalking game at night for long hours."[2] While reflecting the ways that deeply embedded patterns of othering shape the discourse around psychedelic plants in general, *V. africana*'s construction as a specifically African ceremonial psychedelic positions it as a curiosity relative to the broader literature.[3] The current semiotic packaging—referring to the layers of repeated images, tropes, and ideas giving meaning to *V. africana* products as commodities on the world market—developed between the 1950s and 1980s as advances in organic chemistry transformed *V. africana* from an obscure rubber adulterant to an important pharmaceutical precursor. This historical process of commodification in turn overlapped with the Western exploration of psychedelic spaces in the postwar era, as well as "real-world" frontiers of colonization, resource extraction, and knowledge production.

The demand to identify and experiment with plants like *V. africana* reflects a desire to recover contact with knowledge imagined as part of ancient, fundamentally human spiritual traditions. Popularized in the 1980s and 1990s by Terence McKenna, the idea that psychedelic or entheogenic substances played a key role in the development of human religion can be traced to the writings in the 1950s of R. Gordon Wasson and Valentina Wasson, who believed that prehistoric religion emerged from the use of hallucinogenic fungi. To support this hypothesis, they pointed to the existence of mushroom ceremonies in what they considered pristine and isolated "primitive" cultural settings.[4] In the Wassons' descriptions of their earliest encounters with the Mazatec people of Northern Oaxaca, they presented the uses of magic mushrooms as survivals of ancient, fundamentally human spiritual practices. Their 1957 article in *Life* magazine describing a mushroom ceremony among the Mazatec emphasized their geographic isolation while downplaying their decades of involvement in the coffee industry, their participation in the Mexican revolution, or their recent wave of migration to the US under the Bracero program.[5]

Mirroring a pattern seen frequently in the discourse about psychedelic plants and fungi, Wasson's article cited as further evidence for his theory about the role of fungi in religion his awareness of "six primitive peoples [from Siberia]—so primitive that anthropologists regard them as precious museum pieces for cultural study—who use an hallucinogenic mushroom in their shamanistic rites," along with the "Dyaks of Borneo and the Mount Hagen natives of New Guinea."[6] The museal interpretation of "primitive" marked the people assigned the label "primitive" as isolated and ahistorical bodies, helpless before the inevitable advance of modernity, in a unilinear metanarrative of human progress.[7] Invoking these peoples' status as primitive intended to convey not only the antiquity of their practices, but also a closeness to the fundamental realities of human nature.[8] In its many retellings by figures like McKenna and others, Wasson's story and his theories provided a powerful guiding metanarrative for future explorers of lesser-known psychedelic plants by presenting them as tools for accessing closed-off worlds of ancient and timeless spiritual wisdom, part of a universal human heritage.[9]

Far from exceptional, the Wassons' rhetoric reflected common ways of thinking about Indigenous people, mirroring the rhetoric of the Mexican Instituto Nacional Indigenista and similar development organizations throughout Latin America aimed at integrating peoples living in areas outside state control into the body politic.[10] The cultural studies scholar Pavel Schlossberg argues that in this discourse, the value of Indigenous people to national society comes from their ability "to produce and showcase . . . so-called traditional works and performances, [conforming] to static and primitivist stereotypes."[11] Outsiders in the twentieth century assumed (and often hoped), often explicitly, that primitive practices like shamanism and the use of hallucinogenic plants would fade before the steady creep of modernity. In the 1970s, for instance, teachers with the New Tribes Mission (today Ethnos360) in Venezuela discouraged Yanomami children from using local hallucinogens by teaching that "to take your dope and contact the evil spirits, you are putting another god before the true God."[12] By this point, the Yanomami, whose territory spans the border between Brazil and Venezuela, had been in contact with the countries claiming sovereignty over their land only for less than two decades.[13] At the same time, the Venezuelan government cooperated with the filmmaker Timothy Asch, the anthropologist Napoleon Chagnon, and the botanist Richard Evans Schultes to document the practices of shamans that the missionaries sought to eradicate.[14] Governments throughout the Americas in the 1950s and 1960s saw hallucinogens as potentially valuable pharmacological tools, either for medical treatments or for enhanced interrogation, and thus frequently sponsored research into their use.[15] Developing within this regional context, the discourse about psychedelic plants has generally centered around the Americas, where late-twentieth-century efforts to understand them were embedded in a hemispheric development project, making a supposedly psychedelic plant from Africa stand out.

Beyond the clear association between Native Americans and substances like peyote, magic mushrooms, or ayahuasca, many psychedelic authors and researchers, including McKenna, spent significant amounts of time in western North America.[16] Their understandings of the psychopolitical struggle surrounding access to the psychedelic frontier (a framing invoked by, among others, Timothy Leary in his 1983 autobiography) thus developed in places that less than a century earlier represented the frontiers of westward expansion, as the US and Canadian governments forced Indigenous peoples off their land into reservations, reserves, and boarding schools.[17] The association of psychedelics with Native Americans and their status as colonized peoples weighed heavily on the way that non-Indigenous users understood them, regardless of their underlying political alignment.[18] In contrast to the assimilationist Indigenista ideology, authors like McKenna have advocated an "Archaic Revival," a return to "primitive" lifeways in an implicit rejection of mainstream society.[19] Schultes, on the other hand, argued that those who "believe they can achieve 'mystic' or 'religious' experience . . . with hallucinogens . . . seldom realiz[e] that they are merely reverting to the age-old practices of primitive societies" and went on to write that such use "may have little or no value and may sometimes even be harmful or dangerous. . . . it is a newly imported and superimposed cultural trait without natural roots in modern Western tradition."[20] Yet the desire to "revert" or regain contact with "primitive" spirituality frequently drove non-Indigenous psychonauts to seek out Indigenous psychedelic plants. Describing his 1972 trip to the Sierra Mazateca to consume magic mushrooms, the Mexican author Enrique Gonzalez Rubio Montoya wrote glowingly about how the Mazatec "have their gods, the *Dueños* of the Earth, who protect them, speak to them, and enlighten them through the sacred mushrooms. The city man has none of this; he's poorer than the people of the Sierra Mazateca."[21] Although expressing opposite understandings of the boundaries between the "primitive" and "modern" spheres, both perceived hallucinogenic plants as belonging to an ancient fundamentally human heritage lost to, or even inaccessible to, "modern" man.

Developing within the historically specific context of the Americas, Africa remained marginal to the concerns of mainstream and countercultural psychedelic discourses. National integration and accompanying drives to document Native American psychiatric knowledge between the 1950s and 1970s coincided with movements for independence in sub-Saharan

Africa, beginning with Ghana in 1957, and a simultaneous reevaluation of once-spurned African medicinal plant knowledge.[22] Although altered states of consciousness played important roles in religious practices across the African continent, most authors accepted the position of Wade Davis, who in 1985 wrote, "While the Amerindian successfully explored his forests for hallucinogens, the African did not . . . If the peoples of Africa did not explore their environment for psychoactive drugs, it is because they felt no need to."[23] This argument extended from colonial stereotypes of Africans as simple-minded and spiritually dangerous.[24] Since the time of the slave trade, Europeans feared the power of African priest-healers, who used their knowledge not only to carve out positions of authority, but to undermine and even kill their masters.[25] Visitors to sub-Saharan Africa in the nineteenth century likewise spoke disdainfully of African spirituality; many outsiders believed that, as supposed "savages," Africans possessed no real science, religion, or philosophy.[26] During the height of colonial rule in the late nineteenth and early twentieth centuries, the British government subjected Akan priest-healers in the Gold Coast (today Ghana) to onerous restrictions, requiring them to register their idols with the government and swear off the use of any "poisonous or noxious medicines" in written letters to the local district commissioner.[27]

Further reinforcing the myth that African societies possessed little to no psychedelic or psychoactive plants, the ecstatic techniques of African priest-healers received little of the veneration that Indigenous shamans like María Sabina or Don Juan Matus received from the North American counterculture. The ambitious leaders of newly independent African states, hoping to set their nations on paths to modernity, internalized colonial rhetoric around Indigenous medicoreligious practices and sought to validate African medicine by downplaying its spiritual aspects.[28] The evidence suggests that scholars have dramatically underestimated the extent and complexity of African knowledge about hallucinogenic plants. In 2002, Jean-François Sobiecki documented thirty-nine different psychoactive plants used in southern Africa alone, including several hallucinogens.[29] More recently, a survey of archeological, ethnobotanical, and historical data by the geographer Chris Duvall provides a convincing argument for a radical revision of the history of cannabis that traces the plant's arrival in the New World to Africa.[30] Diviners and medicine men among the Igbo of southeastern Nigeria reportedly have "certain hallucinogenic herbs crushed and squeezed into [their] eyes to make [them] see double—to see both spirit and men, and to hear the message of the spirit world."[31] Similarly, the Ghanaian author Kofi Appiah-Kubi wrote that in the first year of an Akan healer's training, the healer "washes his eyes and ears with herbs that help him to see the normally unseen and to hear the normally unheard."[32] Knowledge of the precise plants used for this purpose generally remains secret, likely owing to a combination of the spiritual power that they afford the user and the colonial repression of "noxious medicines." Research by Samuel Ntewusu into the social history of *Datura* in Ghana suggests that the healers and diviners who use this anticholinergic nightshade plant do so privately before sleeping rather than during their interactions with clients, suggesting a desire to keep the use of such plants out of public view.[33]

Labeling *V. africana* as an underexplored "ceremonial psychedelic" from Africa not only promises the Western consumer a novel and meaningful experience, but also serves as a rejoinder to dominant narratives about the scarcity of African psychoactive plants, fitting into an underlying countercultural desire to challenge the global capitalist status quo. Despite significant evidence that ceremonial psychedelics exist on the African continent, however, the idea that the people of Ghana use *V. africana* in such a way stands on much shakier ground. An alkaloid-rich tree from the dogbane (Apocynaceae) family, *V. africana* produces green speckled fruits that, when ripe, open to expose wrinkled, elliptical seeds in sticky orange pulp. Prior to the discovery of medicinally useful alkaloids in its seeds in 1956, colonial botanists and foresters labeled the tree a "rubber adulterant," one of many "waste plants" that Britain's Gold Coast Forestry Department hoped to eventually cleanse from the forest in favor of economically valuable species.[34] Yet by the 1950s, the department's own internal reports indicated a surge in pharmaceutical interest in Apocynaceous plants, although foresters lamented the rarity of many requested species.[35]

The spike in demand for African dogbanes fit into the context of an international search for healing plants across the Global South, enabled by new understandings of organic chemistry and breakthroughs in scientific understandings of atoms and molecules.[36] By 1943, pharmacologists at the School of Tropical Medicine in Calcutta had published case reports describing the successful treatment of schizophrenics with reserpine, an alkaloid isolated by Gananth Sen and Kartick Chandra Bose from Rauwolfia serpentina in 1931.[37] By the early 1950s, psychiatrists outside India had started to integrate reserpine into models for the treatment of mental illnesses.[38] Alongside other valuable medicinal alkaloids found in dogbane plants like *Tabernanthe iboga, Catharanthus roseus,* and *Strophanthus kombe,* the discovery of reserpine had positioned the Apocynaceae family as a promising frontier for further exploration.[39] As part of a larger project evaluating a range of dogbane plants, including some African *Rauwolfia* species, the French chemists Robert Goutarel and Maurice Marie-Janot patented a process for the extraction of three potential cardiotonic alkaloids in 1956 on behalf of France's Institute for the Chemistry of Natural Substances (ICNS).[40] In doing so, they asserted an intellectual and economic claim to a distant colonial landscape where French colonial power seemed threatened by an increasingly powerful pan-African movement for citizenship outside the four communes in present-day Senegal, eventually growing into calls for independence.[41] Just as the inscription of the plant as a rubber adulterant reflected the ways that the colonial state rendered the landscape legible in past centuries, the inscription of intellectual property claims to dogbane alkaloids reflected colonial administrative efforts to deepen economic claims to African landscapes even as independence movements gained steam.

Even as it gained new economic value, the consequences of the plant's 1896 identification as a rubber adulterant and the ensuing taxonomic ambiguity lingered as palimpsests in the scientific discourse surrounding its exploitation. For instance, the French chemist Jacque Poisson filed a patent for the process of obtaining tabersonine, an important precursor for the chemotherapy drug vinblastine, from *V. africana* with the patent office in Yaounde, Cameroon, in 1968.[42] The Cameroonian patent acknowledged that "several alkaloids have been extracted from various Voacanga" and asserted that "[t]he present invention consists of the use of the seeds of Voacanga as a source of an alkaloid other than those isolated so far from this Apocynaceae."[43] An application for a US patent filed in 1969 had to be abandoned; the patent ultimately granted in 1973 indicated a further reckoning with the plant's taxonomic ambiguity, adding a claim to "the process for obtaining the alkaloid tabersonine from plants of the Voacanga genus," naming *V. africana*, *Voacanga thouarsii*, *Voacanga bracteate*, *Voacanga candiflora*, *Voacanga glabra*, and *Voacanga obtusa*.[44] With this claim, they asserted the rights to the process of "harvesting the seeds of Voacanga plant [and] freeing the seeds from foreign bodies," suggesting ownership over not just the laboratory process, but the knowledge and labor of the purchasing agents and plant collectors, whose collection of the seeds would necessarily utilize local categories rather than the ambiguous binomial nomenclature.[45] Indeed, a 2009 analysis by Japanese researchers of *V. africana* seed material sold online suggested the products entering the market often contain a mixture of similar species.[46] The local collectors I spoke with while in Ghana primarily called the plant *bonawa*, and despite acknowledging multiple kinds of *bonawa*, they saw the differences between varieties as largely irrelevant for the export business, further suggesting that the plants entering the only ethnobotanical market may represent multiple distinct species.

The taxonomic uncertainty arose from the problematic history of the currently accepted Linnean name for almost all the plants claimed in Poisson's patent—*V. africana*. The Austrian botanist Otto Stapf created the name after receiving a specimen from his colleague George Scott-Elliot. Scott-Elliot sent him the plant after traveling through the interior of Sierra Leone with the boundary commission, tasked with charting the border between Sierra Leone and its neighbors, for about a year.[47] Describing the expedition as "most disappointing," Scott-Elliot later depicted Sierra Leone in his 1919 book *Stories of Savage Life* as a "miserable" place dominated by "poverty and filth indescribable."[48] Stapf, an Austrian botanist then in charge of the collection of South Asian plants housed in the Royal Botanic Gardens at Kew, compared Scott-Elliot's specimen with thirteen other plants gathered by preceding nineteenth century plant collectors and suggested the name as a catch-all for a range of similar and evidently useless plants.[49] The botanical community did not readily accept Stapf's new description, embracing more locally specific names for species and sometimes placed specimens later categorized as *V. africana* in different genera entirely. By 1947, the French taxonomist Marcel Pichon even suggested dividing the species *V. africana* into five varieties, citing irregularities in the herbarium specimens that he had examined and the ambiguities of Stapf's original description.[50] Yet beginning in 1970, the Wageningen Agricultural University–based botanist Antony J. M. Leeuwenberg eliminated more than twenty locally specific varieties in a sweeping revision of the Apocynaceae family, going through the collection of herbariums from St. Louis to London to Cameroon and relabeling plants as *V. africana*.[51] The specimens verified by Leeuwenberg proceeded to circulate to research institutions in Brazil, Japan, China, Australia, and elsewhere, until eventually the name *V. africana* predominated. Beyond simplifying the complex taxonomy of the genus, the revision also strengthened intellectual property claims to Voacanga alkaloids and enabled them to transcend local boundaries.

Prior to the mid-2000s, rumors of the plant's psychoactivity revolved less around the *V. africana* species and more around the genus as a whole, rarely mentioning Ghana.[52] Frederick R. Irvine's 1960 book *Woody Plants of Ghana*, a revision of an earlier text compiled with the help of his African students at Achimota College in the 1930s, lent limited credence to the idea that a few (but not all) of the plants referred to by the names *V. bonawa, V. kakapempe,* or *V. ofuruma* possessed psychoactive properties.[53] For instance, he identified *Rauwolfia vomitoria*, noted elsewhere as an herb used to anoint the heads of dying patients, as a "sedative for madness."[54] In 1985, a researcher at the Chelsea College Department of Pharmacy in London named Norman Bisset published a sweeping review of the uses of the Voacanga genus across the African continent, which multiple authors later cited to support claims of *V. africana*'s psychoactivity.[55] Mindful of Leeuwenberg's ongoing revision of the genus and its complicated taxonomy, Bisset carefully listed the first species in the review as "*Voacanga africana (Angustifolia?, Lutescens, Puberula)*" and noted its use in a decoction of the leaves consumed "as a tonic and against fatigue due to breathlessness," in Senegal, alongside two full pages of additional uses ranging from "making ropes" in Mozambique to a liquor "drunk to cure gonorrhoea" in Ghana.[56] Tellingly, he speculated that the plant's use in cases of madness among certain peoples of the Ivory Coast occured "possibly through confusion with other Apocynaceae—*Rauwolfia vomitoria* or *Tabernaemontana crassa*." Citing a herbarium specimen collected by F. J. Breteler in 1970, he mentioned that people in Gabon use *V. bracteate*, meanwhile, "to become 'high.'"[57] Yet the psychoactivity of the plant figured as being peripheral to Bisset's work, appearing alongside a diverse list of uses extending across sub-Saharan Africa.

Rumors of the plant's psychoactivity nonetheless continued to gain traction. By 1995, *Psychoaktive Planzen*, a book by the German author Bert Marco Schuldes, featured an entry on *V. africana*, claiming without a citation that "West African natives" use "[t]he bark . . . as a stimulant [to] withstand tribal festivals . . . dances and strenuous hunting expeditions," while "shamans" use the seeds "to create visionary experiences."[58] Christian Rätsch cited both Bisset and Schuldes in his 1998 *Encyclopedia of Psychoactive Plants*, reporting that the "bark and seeds [of *V. africana*] reportedly induce stimulating and hallucinogenic effects." He went on to mention several other species of Voacanga with alleged hallucinogenic or psychoactive properties, including the claim that "West African sorcerers ingest the seeds of *Voacanga grandiflora* . . . for visionary purposes. Unfortunately, the details of this use are still unknown, as the sorcerers keep their knowledge secret."[59] Rätsch and Schuldes's descriptions dominated most online storefronts that carried *V. africana* seeds and root bark in the first decade of the twenty-first century, and they likewise appeared on harm-reduction sites like Erowid. Experience reports from the period suggest that certain retailers occasionally included free samples of *V. africana* alongside shipments of more well-established and popular "legal highs," like *Salvia divinorum*.[60] Although most who tried it reported mixed results, the idea of encountering an uncharted realm of psychedelic space formed a core part of *V. africana*'s appeal to Western consumers as it drifted from the pharmaceutical sector and into the online market for legal entheogens and psychedelics. One author of a trip report described the thrill of being "on a 'seldom walked trail' . . . thinking of [the] origin and traditional use of ethnobotanicals and following a 'traditiona' [sic] that few people have the opportunity to do."[61] The lack of taxonomic clarity and the obscurity of its local usage thus formed a core part of its appeal, wrapping the plant in an aura of mystery.

The market for *V. africana* saw its biggest bump when a 2007 Wikipedia article created by a user named MrGoodGuy introduced highly specific verbiage about the plant's use "in Ghana as a poison, stimulant, aphrodisiac, and ceremonial psychedelic." The claim spread quickly, supplanting descriptions taken from Rätsch and Schuldes on several websites. For a citation, MrGoodGuy embedded a link to his business offering *V. africana* seeds, along with a handful of other Ghanaian botanicals. The moderator removed the link, although MrGoodGuy reintroduced it several times before being threatened with a ban. Evidence for the claim remains thin, and though it is tempting to assume the worst of MrGoodGuy's motivations, the possibility cannot be ruled out that he simply reported knowledge that had otherwise escaped the attention of the literature. When I reached out to one Ghanaian historian, they replied that the plant *V. ofuruma* was "given out to devotees of some cults" in northern Ghana, a relatively poorer region of the country. Yet issues of translation become still more complicated here, as the word *ofuruma* comes from the Akan language, not spoken by most groups in northern Ghana. Moreover, plants produce alkaloids as secondary metabolites in response to ecological conditions, allowing the sessile and pollinator-dependent organisms to mediate their interactions with insects, birds, and mammals in their environment.[62] *V. africana* trees, even if genetically identical, confront drier and relatively less competitive environments in the northern savannahs than they do in the hilly southern rain forests or the coastal swamps, and thus likely produce different levels of various secondary metabolites in each environment.

Online trip reports reflect the taxonomic and chemical variability of plant material sold under the label *V. africana*. One 2007 report by a 185-pound male described taking 250 seeds and speculated about the presence of "several chemicals with dissimilar effects."[63] The effects manifested at first as a "strong sense of lethargy and sleepiness," and then progressed after an hour to an intensification of sensitivity to auditory stimuli, including the apparently "inane" conversations of his neighbors, and the inability "to count above 30something [sic]."[64] However, a 2008 experience, written by a 130-pound male, reported that eating two seeds and taking forty-three more in tea caused, after two hours, "a very mild change in awareness," followed by vomiting, weakness, and "gut pains" that "persisted for days."[65] Many find the plant merely underwhelming; one individual, who in 2009 experimented with both the seeds and root bark with few noticeable effects, wrote that "this stuff was neither recreational nor spiritual . . . it was an obvious let-down."[66] Yet another report from 2005, involving tea made with seventy-five seeds accompanied by cannabis consumed at the rate of "about a bowl an hour" described "a centered alertness," followed by "San Pedro/morning glory visuals—very colorful, twisting undulating [sic] shapes." They went on to describe it as "the most lucid, clear-headed trip I've experienced," accompanied by "a warm psychedelic after-glow for four or five hours thereafter."[67] In all, a qualitative analysis of forty-six online experience reports conducted for my research found little correlation between reported quantities of seeds and the reported effects.

The 1894 invention of the name *V. africana* allowed a diverse and far-flung set of plants to enter the colonial gaze as European states sought to extend their power beyond coastal areas into the interior of the continent.[68] Detached from their ecological contexts, samples of plant material carefully arranged on herbarium plates allowed taxonomists like Pichon and Leeuwenberg to observe, describe, and make judgments about aspects of a distant frontier landscape, which remained authoritative even in the absence of overt colonial control. By 1956, new technologies allowed deeper levels of legibility and power over the environments of colonies on the brink of independence. The plant itself grew increasingly unrecognizable and distant from its ecological context as chemists crushed, dissolved, and manipulated the seeds and root bark in laboratories, allowing pharmaceutical companies to assert sweeping claims over the tree in the form of patents. The more recent casting of the plant as a ceremonial psychedelic extended from this historical process of exploitation, promising contact with a carefully protected, mysterious body of Indigenous knowledge that Wasson and others have construed as rooted in ancient, universally human traditions. Although intended to exalt and romanticize the Indigenous, the image of priest-healers and shamans circulated in storefronts, trip reports, and some literature still utilizes them primarily as a narrative foil to modernity.

On a biological level, the production of secondary metabolites and other chemical signals by plants reflect underlying processes of mutual construction unfolding between the organism and its environment. Similarly, legible, speakable phrases like "*bonawa*," "rubber adulterant," "ceremonial psychedelic," or "*V. africana*" exist materially as tangles of neurons attached to countless sensory cues, memories, and meanings.[69] On the level of macro-organic (species-level) behavior, the utility of such constructs comes in their ability to allow bodies to coordinate their behavior, although the understanding of the world that they sustain does not necessarily offer an unproblematic or unbiased perception of reality.[70] Over time, useful shared meanings accrete into increasingly stable and information-dense semiotic constructs embedded in the environment so as to outlive generations, with many of their underlying irrationalities or contradictions concealed by the appearance of stability.[71] The term "psychedelic" indicates not a clearly established quality inherent to specific compounds, but rather one of many ways that the human brain can read the response of the rest of the body to foreign chemical signals, and by extension interpret its relationships with the organisms producing said signals. The word "psychedelic" emerged from the context of an individualistic North American frontier culture undergoing a generational rebellion after hundreds of years of violent settler-colonialism and is deeply connected with discourses surrounding indigeneity. Labeling *V. africana* as an African psychedelic extends the frontiers of psychedelic exploration beyond its usual Americentric frame of reference, and yet its staying power reflects less the grassroots realities of African religious practices and more the desires of consumers for contact with something that they imagine is a lost spiritual heritage.

NOTES

1.   A sample of fifty online retailers and forty-six online trip reports was collected by the author for this chapter. The data was analyzed in NVIVO Qualitative Analysis software and in Microsoft Excel. Because the online retailers sometimes operate in a "gray market," I have not attributed any quotes from their websites to specific companies.

2.   AluminumFoilRobots, "V. africana Root Bark," *DMT-Nexus* (website), December 26, 2010, https://www.dmt-nexus.me/forum/default.aspx?g=posts&m=207136.

3.   Edward Said, *Orientalism* (New York: Pantheon Books, 1978). Obioma Nnaemeka, "Racialization and the Colonial Architecture: Othering and the Order of Things," *PMLA: Publications of the Modern Language Association of America* 123, no. 5 (2008): 1748–1751.

4.   R. Gordon Wasson and Valentina Wasson, *Mushrooms, Russia, and History* (New York: Pantheon Books, 1957). Peter Frust, *Flesh of the Gods: The Ritual Use of Hallucinogens* (New York: Praeger Publications, 1972), viii–ix. Terence McKenna, *Food of the Gods: The Search for the Original Tree of Knowledge* (New York: Random House, 1993). Robert Kohler, *Landscapes and Labscapes* (Chicago and London: University of Chicago Press, 2002), 13.

5.   Juan Carrera, *La Otra Vida de María Sabina* (Mexico, DF: Universidad Autonoma del Estado de Mexico, 1986). Benjamin Feinberg, *The Devil's Book of Culture: History, Mushrooms, and Caves in Southern Mexico* (Austin: University of Texas Press, 2003).

6.   R. Gordon Wasson, "Seeking the Magic Mushroom," *Life Magazine,* May 13, 1957.

7.   Franz Boas, *The Mind of Primitive Man* (London: MacMillan, 1911).

8.   Antonio Ceraso, "Entheogens and the Public Mystery: The Rhetoric of R. Gordon Wasson," *Configurations* 16 (2008): 215–243.

9.   Terence McKenna et al., *The Sacred Mushroom Seeker: Tributes to R. Gordon Wasson* (Rochester, NY: Inner Traditions, 1997).

10. Jens Andermann, *Optic of the State: Visuality and Power in Argentina and Brazil* (Pittsburgh: University of Pittsburgh Press, 2007). Stephen Lewis, "Indigenista Dreams Meet Sober Realities: The Slow Demise of Federal Indian Policy in Chiapas, Mexico, 1951–1970," *Latin American Perspectives: Rethinking Indigenismo on the American Continent* 39, no. 5 (2012): 63–79.

11. Pavel Schlossberg, "Heritage Practices, Indigenismo, and Coloniality: Studying-up into Racism in Contemporary Mexico," *Cultural Studies* 32, no. 3 (2018): 414–437.

12. Napoleon Chagnon and Timothy Asch, "New Tribes Mission" *Yanomamö Series* (Watertown, MA: Documentary Educational Resources, 1975), 5:50–6:57.

13. Davi Kopenawa and Bruce Albert, *The Falling Sky: Words of a Yanomami Shaman* (Cambridge, MA: Harvard University Press, 2013).

14. Napoleon Chagnon, Philip Le Quesne, and James Cook, "Yanomamo Hallucinogens: Anthropological, Botanical, and Chemical Findings," *Current Anthropology* 12, no. 1 (1971): 72–74.

15. Alexander Dawson, "Salvador Roquet, María Sabina, and the Trouble with Jipis," *Hispanic American Historical Review* 95, no. 1 (2015): 103–118.

16. Erika Dyck, *Psychedelic Psychiatry: LSD from Clinic to Campus* (Baltimore: Johns Hopkins University Press, 2008). Avi Solomon, "Interview: Dennis McKenna," *Boing* (website), June 9, 2011. https://boingboing.net/2011/06/09/mck.html; Jay Stevens, *Storming Heaven: LSD and the American Dream* (New York: Perennial Library, 1998).

17. Timothy Leary, *Flashbacks: An Autobiography* (Los Angeles: Tereny P. Torcher, 1983), 48; Andrea Ens, "Silencing Indigenous Pasts: Critical Indigenous Theory and the History of Psychedelics," *International Journal of Qualitative Studies in Education* 34, no. 10 (2021): 904–914.

18. Alexander Dawson, *The Peyote Effect: From the Inquisition to the War on Drugs* (Oakland: University of California Press, 2018).

19. Ananda Das, "Terence McKenna in Maui Hawaii 1994—Axiom Production," March 2, 2016, video, 2:04:30, https://www.youtube.com/watch?v=ANosz9vVRlI.

20. Richard Schultes, *A Golden Guide: Hallucinogenic Plants* (Racine, WI: Western Publishing, 1976), 10–11.

21. E. Franz Val. G, *Conversaciones con María Sabina y otros curanderos* (Mexico: Publicaciones Cruz O.S.A, 1996), 17. Translation from Spanish by author.

22. Abena Osseo-Asare, *Bitter Roots: The Search for Healing Plants in Africa* (Chicago: University of Chicago Press, 2014).

23. Wade Davis, "Hallucinogenic Plants and Their Use in Traditional Societies—An Overview," *Cultural Survival Quarterly Magazine* 9, no. 4 (1985), https://www.culturalsurvival .org/publications/cultural-survival-quarterly/hallucinogenic-plants-and-their-use-traditional -societieseportedly. Davis echoed the position of his advisor, expressed in Schultes, *Golden Guide*, 22.

24. Sandra Greene, *Sacred Sites and the Colonial Encounter: A History of Meaning and Memory in Ghana* (Bloomington: Indiana University Press, 2002). Kwasi Konadu, *Indigenous Medicine and Knowledge in African Society* (Routledge, 2007).

25. James Sweet, *Domingos Álvares: African Healing, and the Intellectual History of the Atlantic World* (Durham, NC: University of North Carolina Press, 2011).

26. Erwin H. Ackerknecht. "Natural Diseases and Rational Treatment in Primitive Medicine," *Bulletin of the History of Medicine* 19, no. 5 (1946), 467–497. E. Bolaji Idowa, *African Traditional Religion. A Definition* (Maryknoll, NY: Orbis Books, 1975). Munyaradzi Mawere, *African Belief and Knowledge Systems: A Critical Perspective* (Mankon, Cameroon: Langaa Research and Publishing Common Initiative Group, 2011).

27. Kojo Kobi to the P. N. D., July 12, 1937, No. 9885/37/Oda; George Barns to the District Commissioner, Western Akim, March 10, 1934, Courtesy of the Public Records and Archives Administration Department, Accra, Ghana. ADM 36, Case No. WA 63/1920 "Fetish 1920–46."

28. Konadu, *Indigenous Medicine and Knowledge in African Society*, 2017.

29. Jean François-Sobiecki, "A Review of Plants Used in Divination in Southern Africa and Their Psychoactive Effects," *Southern African Humanities* 20 (2008): 333–351. This review encompasses South Africa, Botswana, Swaziland, Lesotho, Zambia, Zimbabwe, and Namibia.

30. Christopher Duvall, *The African Roots of Marijuana* (Durham, NC: Duke University Press, 2019).

31. Agwu Christopher Agqu, *A Philosophical Concept of Agwu in Igbo Land* (Bloomington, IN: Trafford Publishing, 2013), 41.

32. Kofi Appiah-Kubi, *Man Cures, God Heals: Religion and Medical Practice among the Akans of Ghana* (Totowa, NJ: Allanheld, Osmun, and Co. Publishers, 1981), 38.

33. Samuel Aniegye Ntewusu, "Labour, Religion and Madness: A Social History of Datura Spp. in Ghana," *Journal of Performing Arts* 5, no. 2 (2017): 39–40.

34. Otto Stapf, "Apocynaceae," *Botanical Journal of the Linnean Society* (London: Oxford University Press, 1894), 87–88. For more, see Timothy Vilgiate, "Forestry and the 'World on Paper': Ideas of Science and Resistance to Forest Reservation on the Gold Coast in the Early Twentieth Century," *Ghana Studies* 23 (2020): 3–27.

35. Gold Coast Forestry Department, *Annual Report, 1955–1956* (Accra: Government Printer, 1957), 43–44.

36. Gabriela Laveaga, *Jungle Laboratories: Mexican Peasants, National Projects, and the Making of the Pill* (Durham, NC: Duke University Press, 2009); Osseo-Asare, *Bitter Roots*, 2014.

37. J. C. Gupta, A. K. Deb, and B. S. Kahali, "Preliminary Observations on the Use of Rauwolfia serpentina Benth. in the Treatment of Mental Disorders," *Indian Medical Gazette* 78, no. 11 (1943), 547–549. Pradipto Roy, "Global Pharma and Local Science: The Untold Tale of Reserpine," *Indian Journal of Psychiatry* 60, Suppl. 2 (2018): S277–S283.

38. David Healy and Marie Savage, "Reserpine Exhumed," *British Journal of Psychiatry* 172 (1998): 376–378.

39. Vincent Ravalec, Mallendi, and Agnès Paicheler, *Iboga: The Visionary Root of African Shamanism* (Rochester, VT: Park Street Press, 2007). Osseo-Asare, *Bitter Roots*, 1–35.

40. J. A. Le Hir Poisson, R. Goutarel, and M. M. Janot, "Isolation of Reserpine from Roots of Rauwolfia Vomitoria Afz," *Comptes Rendus Hebdomadaires des Séances de l'Académie des Sciences* 238, no. 15 (1954): 1607–1609. M. M. Janot and R. Goutarel, "A Process for the Preparation of Novel Ibogainabkoemmlingen," German Patent DE1039068B, filed October 9, 1956, and issued September 18, 1958; M. M. Janot and R. Goutarel, "Alkaloids of Voacanga," US Patent 2823204, filed March 30, 1956, and issued February 11, 1958.

41. Janot and Goutarel, "Alkaloids of Voacanga"; Frederick Cooper, *Citizenship between Empire and Nation: Remaking France and French Africa, 1945–1960* (Princeton, NJ: Princeton University Press, 2014).

42. Jacques Poisson, "Procédé d'obtention de la tabersonine," Cameroonian Patent C07–03025, filed March 22, 1969, and issued December 15, 1970; Cites Belgian Patent 712841, issued March 27, 1968.

43. Poisson, "Procédé d'obtention de la tabersonine."

44. Jacques Poisson, "Process of Obtaining Tabersonine," US Patent 3754478, filed July 16, 1971, and issued September 11, 1973.

45. Poisson, "Process of Obtaining Tabersonine." All pharmaceutical companies that I reached out to over the course of this research declined to answer any questions about their collection procedures.

46. Yukihiro Goda, Ruri Kikura-Hanajir, Takuro Muruyama, and Akinori Miyashita, "Chemical and DNA Analyses for the Products of a Psychoactive Plant, *Voacanga africana*," *Yakugaku Zasshi* 129, no. 8 (2009): 975–983.

47. George Scott-Elliot, "On the Botanical Results of the Sierra Leone Boundary Commission," *Botanical Journal of the Linnean Society* (London: Oxford University Press, 1894): 64–65.

48. Scott-Elliot, "On the Botanical Results of the Sierra Leone Boundary Commission," 64; George Scott-Elliot, *Stories of Savage Life* (London: Seeley, Service and Co., 1919), 205.

49. Stapf, "Apocynaceae," 87–88; Dr. Otto Stapf, F.R.S. *Nature* 132 (1933): 305. https://doi.org /10.1038/132305a0.

50. Marcel Pichon, "Classification of Apocynacees: VIII, The Voacanga of Africa," *Bulletin du Muséum national d'histoire naturelle* 14, no. 5 (1947): 409–410.

51. Henk Beetje, "Review: A Revision of Tabernaemontana. The Old World Species by A. J. M. Leeuwenberg," *Kew Bulletin* 47, no. 3 (Berlin: Springer, 1992): 548.

52. P. A. G. M. De Smet, "Some Ethnopharmacological Notes on African Hallucinogens," *Journal of Ethnopharmacology* 50 (1996): 144–145.

53. Frederick Irvine, *Woody Plants of Ghana: With Special Reference to Their Uses* (London: Oxford University Press, 1961).

54. Irvine, *Woody Plants*, 633. Appiah-Kubi, *Man Cures, God Heals*, 157.

55. De Smet, "African Hallucinogens," 146.

56. Norman Bisset, "Uses of *Voacanga* Species," *Agricultural University of Wageningen Papers* 85, no. 3 (1985): 116–122.

57. Bisset, "Uses of Voacanga Species," 118.

58. Bert Marco Schuldes, *Psychoaktive Pflanzen: Mehr ais 65 Pflanzen mit anregender, euphorisierender, beruhigender, sexuell erregender, oder halluzinogener Wirkung* (Lohrbach, Germany: Medienxperimente, 1995), 77.

59. Christian Rätsch, *The Encyclopedia of Psychoactive Plants: Ethnopharmacology and Its Applications,* trans. John R. Baker (Rochester, NY: Park Street Press, 2005).

60. Isana, "A World of Plastic Chicklets: An Experience with Voacanga africana, Salvia divinorum (5x extract) & Cannabis," *Erowid* (website), September 12, 2007, http://www.erowid.org /exp/43231.

61. Shamsu, "Very Interesting Seeds: An Experience with Voacanga africana," *Erowid* (website), August 4, 2005, http://www.erowid.org/exp/43102.

62. Li Yang et al., "Response of Plant Secondary Metabolites to Environmental Factors," *Molecules* 23, no. 4 (2018): 762.

63. As, "Ibogainish? An Experience with Voacanga Africana," *Erowid* (website), December 15, 2009, http://www.erowid.org/exp/61486.

64. As, "Ibogainish? An Experience with Voacanga Africana."

65. Hempeater. "This Is Poison: An Experience with Voacanga africana," *Erowid* (website), December 15, 2009, http://www.erowid.org/exp/70018.

66. bry-bry w., "Booooo! An Experience with Voacanga africana & Morning Glory Seeds," *Erowid* (website), February 21, 2018, http://www.erowid.org/exp/85140.

67. DiscipulusMentis, "First Glimpse of Paradise: An Experience with Voacanga africana & Cannabis (exp43493)," *Erowid* (website), December 15, 2009. erowid.org/exp/43493; Since *V. africana* contains three cannabinoid receptor antagonists, it likely interacts in a significant way with cannabis; a full discussion of this fact lies outside the scope of this chapter, but the role of CB1 antagonists, which reduce appetite and induce a feeling described as dysphoric, may account for the use of some *V. africana* varieties in African shamanic practices where fasting plays an important role, and for the negative responses of some users. Yukihiro Goda et al., "Discovery of Indole Alkaloids with Cannabinoid CB1 Receptor Antagonistic Activity," *Bioorganic & Medicinal Chemistry Letters* 21, no. 7 (2011): 1962–1964. Balapal Basvaraj-appa, "Cannabinoid Receptors and Their Signaling Mechanisms," in *The Endocannabi-noid System: Genetics, Biochemistry, Brain Disorders, and Therapy,* ed. Eric Murillo-Rodríguez (Amsterdam: Elsevier, 2017), 28.

68. Helen Tilley, *Africa as a Living Laboratory: Empire, Development, and the Problem of Scientific Knowledge, 1870–1950* (Chicago: Chicago University Press, 2011).

69. Danilyn Rutherford, "Affect Theory and the Empirical," *Annual Review of Anthropology* 45 (2016): 285–300.

70. Kim Fortun, "From Latour to Late Industrialism," *Hau: Journal of Ethnographic Theory* 4 (2014): 309–329.

71. Marcello Barbieri, "Biosemiotics: A New Understanding of Life," *Naturwissenschaften* 95, no. 7 (2008): 577–599.

BIBLIOGRAPHY

Primary Sources

Aluminum Foil Robots. "V. africana Root Bark." *DMT-Nexus* (website). Accessed December 26, 2010. https://www.dmt-nexus.me/forum/default.aspx?g=posts&m=207136.

As. "Ibogainish? An Experience with Voacanga Africana." *Erowid* (website). December 15, 2009. http://www.erowid.org/exp/61486.

bry-bry w. "Booooo! An Experience with Voacanga africana & Morning Glory Seeds." *Erowid* (website). February 21, 2018, http://www.erowid.org/exp/85140.

Das, Ananda. "Terence McKenna in Maui Hawaii 1994—Axiom Production." March 2, 2016, video, 2:04:30. https://www.youtube.com/watch?v=ANosz9vVRlI.

Discipulus Mentis. "First Glimpse of Paradise: An Experience with Voacanga africana & Cannabis (exp43493)." *Erowid* (website), December 15, 2009. erowid.org/exp/43493.

Gold Coast Forestry Department. *Annual Report, 1955–1956* (Accra: Government Printer, 1957), 43–44.

Hempeater. "This Is Poison: An Experience with Voacanga africana." *Erowid* (website). December 15, 2009, http://www.erowid.org/exp/70018.

Isana. "A World of Plastic Chicklets: An Experience with Voacanga africana, Salvia divinorum (5x extract) & Cannabis." *Erowid* (website), September 12, 2007, http://www.erowid.org/exp/43231.

Janot, M. M., and R. Goutarel. "Alkaloids of Voacanga." US Patent 2823204, filed March 30, 1956, and issued February 11, 1958.

Janot, M. M., and R. Goutarel. "A Process for the Preparation of Novel Ibogainabkoemmlingen." German Patent DE1039068B, filed October 9, 1956, and issued September 18, 1958.

Kojo Kobi to the P. N. D., July 12, 1937, No. 9885/37/Oda; George Barns to the District Commissioner, Western Akim, March 10, 1934, Courtesy of the Public Records and Archives Administration Department, Accra, Ghana. ADM 36, Case No. WA 63/1920 "Fetish 1920–46."

Poisson, Jacques. "Procédé d'obtention de la tabersonine," Cameroonian Patent C07–03025, filed March 22, 1969, and issued December 15, 1970; Cites Belgian Patent 712841, issued March 27, 1968.

Poisson, Jacques. "Process of Obtaining Tabersonine." US Patent 3754478, filed July 16, 1971, and issued September 11, 1973.

Shamsu. "Very Interesting Seeds: An Experience with Voacanga africana." *Erowid* (website). August 4, 2005, http://www.erowid.org/exp/43102.

Solomon, Avi. "Interview: Dennis McKenna." *Boing Boing* (website). June 9, 2011. https://boingboing.net/.

Stapf. "Apocynaceae." 1894, 87–88; Dr. Otto Stapf, F.R.S. *Nature* 132 (1933): 305. https://doi.org/10.1038/132305a0.

Wasson, R. Gordon. "Seeking the Magic Mushroom." *Life Magazine*, May 13, 1957.

Secondary Sources

Agwu, A. Christopher. *A Philosophical Concept of Agwu in Igbo Land*. Bloomington, IN: Trafford Publishing, 2013.

Andermann, Jens. *Optic of the State: Visuality and Power in Argentina and Brazil*. Pittsburgh: University of Pittsburgh Press, 2007.

Aniegye Ntewusu, Samuel. "Labour, Religion and Madness: A Social History of Datura Spp. in Ghana." *Journal of Performing Arts* 5, no. 2 (2017): 39–40.

Appiah-Kubi, Kofi. *Man Cures God Heals: Religion and Medical Practice among the Akans of Ghana*. Totowa, NJ: Allanheld, Osmun, and Co. Publishers, 1981.

Barbieri, Marcello. "Biosemiotics: A New Understanding of Life." *Naturwissenschaften* 95, no. 7 (2008): 577–99.

Basavarajappa, Balapal S. "Cannabinoid Receptors and Their Signaling Mechanisms." In *The Endocannabinoid System*, 25–62. Cambridge, MA: Academic Press, 2017.

Beetje, Henk. "Review: A Revision of Tabernaemontana. The Old World Species by A. J. M. Leeuwenberg." *Kew Bulletin* 47, no. 3 (1992): 548.

Bisset, Norman. "Uses of Voacanga Species." *Agricultural University of Wageningen Papers* 85, no. 3 (1985): 116–122.

Boas, Franz. *The Mind of Primitive Man*. London: MacMillan, 1911.

Carrera, Juan. *La Otra Vida de María Sabina*. Mexico City: Universidad Autonoma del Estado de Mexico, 1986.

Ceraso, Antonio. "Entheogens and the Public Mystery: The Rhetoric of R. Gordon Wasson." *Configurations* 16 (2008): 215–243.

Chagnon, Napoleon, and Timothy Asch. *"New Tribes Mission" Yanomamö Series*. Watertown, MA: Documentary Educational Resources, 1975.

Chagnon, Napoleon, Philip Le Quesne, and James Cook. "Yanomamo Hallucinogens: Anthropological, Botanical, and Chemical Findings." *Current Anthropology* 12, no. 1 (1971): 72–74.

Cooper, Frederick. *Citizenship between Empire and Nation: Remaking France and French Africa, 1945–1960*. Princeton, NJ: Princeton University Press, 2014.

Davis, Wade. "Hallucinogenic Plants and Their Use in Traditional Societies—An Overview." *Cultural Survival Quarterly Magazine* 9, no. 4 (1985). https://www.culturalsurvival.org/publications/cultural-survival-quarterly/hallucinogenic-plants-and-their-use-traditional-societieseportedly.

Dawson, Alexander. *The Peyote Effect: From the Inquisition to the War on Drugs*. Oakland: University of California Press, 2018.

Dawson, Alexander. "Salvador Roquet, María Sabina, and the Trouble with Jipis." *Hispanic American Historical Review* 95, no. 1 (2015): 103–118.

Duvall, Christopher. *The African Roots of Marijuana*. Durham, NC: Duke University Press, 2019.

Dyck, Erika. *Psychedelic Psychiatry: LSD from Clinic to Campus*. Baltimore: Johns Hopkins University Press, 2008.

Ens, Andrea. "Silencing Indigenous Pasts: Critical Indigenous Theory and the History of Psychedelics." *International Journal of Qualitative Studies in Education* 34, no. 10 (2021): 904–914.

Feinberg, Benjamin. *The Devil's Book of Culture: History, Mushrooms, and Caves in Southern Mexico*. Austin: University of Texas Press, 2003.

Fortun, Kim. "From Latour to Late Industrialism." *Hau: Journal of Ethnographic Theory* 4 (2014): 309–329.

François-Sobiecki, Jean. "A Review of Plants Used in Divination in Southern Africa and Their Psychoactive Effects." *Southern African Humanities* 20 (2008): 333–351.

Frust, Peter. *Flesh of the Gods: The Ritual Use of Hallucinogens*. New York: Praeger Publications, 1972.

Goda, Yukihiro, Masumi Iwai, Ruri Kikura-Hanajir, Mariko Kitujima, Mitsuru Lida, and Hiromitsu Takayama. "Discovery of Indole Alkaloids with Cannabinoid CB1 Receptor Antagonistic Activity." *Bioorganic & Medicinal Chemistry Letters* 21, no. 7 (2011): 1962–1964.

Goda, Yukihiro, Ruri Kikura-Hanajir, Takuro Muruyama, and Akinori Miyashita. "Chemical and DNA Analyses for the Products of a Psychoactive Plant, Voacanga Africana." *Yakugaku Zasshi* 129, no. 8 (2009): 975–983.

Greene, Sandra. *Sacred Sites and the Colonial Encounter: A History of Meaning and Memory in Ghana.* Bloomington: Indiana University Press, 2002.

Idowa, E. Bolaji. *African Traditional Religion: A Definition.* Maryknoll, NY: Orbis Books, 1975.

Irvine, Frederick. *Woody Plants of Ghana: With Special Reference to Their Uses.* London: Oxford University Press, 1961.

Kohler, Robert. *Landscapes and Labscapes.* Chicago and London: University of Chicago Press, 2002.

Konadu, Kwasi. *Indigenous Medicine and Knowledge in African Society.* Abindgon: Routledge, 2007.

Kopenawa, Davi, and Bruce Albert. *The Falling Sky: Words of a Yanomami Shaman.* Cambridge, MA: Harvard University Press, 2013.

Laveaga, Gabriela. *Jungle Laboratories: Mexican Peasants, National Projects, and the Making of the Pill.* Durham, NC: Duke University Press, 2009.

Leary, Timothy. *Flashbacks: An Autobiography.* Los Angeles: Tereny P. Torcher, 1983.

Lewis, Stephen. "Indigenista Dreams Meet Sober Realities: The Slow Demise of Federal Indian Policy in Chiapas, Mexico, 1951–1970." *Latin American Perspectives: Rethinking Indigenismo on the American Continent* 39, no. 5 (2012): 63–79.

Mawere, Munyaradzi. *African Belief and Knowledge Systems: A Critical Perspective.* Mankon, Cameroon: Langaa Research and Publishing Common Initiative Group, 2011.

McKenna, Terence. *Food of the Gods: The Search for the Original Tree of Knowledge.* New York: Random House, 1993.

McKenna, Terence, Joan Halifax, Peter T. Furst, Albert Hofmann, and Richard Evans Schultes. *The Sacred Mushroom Seeker: Tributes to R. Gordon Wasson.* Rochester, NY: Inner Traditions, 1997.

Nnaemeka, Obioma. "Racialization and the Colonial Architecture: Othering and the Order of Things." *PMLA: Publications of the Modern Language Association of America* 123, no. 5 (2008): 1748–1751.

Osseo-Asare, Abena. *Bitter Roots: The Search for Healing Plants in Africa.* Chicago: University of Chicago Press, 2014.

Pichon, Marcel. "Classification of Apocynacees: VIII, The Voacanga of Africa." *Bulletin du Muséum national d'histoire naturelle* 14, no. 5 (1947): 409–410.

Rätsch, Christian. *The Encyclopedia of Psychoactive Plants: Ethnopharmacology and its Applications.* Translated by John R. Baker. Rochester, NY: Park Street Press, 2005.

Ravalec, V., Mallendi, and Agnès Paicheler. *Iboga: The Visionary Root of African Shamanism*. Rochester, VT: Park Street Press, 2007.

Rutherford, Danilyn. "Affect Theory and the Empirical." *Annual Review of Anthropology* 45 (2016): 285–300.

Said, Edward. *Orientalism*. New York: Pantheon Books, 1978.

Schlossberg, Pavel. "Heritage Practices, Indigenismo, and Coloniality: Studying-up into Racism in Contemporary Mexico." *Cultural Studies* 32, no. 3 (2018): 414–437.

Schuldes, Bert Marco. *Psychoaktive Pflanzen: Mehr ais 65 Pflanzen mit anregender, euphorisierender, beruhigender, sexuell erregender, oder halluzinogener Wirkung*. Lohrbach, Germany: Medienxperimente, 1995.

Schultes, Richard. *A Golden Guide: Hallucinogenic Plants*. Racine, WI: Western Publishing, 1976.

Scott-Elliot, George. "On the Botanical Results of the Sierra Leone Boundary Commission." *Botanical Journal of the Linnean Society*. London: Oxford University Press, 1894.

Scott-Elliot, George. *Stories of Savage Life*. London: Seeley, Service and Co., 1919.

Smet, P. A. G. M. De. "Some Ethnopharmacological Notes on African Hallucinogens." *Journal of Ethnopharmacology* 50 (1996): 144–145.

Stapf, Otto. *"Apocynaceae," Botanical Journal of the Linnean Society*. London: Oxford University Press, 1894.

Stevens, Jay. *Storming Heaven: LSD and the American Dream*. New York: Perennial Library, 1998.

Sweet, James. *Domingos Álvares: African Healing, and the Intellectual History of the Atlantic World*. Durham, NC: University of North Carolina Press, 2011.

Val, E. Franz. G. *Conversaciones con María Sabina y otros curanderos*. Patriotismo, Mexico: Publicaciones Cruz O.S.A, 1996.

Vilgiate, Timothy. "Forestry and the 'World on Paper': Ideas of Science and Resistance to Forest Reservation on the Gold Coast in the Early Twentieth Century." *Ghana Studies* 23 (2020): 3–27.

Wasson, R. Gordon, and Valentina Wasson. *Mushrooms, Russia, and History*. New York: Pantheon Books, 1957.

Yang, Li, Kui-Shan Wen, Xiao Ruan, Ying-Xian Zhao, Feng Wei, and Qiang Wang. "Response of Plant Secondary Metabolites to Environmental Factors." *Molecules* 23, no. 4 (2018): 762.

8 FROM BWITI TO IBOGAINE AND BACK: A TRANSNATIONAL HISTORY OF *TABERNANTHE IBOGA*

Julien Bonhomme

In 2007, ibogaine was added to the list of illegal narcotics in France "due to its hallucinogenic properties and its high level of toxicity," according to the conclusions of the Ministry of Health. This decision followed the suspicious death of a young man who had taken ibogaine during a "detoxification program" run by an organization that was also providing personal development courses. *Tabernanthe iboga* is a shrub from the Apocynaceae family, and its roots have been used for centuries in Bwiti, a Gabonese initiation ritual. From the 1990s onward, ibogaine became increasingly popular in France and across Europe and the Americas, and it was consumed as part of courses and detox programs often inspired by Bwiti practices. This plant, originally from Africa, subsequently drew the attention of the French Agency for the Safety of Health Products, as well as the Interministerial Mission for Vigilance and Combating Sectarian Aberrations. Merely two years after ayahuasca was banned, the French prohibition of ibogaine occurred in the context of public policies surrounding "drugs" and the consumption of psychotropic substances, "cults" and new religious movements, "alternative therapies," and illegal medicine. Moreover, ibogaine's prohibition was proof that a growing segment of the population was drawn to these psychoactive plants and the religious traditions with which they were associated.

In what context and conceptual framework did these new uses of ibogaine emerge? To answer this question, this chapter compares Western uses of ibogaine with its ritual uses in Gabon. However, this comparative approach does not imply a great divide between "us" and "them." African initiation rituals have had a significant and direct influence on both European and American ibogaine consumption. The rise of transnational networks allowed stakeholders, substances, concepts, and uses to circulate among Africa, Europe, and the Americas. However, the mediation carried out by American, European, and African cultural brokers also involved a process of intercultural translation. A series of reinterpretations took place in the Euro-American adaptation of ibogaine, as well as "working misunderstandings," to use the anthropologist Marshall Sahlins' concept.[1] For instance, American treatments focus on ibogaine, the chemical molecule, and its psychoactive properties, whereas in Gabon, the emphasis is placed on the iboga root itself, the plant in its natural state.[2] This chapter, therefore, explores the liminal nature of the cultural practices that lie at the heart of Western uses of ibogaine.

A DRUG TO END DRUG ABUSE?

In 1889, the botanist Henri Baillon identified *Tabernanthe iboga* thanks to a Navy doctor, Marie-Théophile Griffon du Bellay, who brought a sample from Gabon. This identification paved the way for pharmacological studies on the plant in Europe, and its main alkaloid, ibogaine, was isolated in 1901. In 1939, an ibogaine-based drug was commercialized in France under the name Lambaréné, as a tribute to Dr. Albert Schweitzer, the main figure of colonial medicine in French Equatorial Africa, and his hospital in Lambaréné, Gabon. The drug was sold as a tonic: although high doses of ibogaine cause hallucinations, smaller amounts have an energizing effect. Lambaréné was classified as a doping agent following reports of athletes using it, and it was discontinued in the late 1960s.

Against this backdrop, a seminal event considerably rekindled interest in ibogaine around the world. In 1962, a young American heroin addict by the name of Howard Lotsof was given some ibogaine by a chemist friend. After a long trip, he woke up feeling fantastic and realized that his urge to take heroin had vanished. The baffled Lotsof then tested ibogaine on his addict friends, and the results were just as striking. In the subsequent decades, he became a vocal proponent of ibogaine and its apparent antiaddictive

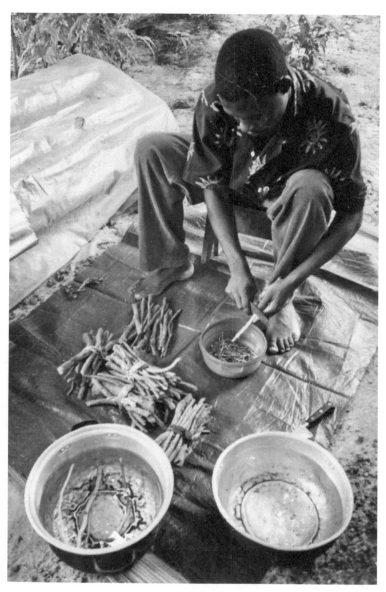

Figure 8.1
Scraping bark from iboga roots in preparation for an initiation in Estuaire Province, Gabon,
2001. Photo: Julien Bonhomme.

properties. This is how ibogaine came to join the postwar drug scene, albeit in an unexpected way—as a drug that actually could end drug addiction.

To demonstrate ibogaine's potential to interrupt addiction, Lotsof sought help from scientists. He turned to the National Institute on Drug Abuse (NIDA), as well as several pharmaceutical companies, but they did not share his enthusiasm. By the late 1960s, ibogaine had been banned in the US, and the World Health Organization (WHO) had classified it as a narcotic. Nonetheless, Lotsof managed to convince pharmacologists and doctors in the US and Europe to study the effects of this alkaloid. He also realized its economic potential; in the 1980s, he filed several patents for the therapeutic use of ibogaine and created NDA International, a for-profit company that marketed its ibogaine-based drug Endabuse. In 1987, he convened an international symposium on ibogaine in Paris, which brought together scientists from various fields, including Otto Gollnhofer, a French ethnologist working on Bwiti ceremonies in Gabon. The same year, Lotsof traveled to Gabon and met President Omar Bongo and one of his scientific advisers, Professor Jean-Noël Gassita, a pharmacologist, pharmacist, and vocal proponent of ibogaine. The Gabonese president then allegedly offered him several kilograms of iboga roots as a "gift from Gabon to America and the world," but subsequently classified the plant as part of the country's national heritage and prohibited its export to ensure that foreign companies would not profit from it at the expense of the country.[3]

To investigate ibogaine's therapeutic potential, clinical trials required prior experimentation on animals, and rats were used to study the biochemical effects of ibogaine on the brain receptors involved in addiction. Scientific researchers working on ibogaine did not investigate the molecule's hallucinogenic properties—indeed, it would not have been possible to examine the visionary dimension of the experience in animals. Instead, they developed a synthetic alkaloid derived from ibogaine and devoid of hallucinogenic effects. Therefore, the coalition between scientists specialized in experimentation on animals and recovered addicts eulogizing ibogaine was flawed on a most basic level. The former were interested in the biochemical effects of the molecule, while the latter emphasized the therapeutic effect of the visions. This opposition reproduced a uniquely Western dichotomy regarding the understanding of psychotropic drugs: the distinction between physical dependence and psychological dependence, which, in the field of drug addiction, reflects the opposition between body and mind—the cornerstone of modern Western naturalism.

In the mid-1990s, the NIDA-driven research was abandoned for scientific, financial, and ideological reasons. Nevertheless, former addicts continued to promote ibogaine's supposed efficacy as an addiction interrupter. They challenged the scientific monopoly on truth by setting themselves up as experts following the user community model. Organizations such as International Addict Self-Help (INTASH) and International Coalition for Addict Self-Help (ICASH) were founded, while treatment centers opened all over the world. These "ibogaine clinics" did not necessarily operate illegally because the drug was still authorized in some countries. To work around the US ban, these centers were housed in neighboring countries. For instance, Lotsof opened one in Panama in 1994, while others were created in St. Kitts, Mexico, and Canada, but also in European countries such as the Netherlands, France, Britain, Italy, and Slovenia.

The treatments were designed to address both psychological and physical dependence. Ibogaine could stop the physical symptoms of withdrawal and therefore facilitate weaning, especially in the case of opiate addiction. However, across all research protocols, visions occupied a central place in the therapeutic rationale; it was not just a chemical-based treatment, but rather a psychological and spiritual therapy as well. For instance, the St. Kitts center was named "Healing Visions." Hence, ibogaine advocates rejected the pejorative word "hallucinogen" in favor of "psychedelic" (for the same reason, they preferred "vision" to "hallucination"). From their perspective, ibogaine was a powerful mind-revealer (per the etymology of the word "psychedelic") and this emphasis on the psychotherapeutic power of visions became a key feature in Euro-American ibogaine use.

These ibogaine-based therapies emerged in the wake of narcoanalysis, a form of psychotherapy using psychoactive substances as adjuncts. Narcoanalysis came into being in the first half of the twentieth century and experienced renewed interest after World War II, following the discovery of LSD by the Swiss chemist Albert Hofmann. The influence of the American counterculture on psychotherapy in the 1960s also contributed to this enthusiasm. Psychoactive substances were administered in varying doses depending on the protocols used and were designed to access the patient's unconscious self. These drugs were catalysts for the psychotherapeutic process, and they significantly shortened the treatment period compared to traditional analytical approaches.[4] Various psychotropic drugs were used—LSD, amphetamines, mescaline, and harmaline, but also ibogaine, which the Chilean psychiatrist Claudio Naranjo had been using to treat his patients since the 1960s. The ibogaine clinics opening in the 1990s followed the narcoanalysis model, and ibogaine became an adjunct to analytical introspection or, in higher doses, allowed someone to relive repressed trauma in the form of cathartic abreaction. According to Lotsof, "It is like going through ten years of psychoanalysis in three days," a catchphrase that was originally created for LSD-based therapies and then was taken up by ibogaine enthusiasts everywhere.

New Age culture, to which narcoanalysis was partly linked, also played a part in the development of ibogaine-based therapies. Indeed, the notion of "personal development," embodied by a transformation of the individual through the awakening of the mind and the expansion of consciousness, greatly appealed to New Agers. This was a decidedly optimistic view of human beings, who were deemed capable of achieving self-mastery through self-improvement. New Age culture operated at the crossroads of psychotherapy and religion, and it was driven by "spirituality," which gave primacy to personal experience over the authority of established religion. One of the recurring features of these spiritual experiences, which borrowed heavily from Christian and Eastern mystical traditions, was the feeling of "cosmic harmony" that many ibogaine users reported having experienced. New Age spirituality was based on a "holistic" understanding of human beings that emphasized a body-mind-spirit trinity. These three dimensions were seen as inseparable—hence the criticism leveled at biomedicine, which was accused of treating only the body at the expense of the mind. This holistic trinity was a central feature of ibogaine-based therapies: a low dose could alleviate physical dependence; a medium dose could favor psychological exploration of personal problems; and a strong dose typically led to a spiritual experience that radically transformed the patient's life.

New Age spirituality was fascinated by non-Western traditions and freely borrowed from Indigenous shamanism by scholars and authors who were highly controversial in their own academic fields, but widely referenced in New Age circles. These included Mircea Eliade and his work on the archaic techniques of ecstasy; Carlos Castañeda on peyote use in Mexico; and Michael Harner and Jeremy Narby on ayahuasca in the Amazon. Such reinterpretations of Indigenous shamanism gave birth to what is colloquially known as "neo-shamanism," in which hallucinogenic plants occupy a central role. A controversial hypothesis defended by scholars such as Weston La Barre and R. Gordon Wasson suggested that these plants formed the basis of a paleolithic brand of shamanism upon which all prehistoric human religions were based. The consumption of these "entheogenic" substances ("which generate the divine within") could therefore offer Westerners access to a spiritual experience they deemed "authentic" due to its "primitive" nature. This visionary experience was said to have the power to "open the doors of perception," to use Aldous Huxley's phrase, by removing the blinkers imposed by modern civilization and revealing the world as it really was.[5] In 1999, against this backdrop, a new religious movement called Sakrament Prehoda (Sacrament of Transition) was officially registered in Slovenia. This movement treated ibogaine as a holy sacrament and taught followers that Jesus had eaten a mixture of ibogaine, cannabis, and wild rue (*Peganum harmala*) during the Last Supper.

Within these networks, New Agers were free to devise their own spiritual toolkits through readings, conferences, personal development courses, and websites. By the end of the 1990s, the Internet had indeed become a critical site for the globalized market for modern spirituality, and the international enthusiasm for ibogaine therefore owes a great deal to the proliferation of websites promoting its mind-altering properties—there were already several dozen by the 2000s. These sites provided information on ibogaine, along with reports of experiences, and most of them also offered access to ibogaine-based treatment or initiation rituals. They were often translated into several languages (one even featured an Esperanto version) and referenced each other with hyperlinks. In this way, a virtual ibogaine community was allowed to flourish, enabling the creation and circulation of beliefs and theories associated with its use. Those interested in ibogaine could tap into this New Age–inspired common trove mixing references to Bwiti, Native American shamanisms, the Tibetan *Book of the Dead*, and Indian chakras in order to make sense of their own visionary experiences.

THE GABONESE CONNECTIONS

Upon discovering ibogaine in the 1960s, Lotsof remained unaware of the plant's history in African initiation rites. It was more recently that ibogaine enthusiasts learned from the anthropological literature on its ritual use. Having carried out ethnographic fieldwork in Gabon just before its independence in 1960, the American anthropologist James Fernandez published a chapter entitled "*Tabernanthe Iboga*: Narcotic Ecstasis and the Work of the Ancestors" in a 1972 book on the ritual uses of psychedelics across the world. Fernandez's chapter was widely read by Western ibogaine users. Various writers discussed Bwiti from the mid-1960s onward, including Otto Gollnhofer and Roger Sillans in France and Stanisław Świderski in Canada. Hence, professional anthropologists played an important role in adapting Bwiti and ibogaine to the Euro-American context, as was also the case with other hallucinogenic substances and religious traditions from Central and South America.[6]

Upon returning from their trip to Gabon, Lotsof and his colleague Bob Sisko delved into the literature on Bwiti and decided to integrate a ritual dimension into their therapeutic model, and in the process, they drew a much clearer line between themselves and the pharmacologists working on ibogaine. Sisko reinterpreted his own experience with ibogaine as an encounter with Bwiti and prophesized: "Bwiti will be alive in thousands of junkies and crackheads."[7] Almost every treatment center adopted this Bwiti-informed ritual approach to therapy, and this reinforced the spiritual component of the ibogaine experience. The attention to the set and setting was a recurring concern in the psychedelic movement, which sought to design supportive frameworks for hallucinogenic experiences by paying close attention to the environmental circumstances and the attitude of the user. This approach was part of a critique of the medicalization of the therapeutic model, as illustrated by Nico Adriaans, who was involved in the Dutch scene:

"I don't believe in clinical settings. We should keep the ritual involved with it"[8]—never mind that the borrowing from Bwiti was often imprecise or tenuous. In one of the Dutch groups, the protocol was described as follows:

> We'd introduce ourselves as Momma and Poppa Iboga, because the addict is the child going through re-birth. We'd tell them about the African ritual the night before the treatment so that they'd totally know what they were going to face. We'd tell them the Africans use it basically to guide people into adulthood so they become more responsible people, and that's what we'd be doing. Making a person more responsible in life, so that he'd have control over drugs instead of drugs over the person.[9]

This introductory discourse was followed by the symbolic destruction of paraphernalia such as syringes and spoons. In the room where treatment took place, there were two doors bearing images of the Moon and the Sun, omnipresent symbols in Gabonese Bwiti rituals. The addition of this African element to ibogaine-based treatments drew the attention of African American associations such as the Black Coalition on Drugs and the African Descendants Awareness Movement, who were eager to bring together the quest for healing and the search for ancestral roots.

The discovery of Bwiti by ibogaine advocates created new connections within transnational ibogaine networks. In addition to the groups that had grown out of American psychedelia, a French-Gabonese network emerged. Its key cultural brokers were French people living in Africa who were initiated into Bwiti by Gabonese guides (locally referred to as "initiators" or "fathers of initiation"). By becoming facilitators themselves, they attracted new Western recruits, who were overwhelmingly white. In the 2000s, the most famous of these guides was Tatayo, a French man initiated into Bwiti in 1979. The first initiation of a European into Bwiti probably goes back to colonial times—Gabon was a French colony until 1960. However, it was only in the 1980s and 1990s that the global phenomenon gained momentum due to Bwiti opening up to outsiders and expanding into urban areas. Hitherto, the cult had remained very closed and secretive, and even clandestine during the colonial period because of animosity from the missionaries and a hostile administration.[10]

The first generation of French converts initially discovered Bwiti in Gabon, and it was only later that they were exposed to American and Dutch ideas regarding the antiaddictive properties of ibogaine, particularly through the Internet. In the 2000s, the two networks nevertheless converged to a large extent, as evidenced by the overlapping of concepts, and occasionally of practices, as well as the way that individuals facilitated these connections between one setting and the other. Several initiation sites were created in France and Gabon (and to a lesser extent in Cameroon and Equatorial Guinea), and these new locations were advertised on various websites. It is worth noting that they all highlighted the antiaddictive properties of ibogaine. The guides included French people who were living or had lived in Gabon, as well as Gabonese individuals in their own country or in France. Indeed, a number of Gabonese facilitators quickly realized the benefits, both symbolic and material, that they could reap from this ibogaine-initiation tourism. It was not uncommon for French and Gabonese guides to practice Bwiti in tandem: the former sought potential recruits in France, Europe, and the Americas, while the latter conducted the ceremonies, thus giving the rituals a feeling of African authenticity. These Gabonese and French guides set up elaborate networks to accompany clients from their arrival at Gabon's Libreville International Airport to the villages in the hinterland, where they would undergo initiation.[11]

With the incorporation of Bwiti, ibogaine-based therapy reestablished a connection with Africa that had been lacking in the initial American and Dutch experiments. This relationship was the case for clients traveling to Gabon to be initiated, where they participated in ceremonies of great aesthetic and emotional intensity, with music, songs, and dances. However, this was also the case for patients taking ibogaine in a more neutral setting. For example, one drug addict received ibogaine treatment in an anonymous room in an Amsterdam hotel in 1989. During the experience, he heard African drums, walked through the heart of the equatorial forest, and met a Pygmy. After his experience, he said that he felt deeply connected to Africa and Africans. These visions of a largely romanticized continent echoed the images of the "White world" that often populated the visions of Gabonese initiates. The visionary experience revealed a desire for otherness and was based on racialized fantasies as much for European and American patients as it was for Gabonese initiates.

HEALING QUESTS

To put Euro-American uses of ibogaine into perspective, the role of visions in Gabonese Bwiti rituals cannot be ignored. This role has varied throughout the ritual's history and in its various forms. *Disumba*, the original form of Bwiti, (or, at least, the oldest known), comes from the Mitsogo, an ethnolinguistic group living in the Chaillu Mountains in southern Gabon. In the 1860s, when Paul Belloni du Chaillu first explored the mountain range that bears his name today, Bwiti *Disumba* was already well established in the region, as remains the case. Initiation served as a rite of passage into adulthood for men. During initiation, the novice, or *banzi*, consumed bark from the iboga root in large quantities. Iboga's extremely bitter taste and its emetic properties made this a grueling ordeal (one of the main reasons why the plant was not used as a recreational drug). A mirror was sometimes used to enhance the visions, with the initiates examining their reflections throughout the night to see various images appear within. To avoid any problems, the guides watched the participants' reactions carefully—looking in particular for vomiting, loss of consciousness, ataxia, or anesthesia.

Iboga was supposed to help the initiate travel to the land of the ancestors to meet the mythical beings present in Tsogo cosmology such as Kombe, the Sun, his wife, Ngonde, the Moon, and the first Mother, Disumba. The experience was intended as a kind of temporary death. The visions were meant to follow a similar pattern for all initiates, who followed in the footsteps of their elders and saw for themselves the truth of the religious knowledge inherited from the ancestors. This homogenization of visions was enhanced by the theatrics surrounding the ritual (scenes from mythology were sometimes played out in front of the initiates using wooden figurines), and also by the way guides reinterpreted the visions after the experience. These rites of passage followed the template of traditional Bwiti visions, and any extraneous elements were considered insignificant. The initiation rituals constrained the iboga visions; the structure of the ritual allowed initiates to connect their personal experiences to a collective mythology. However, most of the initiatory knowledge came not directly from the visions, but from the elders, who controlled access to this knowledge and shared it sparingly during the years following the initiation. Indeed, a career in Bwiti lasts well beyond the rites of passage: it continues for years and involves several initiatory grades, as well as the never-ending learning of religious knowledge.

At the beginning of the twentieth century, the Fang, Gabon's main ethnic group, adopted Bwiti from the Mitsogo when the two groups made contact at logging sites in the center of the country.[12] Under the influence of missionary evangelism, they turned it into a syncretic religion that combined visions of the ancestors and encounters with Christian heroes—particularly Jesus Christ, the Virgin Mary, and Saint Michael.[13] The visionary experience became a window into a future paradise. A central feature of Fang Bwiti was an easing of the constraints of initiatory teachings in favor of prophetic revelations. Initiatory knowledge, which had hitherto been strictly controlled, became a more personal form of mystical knowledge, which led to the emergence of many chapels of Bwiti revolving around minor prophets. In the second half of the century, Fang Bwiti merged with Ombwiri, a possession cult that originated among the Myene-speaking people living along Gabon's coast. Iboga visions were then used to uncover the origins of personal misfortune. The quest for salvation and the quest for healing became intimately connected.

A move toward a more therapeutic approach was also found in Bwiti Misoko, another variation of the initiation ritual, which originated in southern Gabon. It spread exponentially across most of the country from the 1990s onward, particularly in suburban areas.[14] It was mainly carried out by *nganga*, specialists in traditional medicine who acted both as diviner-healers and guides. The Bwiti Misoko initiation ritual was aimed at guarding against illness, misfortune, and witchcraft.[15] As initiates turned to iboga to solve their problems, the visions became increasingly personal, as they closely mirrored the individual's personal experience. However, individuals' accounts of their visions remained somewhat homogenous: they focused on discovering the root of their misfortune and identifying the witch or witches who may be responsible. This realization was followed by a deliverance, generally involving imaginary reprisals against the persecutors. The vision was a

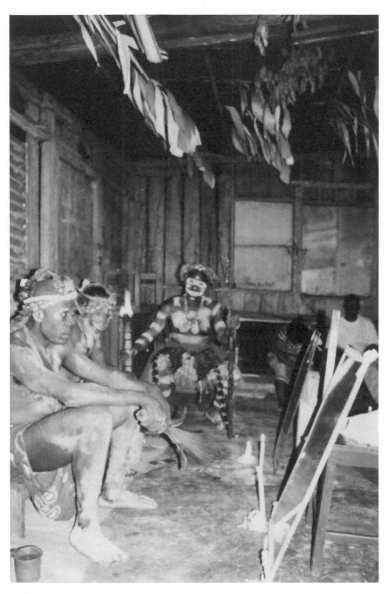

Figure 8.2
Initiation to Bwiti Misoko in Estuaire Province, Gabon, 2001. Thanks to iboga, the two men see visions in the mirror. Photo: Julien Bonhomme.

dramatization of the unfortunate event and the precipitating social conflict. Compared to Bwiti Disumba or even Fang Bwiti, Bwiti Misoko was thus characterized by more personal visions, which were used to solve problems.

Over the past century, Bwiti transformed the role of iboga visions in initiation rituals. These visions were increasingly disconnected from the idea of initiatory knowledge controlled by male elders, allowing a personal quest for mystical knowledge. Within this more individualized approach emerged a "therapeutization" of the rituals, where visions became part of a quest to alleviate illness and misfortune. From its origins among the Mitsogo, for whom it was a way of seeking out ancestral encounters, Bwiti became a quest for salvation in Fang syncretism, and subsequently a quest for healing in Misoko. These transformations within Gabonese Bwiti were instrumental in the Western adaptation of ibogaine use. Instances of the latter did not involve any major departure from contemporary iboga use in Bwiti; on the contrary, it was an extension of these practices. It is no coincidence that the first generation of Europeans to discover Bwiti were initiated by the Fang rather than the Mitsogo, and the nganga of the Misoko took over in more recent decades: because of their spiritual and healing orientation, these versions of the initiation ritual were more in tune with a Western audience than the Bwiti Disumba as it was (and still is) practiced among the Mitsogo. In Europe and the Americas, ibogaine was used to pursue a spiritual journey that made a strong connection between the quest for healing and the quest for oneself: it was about curing addiction, but above all, it was about "finding yourself"—the well-known personal growth mantra.

There are significant connections between Gabonese Bwiti rituals and Western treatments. As one of the websites promoting Bwiti to a European audience stated: "For years, we Europeans and Africans who took the Iboga trip had come to the conclusion that the Bwiti sect, whether Mitsogo or Fang, syncretic or not, was designed to care for the spirit in ways which perpetually readapted to the new mythological imaginaries born out of cultural encounters." [16] Notions of rebirth and purification, which were ubiquitous in Bwiti initiation rituals, were also used in European and American therapies. The ibogaine ordeal was often compared to a "near-death experience." Detoxification programs justified a therapeutic perspective, the idea being that the addict should die in order to be reborn, free from addiction. Facilitators used puns to highlight this idea of rebirth through ibogaine: "I am BOrn aGAin" or "IBEGIN AGAIN." James and Renate Fernandez[17] note that the initiation ritual metaphor of disoriented individuals who "find their way" with the help of iboga visions was also very much in keeping with the spirit of European and American therapies. The visionary experience gave hope for the future and allowed individuals to undergo spiritual rebirth.

The idea of meeting ancestors during initiation rituals was also reinterpreted and integrated into Western therapies. Ibogaine was thought to allow access to one's own subconscious, but also to "genetic ancestral memory." According to one user, "you gain access to the information contained in your individual hereditary archive: you meet your ancestors."[18] "Ibogaine turns the serotoninergic and cholinergic pathways into a super-augmented, stereoscopic entity, capable of scanning ancestral memory in the non-nucleated genetic material of your cells: the ancestors," write Paul De Rienzo and Dana Beal in their 1997 study of Ibogaine use in Staten Island, New York.[19] According to Geerte Frenken, a Dutch ibogaine enthusiast, the visionary experience offered "a journey into one's DNA." This pseudoscientific view of the hallucinogenic experience, popularized by the Canadian anthropologist Jeremy Narby, was inspired by Jungian speculations on the universal unconscious and reinterpreted through the lens of genetic biology. The recycling of the idea of ancestors in Euro-American approaches to the hallucinogenic experience belied a trait typical of New Age culture—namely, combining scientific and primitivist fantasies.

By skillfully playing on these connections, Gabonese guides from transnational Bwiti networks adapted their discourse and practices to suit the expectations of their new European and American clients. This process was facilitated by the import of European esotericism and New Age culture in Africa. The writings of Atome Ribenga,[20] a specialist in Fang Bwiti who was in the public eye and who initiated a number of Europeans in Gabon, epitomizes this adaptation. In Gabon's urban and intellectual circles, the influence of these ideas was already decades old. For instance, in a book published in 1952, "Prince" Birinda, a Gabonese man who had rubbed shoulders with the French surrealists, highlighted the crossovers between occultism and Bwiti, viewing the latter as the "Secret Bible of Black People."[21]

A typical Gabonese facilitator in the early 2000s was Mallendi, a young *nganga* man married to a Frenchwoman and living in France, where he used his talents as a guide until ibogaine was officially banned. In 2004, along with the writer Vincent Ravalec, Mallendi coauthored one of the first books to promote ibogaine to a wider French audience. He thought of himself as a "Whiteologist" (*blancologue*);[22] with this humorous title, he assumed his status as a facilitator for white people. His success resided in his understanding of their culture and expectations. He molded his approach to fit the framework of Western psychotherapy, taking up Lotsof's credo word for word: "In three days, someone can achieve the equivalent of several years of psychoanalysis."[23] He also highlighted the spiritual dimension provided by the African initiation ritual: "Western treatments with ibogaine are limited to physical detoxification, whereas the iboga root and everything that goes with it brings about psychological detoxification by allowing the addict to understand the life events that have led them to take drugs."[24] While the American and Dutch networks were mainly interested in ibogaine, the French-Gabonese networks placed the emphasis on the iboga root, highlighting the value of the plant in its natural state rather than the isolated chemical molecule. This reordering of plants and chemicals also reestablished the hierarchy between body and spirit that lies at the heart of New Age culture. The insistence on the iboga root rather than ibogaine also meant that therapies could be associated with an exotic religious tradition, Bwiti, and with a natural environment, the equatorial forest, as well as the primitivist fantasy that was associated with them. In fact, the Pygmies, the first inhabitants of the equatorial forest before the arrival of the Bantu people, were thought to have discovered the iboga root and laid the foundations for Bwiti rituals.[25] According to the promoters of iboga, eating the plant therefore could be compared to coming back to the "cradle of humanity."

BLACK AND WHITE VISIONS

Although iboga visions were central to Bwiti's success with Westerners, visions were also the source of some divergence between Gabonese rituals and Western detoxification programs. In Western therapies, the entire focus was on taking ibogaine and experiencing visions. This "accelerated psycho-analysis" took place over a much shorter time period than initiation rituals. In Bwiti rituals, visions were only the first step in a journey that could take years to complete. The iboga visions remained secondary to the elders' religious knowledge. Initiation rituals reasserted the elders' authority over the initiates, whereas in Western detoxification programs, the patients had more leeway to make sense of their own personal experiences.

An emphasis on personal visions went hand in hand with the focus on iboga itself. Western programs cut out initiatory teaching, thus placing the plant at the heart of mystical knowledge. This emphasis on the plant led to Bwiti, a ritual tradition managed by a community, being put aside in favor of the "sacred wood," the name often given to the iboga root in Gabon. This shift in priorities is reflected in the titles of various publications; while the scholarship of professional anthropologists refers to Bwiti, promotional material intended for the general public refers to iboga.[26] Tellingly, the authors write about iboga initiation, not Bwiti initiation. The plant is personified as though it has agency: the visions are a vehicle for the wisdom of Iboga (the word is often capitalized to emphasize the personification).[27] In Gabon, however, iboga was merely a mouthpiece for Bwiti. It was not the plant that spoke to the initiates, but Bwiti—in other words, the ancestors. The worshipping of the substance was typical of Western views surrounding psychotropic drugs. The idea was also shared by opponents of ibogaine: the president of the Psychothérapie Vigilance association, for example, charged that ibogaine and ayahuasca encouraged sectarian aberrations, thus positing a strong correlation between natural substances and a form of socioreligious organization.[28]

In Bwiti, visions were shared with guides, as they were messages that concerned the whole community. Initiates made public declarations and guides intervened to manage the initiates' visions. In European and American detoxification programs, however, therapists intervened as little as possible; the vision was seen as an intimate experience requiring introspective contemplation by the patient. This difference in the way that visions were managed may have been the source of cultural misunderstandings. For example, an American journalist who traveled to Gabon to be initiated recounted his discomfort with his guide's intrusive attitude: "The Bwiti insisted I should relate my visions out loud. I was not prepared for that. I had expected whatever I saw to be my own concern. But the Bwiti didn't sympathize with my ideas about privacy. 'Everything you see must be shared,' the king urged. 'You might have a message for the tribe'."[29] To satisfy these new clients who were reluctant to endure "an outdated discipline and hierarchy," some facilitators put forward a form of Bwiti "without prohibitions and without obligations"—one very different from traditional initiation rituals.

Bwiti initiation made the new initiate a member of the community. The metaphor of spiritual kinship highlighted this affiliation: the guide became the initiate's "father." The initiated people became his older brothers. He was required to treat them all with respect and to obey them. The initiatory tradition reproduced social hierarchies largely based on gender and age. Conversely, Western therapies did not require any lasting community involvement—hence the absurdity of the accusations of sectarian aberration made against them. Although they may have been convinced of the miraculous benefits of ibogaine, European and American users were clients rather than followers: only a handful of individuals made the effort to commit to Bwiti for the long term.

In New Age parlance, Bwiti was sometimes described as "African shamanism," a concept, however, that is little used in anthropology in reference to African religious traditions. New World hallucinogen-based shamanism—particularly traditions involving ayahuasca, peyote, and psilocybin mushrooms—became part of transnational religious movements earlier than in the case of iboga.[30] It was this model upon which the reinterpretation of Bwiti was based, as illustrated in the 2008 book by Jan Kounen, Jeremy Narby, and Vincent Ravalec on shamanism, ayahuasca, and ibogaine.[31] Before trying ibogaine, many Westerners had already experienced ayahuasca in a shamanic setting, whether in the Amazon or elsewhere. Westerners approached shamanism exclusively from the perspective of the shaman's spiritual experience rather than as an institution with specific rituals. This—misguided—approach to shamanism was therefore better suited to Western individualism. African initiation, on the other hand, was an extremely hierarchical institution where authority and dependence in relationships were expressed more bluntly (as can be seen in initiatory hazing, a common feature in initiation rituals in Gabon, as elsewhere). "Shamanism" thus served as a way of interpreting Bwiti while excising the social connections surrounding the ritual.

These differences between Gabonese Bwiti and Euro-American detoxification programs also had an impact on the content of the visions. Western programs, with their emphasis on psychotherapy, focused on the idiosyncratic nature of the visions. Like dreams, visions emanated from the individual, and yet they were always expressed in a fantasy world shaped by culture. European and American users' visions were therefore shaped by culture just as much as the visions of Gabonese initiates. In Western detoxification programs, ibogaine visions centered around a form of "regression": "You will relive your childhood experiences to get to the root of your addictions." The parent-child relationship was central to the experience, in line with the triangular nuclear family blueprint that Western psychoanalysis has placed at the heart of personal destiny. Its corresponding visionary experience was seen as an "inner journey" into one's own memory. This idea was a departure from Gabonese Bwiti rituals: Bwiti Misoko initiates did not evoke childhood memories involving their parents; instead, they used iboga to find out what their relatives may have been plotting against them using witchcraft. The visions experienced by Gabonese initiates almost always revolved around the ties between kinship and witchcraft. While not entirely absent, persecution through witchcraft was a minor theme in the visions of European and American users, who instead placed the emphasis on self-reflection. It was all about "reconnecting with yourself," "finding yourself," or "becoming yourself."

This introspection was facilitated by the reflexive duplication typical of the hallucinogenic experience: the patients could observe themselves from the outside. This view enabled them to reassess the past behaviors that had led them down the path of addiction; a process of self-examination that "[led] them to understand their addiction and [showed] them a way out of it." It offered them "the opportunity to rechoose each decision" in order to overcome the problems ensnaring them. [32] This narrative emphasized personal autonomy, an idea at the heart of Western individualism. Ibogaine visions allowed patients to reclaim the agency that addiction had taken from them, in a context where drug abuse was seen as an illness affecting free will.

The same image appeared time and again in European and American patients' visions: the introspective examination was compared to rebooting a hard drive. Ibogaine appeared to reset the brain's memory. As Ravalec and colleagues (2004) put it, "To use a computer analogy, ibogaine clears your memories by showing them to you so that you can gain a better understanding of yourself."[33] As another user recalled, "A powerful cleansing was taking place throughout my whole system. . . . I compare the sensation to a 'defrag of the hard drive.' Any memories of experiences stored in my brain that were incomplete or stuck in some way were being systematically cleared out."[34] The idea, according to De Rienzo and Beal (1997), was to "reboot the consciousness patterns with a new autoexec.bat file for habits, needs, and desires."[35] The following, from a Frenchman who took ibogaine alone, is one of the most eloquent accounts:

> Something which looked a lot like a Windows 98 explorer appeared in my field of vision, with the entire contents and structure of the hard drive accessible on the left, every last detail. On the right-hand side of the screen was a section where I could see the contents of any folder or file I chose in detail, and at the bottom on the right was a kind of hole which symbolized the recycle bin. This virtual hard drive—that was me, my entire history and memories, all of my consciousness and subconsciousness, my thoughts, feelings, emotions, pain, and joy, all my trauma. Absolutely everything that had happened to me from the beginning of my life up until that moment could be accessed from the explorer. I could navigate around my own internal structure and click on any file to examine its contents. I could visualize it on the right-hand side of the screen whenever I wanted, really feel it, analyze the material and emotional content, observe and understand the ramifications, and what it meant for the genesis of my character and my current psychological state. Not only could I read all of this information, but what's more, I could do whatever I wanted with it once I had looked at it, experienced it, analyzed, and dissected it. I could keep it intact or change it as I pleased, delete it by dragging it toward the recycle bin, change the order by modifying the structure of the hard drive, reorganize the tree view and folders. I basically had access to absolutely everything, including

the most fundamental, hidden system files, and I could do whatever I wanted with them. And that is exactly what I did throughout this whole endless episode: I completely reorganized and updated my entire neuronal hard drive. It was an amazing feeling, at that moment it was like being my own creator, my own sculptor, my own progenitor in a way.[36]

As this account shows, the computer metaphor fed into an autopoietic fantasy: ibogaine visions allowed individuals to see through themselves and re-create themselves as they desired in order to overcome their existential problems. While the Gabonese initiates' mirror reflected the images of mythical ancestors or relatives practicing witchcraft, the computers of the Euro-American patients served as mirror-images of themselves. Gabonese initiation rites and Western detoxification programs both used ibogaine; yet these two cultural settings diverged in the content and purpose of the visionary experience. Ultimately, from initiatory knowledge to modern spirituality, from witch doctors to personal development, from mythical ancestors to DNA, a whole series of connections, reinterpretations, and adaptations made it possible for ibogaine to be accepted in the West and gave rise to a form of transnational Bwiti, with links to Africa, Europe, and the Americas.

NOTES

This chapter is a translated and updated version of a paper originally published as Julien Bonhomme, "Les ancêtres et le disque dur: Visions d'Iboga en Noir et Blanc," in *Des plantes psychotropes: initiations, thérapies et quêtes de soi*, ed. Sébastien Baud and Christian Ghasarian (Paris and Toulouse: Imago; Auzas Éditeurs, 2010), 313–336.

1. Marshall Sahlins, *Historical Metaphors and Mythical Realities* (Ann Arbor: University of Michigan Press, 1981). For Sahlins, "working misunderstanding" refers to the unintended consequences produced by shifts in interpretation in intercultural situations.

2. In line with these local understandings, I use the term "ibogaine" when referring to the Euro-American contexts, whereas I use "iboga" when referring to Gabonese Bwiti (or to Western settings that emphasize the importance of the African ritual).

3. On the issue of national heritage in relation to iboga and Gabonese Bwiti, see Julien Bonhomme, "Anthropologue et/ou Initié: L'Anthropologie Gabonaise à l'Épreuve du Bwiti," *Journal des anthropologues* 110–111 (2007): 207–226.

4. On this topic, see Erika Dyck, "'Hitting Highs at Rock Bottom': LSD Treatment for Alcoholism, 1950–1970," *Social History of Medicine* 19, no. 2 (2006): 313–229.

5. Aldous Huxley, *The Doors of Perception* (London: Chatto and Windus, 1954).

6. See, for instance, Richard Evans Schultes's pioneering ethnobotanic work on Mexican peyote and Amazonian ayahuasca.

7. Paul De Rienzo and Dana Beal, *Report on the Staten Island Project: The Ibogaine Story* (Brooklyn, NY: Autonomedia, 1997), 124.

8. De Rienzo and Beal, *Report on the Staten Island Project*, 106.

9. De Rienzo and Beal, *Report on the Staten Island Project*, 104.

10. James W. Fernandez, *Bwiti: An Ethnography of the Religious Imagination in Africa* (Princeton, Princeton University Press, 1982), ch. 14.

11. On initiatory tourism, see Nadège Chabloz, *Peaux Blanches, Racines Noires: Le Tourisme Chamanique de l'Iboga au Gabon* (Louvain-la-Neuve, Belgium: Academia-L'Harmattan, 2014).

12. James W. Fernandez and Renate L. Fernandez, "'Returning to the Path': The Use of Iboga(ine) in an Equatorial African Ritual Context and the Binding of Time, Space, and Social Relationships," *The Alkaloids* 56 (2001): 235–247.

13. André Mary, *Le Défi du Syncrétisme: Le Travail Symbolique de la Religion d'Eboga (Gabon)* (Paris: Éditions de l'EHESS, 1999).

14. Julien Bonhomme, *Le Miroir et le Crâne: Parcours Initiatique du Bwete Misoko (Gabon)* (Paris: CNRS Éditions, 2006).

15. Many situations of illness or misfortune are supposed to have been caused by a witch (i.e., a malevolent person who, out of jealousy, seeks to harm his or her victim by occult means). The suspected witch is most often a close relative, so witchcraft thus reflects tensions within the family.

16. Formerly available at http://www.iboga.org/fr/meyaya.htm (website no longer active).

17. Fernandez and Fernandez, "Returning to the Path."

18. Account available at https://erowid.org/chemicals/ibogaine/ibogaine_writings1.shtml (accessed May 26, 2021).

19. De Rienzo and Beal, *Report on the Staten Island Project*, 121.

20. Atome Ribenga, *La Tradition Bwitiste au Gabon: Voie Directe de Communication avec le Divin* (Libreville: Maison gabonaise du livre, 2004).

21. Mathieu Birinda, *La Bible secrète des noirs selon le bouity* (Paris: Omnium littéraire, 1952).

22. Chabloz, *Peaux Blanches, Racines Noires*, 28–29.

23. Vincent Ravalec, Mallendi, and Agnès Paicheler, *Bois Sacré: Initiation à l'Iboga* (Vauvert, France: Au diable Vauvert, 2004), 115.

24. Ravalec et al., *Bois Sacré*, 118.

25. Julien Bonhomme, Magali De Ruyter, and Guy-Max Moussavou, "Blurring the Lines: Ritual and Relationships between Babongo Pygmies and their Neighbours (Gabon)," *Anthropos* 107, no 2 (2012): 387–406.

26. Ravalec et al, *Bois Sacré*; Marion Laval-Jeantet, *Iboga, Invisible et Guérison: Une Approche Ethnopsychiatrique* (Montreuil, France: CQFD, 2006); Mélanie Navarro, *Une Occidentale Initiée à l'Iboga chez les Pygmées: La Racine Doit Rester Secrète* (Monaco: Alphée, 2007).

27. Marion Laval-Jeantet, *Paroles d'un Enfant du Bwiti: Les Enseignements d'Iboga* (Paris: L'Originel, 2005).

28. "Ayahuasca, iboga, même combat," *Psychothérapie Vigilance*, August 7, 2006, available at http://www.psyvig.com/doc/doc_225.pdf (accessed May 26, 2021).

29. Daniel Pinchbeck, "Tripping on Iboga," *Salon*, November 3, 1999, available at https://www.salon.com/1999/11/03/iboga (accessed May 26, 2021).

30. Beatriz Caiuby Labate and Henrik Jungaberle, *The Internationalization of Ayahuasca* (Vienna: Lit Verlag, 2011).

31. Jan Kounen, Jeremy Narby, and Vincent Ravalec, *Plantes & Chamanisme: Conversations autour de l'Ayahuasca & de l'Iboga* (Paris: Mama Éditions, 2008).

32. Account available at https://ibogainedossier.com/experience-male-1297.html (accessed May 26, 2021).

33. Ravalec et al., *Bois Sacré*, 49.

34. Account available at http://acmc.ie/ibogaine-treatment/experiences/defragging (accessed May 26, 2021).

35. De Rienzo and Beal, *Report on the Staten Island Project*, 150.

36. Account available at http://www.ibogaine.co.uk/exp16.htm (accessed May 26, 2021).

BIBLIOGRAPHY

Primary Sources

"Ayahuasca, iboga, même combat." Psychothérapie Vigilance, August 7, 2006. Accessed May 26, 2021. http://www.psyvig.com/doc/doc_225.pdf.

Account available at http://acmc.ie/ibogaine-treatment/experiences/defragging (accessed May 26, 2021).

Conrad Rob. "The Grinder, the Powerful Woman, the Monkey Tribe and Me." The Vaults of Erowid. Accessed May 26, 2021. https://erowid.org/chemicals/ibogaine/ibogaine_writings1.shtml.

"Ibogaine experience." Account available at https://ibogainedossier.com/experience-male-1297 .html (accessed May 26, 2021).

Pinchbeck, Daniel. "Tripping on Iboga." *Salon*. November 3, 1999. Accessed May 26, 2021. https://www.salon.com/1999/11/03/iboga.

Xavier. "Xavier's Third Iboga Experience (and His Commentary on Indra's Product) (around 1998)." Ibogaine UK. Accessed May 26, 2021. http://www.ibogaine.co.uk/exp16.htm.

Secondary Sources

Birinda, Mathieu. *La Bible secrète des noirs selon le bouity*. Paris: Omnium littéraire, 1952.

Bonhomme, Julien, Magali De Ruyter, and Guy-Max Moussavou. "Blurring the Lines: Ritual and Relationships between Babongo Pygmies and Their Neighbours (Gabon)." *Anthropos* 107, no. 2 (2012): 387–406.

Bonhomme, Julien. "Anthropologue et/ou Initié: L'Anthropologie Gabonaise à l'Épreuve du Bwiti." *Journal des anthropologues* 110–111 (2007): 207–226.

Bonhomme, Julien. "Les ancêtres et le disque dur: Visions d'Iboga en Noir et Blanc." In *Des plantes psychotropes: initiations, thérapies et quêtes de soi*, ed. Sébastien Baud and Christian Ghasarian, 313–36. Paris, Toulouse: Imago Auzas Éditeurs, 2010.

Bonhomme, Julien. *Le Miroir et le Crâne: Parcours Initiatique du Bwete Misoko (Gabon)*. Paris: CNRS éditions, 2006.

Chabloz, Nadège. *Peaux Blanches, Racines Noires: Le Tourisme Chamanique de l'Iboga au Gabon*. Louvain-la-Neuve, Belgium: Academia-L'Harmattan, 2014.

De Rienzo, Paul, and Dana Beal. *Report on the Staten Island Project: The Ibogaine Story*. Brooklyn, NY: Autonomedia, 1997.

Dyck, Erika. "'Hitting Highs at Rock Bottom': LSD Treatment for Alcoholism, 1950–1970." *Social History of Medicine* 19, no. 2 (2006): 313–329.

Fernandez, James W., and Renate L. Fernandez. "'Returning to the Path': The Use of Iboga(ine) in an Equatorial African Ritual Context and the Binding of Time, Space, and Social Relationships." *The Alkaloids* 56 (2001): 235–247.

Fernandez, James W. *Bwiti: An Ethnography of the Religious Imagination in Africa*. Princeton, NJ: Princeton University Press, 1982.

Kounen, Jan, Jeremy Narby, and Vincent Ravalec. *Plantes & Chamanisme: Conversations autour de l'Ayahuasca & de l'Iboga*. Paris: Mama Éditions, 2008.

Labate, Beatriz Caiuby, and Henrik Jungaberle. *The Internationalization of Ayahuasca*. Vienna: Lit Verlag, 2011.

Laval-Jeantet, Marion. *Paroles d'un Enfant du Bwiti: Les Enseignements d'Iboga*. Paris: L'Originel, 2005.

Laval-Jeantet, Marion. *Iboga: Invisible et Guérison: Une Approche Ethnopsychiatrique*. Montreuil, France: CQFD, 2006.

Mary, André. *Le Défi du Syncrétisme: Le Travail Symbolique de la Religion d'Eboga (Gabon)*. Paris: Éditions de l'EHESS, 1999.

Navarro, Mélanie. *Une Occidentale Initiée à l'Iboga chez les Pygmées: La Racine Doit Rester Secrète.* Monaco: Alphée, 2007.

Ravalec, Vincent, Mallendi, and Agnès Paicheler. *Bois Sacré: Initiation à l'Iboga.* Vauvert, France: Au diable Vauvert, 2004.

Ribenga, Atome. *La Tradition Bwitiste au Gabon: Voie Directe de Communication avec le Divin.* Libreville: Maison gabonaise du livre, 2004.

Sahlins, Marshall. *Historical Metaphors and Mythical Realities.* Ann Arbor: University of Michigan Press, 1981.

9 PSYCHOTROPIC DRUGS FROM AND IN THE FIELDS: RURAL ROOTS AND COLLECTIVE EFFECTS OF LSD

Beat Bächi

INTRODUCTION

LSD is an almost immaterial substance, nearly a nonmatter. Odorless, tasteless, and colorless, it is not perceptible by human senses without direct contact. When there is contact, it produces unprecedented effects in incredibly small doses. It was precisely this minimum materiality that fascinated Albert Hofmann (1906–2008), and he attributed its spiritual effects to these exact nonmaterial characteristics of his later "problem child." Hence, as LSD hardly requires any material substrates for its individual effects, it thereby seemed, at least for his inventor, to strike materialism to its core. Gottfried Benn's saying "God is a substance, a drug!" gained in chemical credibility by LSD. That's why Hofmann quoted this crucial slogan for his critique of materialism, which holds matter to be the fundamental substance in nature, in a letter.[1]

The history of drugs usually focuses on consumption. If one looks instead at the production of drugs, it becomes apparent how their creation mobilizes enormous material flows on various levels. First, the raw material for LSD, ergot, had to be produced on rye grown on farmers' fields. In the process, ergot was not only a key element of the industrialization of agriculture and the introduction of fertilizers and pesticides, but it also transformed the epistemic culture of plant breeding in the Swiss context. Finally, ergot production contributed to a vision of plants and living organisms as a potential property. Thereby it prepared the breakthrough of new property regimes in the realm of agriculture.[2] However, whereas LSD commonly stands as the trigger for a disturbing revolution on the side of its consumers, as part of the counterculture in the 1960s, the production of ergot as raw material for lysergic acid from the 1930s onward sheds light on how these substances prepared the extension of capitalism into a new, neoliberal epoch. Furthermore, from a production perspective, the story of discovery also appears different from the one described by Hofmann himself. Contrasting his discovery story, this chapter argues that this opportunity had been given to synthesize LSD-25[3] mainly by the large-scale production of ergot, which had massively lowered the price of this previously extremely expensive substance and made new experiments with lysergic acid feasible. The story of LSD is told here from the perspective of ergot production in Switzerland using source material from the estate of Hofmann, which has only recently become accessible, and sources from the Novartis Historical Company Archives.

First, this chapter shows how ergot production defied a "cultivation battle" being waged in Switzerland during World War II, how the mass production of ergot made the discovery of LSD-25 possible, and how Hofmann made a first central reinterpretation of the effect of LSD in the field. It then focuses on how ergot drove the industrialization of agriculture and the introduction of chemical pesticides and fertilizers to Swiss fields after World War II; and what significance ergot production had for the reorganization of seed breeding. Furthermore, ergot also brought the "Flesh of the Gods" to the Sandoz laboratories in Basel. The central question of this chapter aims to explore the links between "flower power," the patenting of living organisms, the use of chemical adjuvants in agricultural production, and the extension of biotechnology.

PRODUCING ERGOT ON THE FIELD

To give birth to LSD, ergot (*Claviceps purpurea*) had to grow on farmers' fields. Ergot is a fungus that grows as a parasite preferably on rye, coating its seed heads with a black crust, or sclerotium. Thereby, it makes the rye inedible for humans and can be fed only to other animals (e.g., pigs) after careful sorting. Bread made from ergot-infested rye led to epidemics of a disease traditionally known as "St. Anthony's Fire" and later described as "ergotism."[4]

Its symptoms include seizures, skin lesions, psychotic disturbances, and a "dry gangrene" that can cause the fingers or toes to lose sensation and rot away. At the turn of the twentieth century, ergot was transformed from a poison into a medicine, particularly for use in gynecology. As it also produces uterine contractions, it came to be used to stop postpartum hemorrhages, speed up childbirth, or trigger abortions. This gave it the German common name *Mutterkorn*—"mother's corn." As its beneficial use was known, it became medically used, but not as a standardized medical specialty. The variations in content of several alkaloids were quite dangerous, as mother's corn contains lysergic acid amide, among other alkaloids, which would later be the starting material for LSD.

For centuries, farmers had done their best to suppress the growth of ergot in their fields, such as by breeding rye varieties that were less susceptible to ergot infestation. Beginning in the 1920s, ergot-infected rye was collected and delivered to the Swiss pharmaceutical company Sandoz, which started researching ergot and its potential use in gynecology. Sandoz (today part of Novartis) had been established in 1886 mainly as a manufacturer of dyestuffs, but soon entering the realm of pharmaceuticals as well. One of the prerequisites for the impressive career of ergot at Sandoz was the founding of the pharmaceutical department in 1917 by Arthur Stoll (1887–1971). The fact that the pharmaceutical department was founded in that year was a direct consequence of World War I, which had given the Swiss chemical companies an enormous boost due to the elimination of German competition, increased hunger for chemical dyes by the Allied powers, and the fact that Switzerland had been spared from the war.[5]

Most of the naturally grown ergot that Sandoz transformed into medical preparations originated in the Emmental Valley in the center of Switzerland, where it infected rye in a relatively humid climate, especially during wet springs. At this point, ergot was a scarce and expensive commodity for chemists, while it remained a pest for farmers. Its use in the Sandoz laboratories was closely controlled. In the mid-1930s, Stoll, as head of the pharmaceutical department, instructed Hofmann to adopt microchemical procedures when working with this costly fungus so as not to waste it.[6] When Hofmann produced LSD-25 on the basis of ergot for the first time in 1938, a small quantity was reserved for testing on animals. It failed to demonstrate any particular vasoconstricting properties on the uteruses of rabbits. Consequently, the new substance risked falling into oblivion until it emerged anew in 1943, when the situation regarding the resource ergot had fundamentally changed.

CULTIVATION BATTLES

The change in question occurred in the shadow of World War II. On the eve of the conflict, the privately run company Sandoz gave the go-ahead for mass ergot production and cultivation in the Swiss countryside. Farmers began as contracting parties, inoculating rye with a special gun that dispersed a chemical treatment into the fields ("Hecht's Revolver," see figure 9.1), in an effort to stimulate systematic, industrial-scale ergot production and sell it to Sandoz, who paid a very good price for it. Indicating the importance of ergot at the time, the fungus was also exhibited at the Swiss national exhibition LANDI in 1939 as a typical Swiss innovation speaking to the national character (in the service of intellectual national defense).[7] The creation of agricultural ergot cultivation required new market regulation, especially with respect to property rights. With this in mind, Sandoz informed the farmers growing ergot for them of the following: "We would like to draw the attention of the farmers to the fact that up to now, the collecting of ergot was free to everyone. But now that ergot is cultivated by artificial culture, one has to take care that it is not stolen. It is in the farmer's interest to take the necessary measures to do so."[8] Even though this came as a rather informal, nonbinding request from Sandoz, it is significant, as it speaks to a change in thinking about plant breeding along the lines of property and control over plant cultures that emerged throughout capitalist economies.

Ergot production, a growing agricultural business branch by then, was in direct competition with the country's food policies during World War II. Switzerland implemented an agricultural multicultivation plan for self-sufficiency. Conceived by Friedrich Traugott Wahlen (1899–1985), at the same time the director of the federal Agricultural Research Station Zurich-Oerlikon and head of agricultural production in the War Nutrition Office

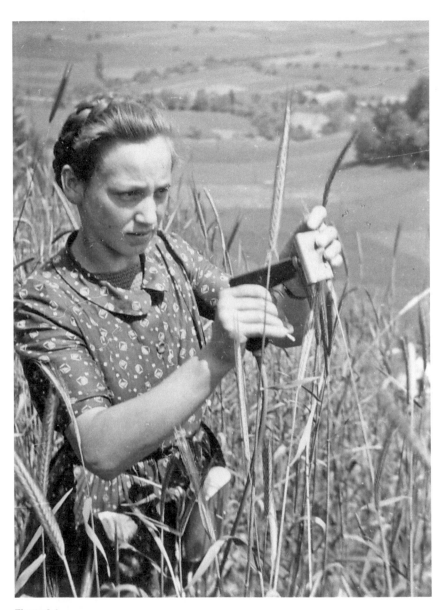

Figure 9.1
Inoculation of ergot mycelium with revolver, 1942. (Photographer: Otto Allemann.) Reproduced with the permission of the Novartis Archives, Basel. Source: FA Novartis, Sandoz: SA_FOT_8.10.

and the country's top bureaucrat involved in agriculture, the plan has come to be known as "Plan Wahlen," or the "cultivation battle." This meant that gardens, parks, soccer fields, and other locations were plowed for food crops. Since ergot cultivation endangered this multiple cultivation, the production of ergot had to be approved by the War Nutrition Office, which set the great national economic importance of ergot for pharmaceutical production against losses in rye production for human nutrition. A closer look into the historical sources reveals that the approval procedure was not a simple matter of paperwork. Wahlen, in his dual role as head of the Federal Research Institute and "Section Head for Agricultural Production and Home Economics in the War Nutrition Office," proposed a deal: it would be "very desirable," he wrote in a letter to Sandoz, to limit the production of ergot "as far as possible" to relatively narrowly defined areas. In return, his research station at Zurich-Oerlikon would be happy to "advise Sandoz on the selection of susceptible rye varieties, and possibly also to carry out comparative infection trials in our trial fields."[9] Sandoz happily accepted this offer and now used the federal research station in Zurich for variety and infection trials. They also used other places, such as Arthur Stoll's garden in Basel, and, maybe more surprisingly, fields in Austria, Czechoslovakia, Bulgaria, and newly built greenhouses in Yugoslavia (where the important Austrian scientist Walter Hecht, the inventor of the abovementioned "Hecht's Revolver," organized comparative infection trials for the Sandoz company).[10]

Ergot cultivation was approved by the War Nutrition Office due to its significant economic benefits. In 1939, ergot cultivation contributed to the gross domestic product a total of 202,000 Swiss francs, which today correspond to roughly 3 million euros. The revenues were divided in the following way: nearly a quarter went to the farmers and the rest went to the other helpers and wage laborers, among them approximately 350 who previously had been unemployed. Since from the outset of its ergot campaign, Sandoz was also cooperating with plant breeders, plant pathologists of the Swiss Federal Institute of Technology, and seed breeding cooperatives, there was a mixture of private, public, and cooperative (farmers') associations in the realm of plant and seed breeding research and multiplication—similar to other Western countries at the eve of what has been called the "Green" Revolution.

While Sandoz succeeded in developing an inoculation machine with about 16,000 needles, in July 1941 the War, Industry and Labor Office informed the company that a very strong "opposition . . . [was forming in] certain circles in agriculture" to the plan to introduce the ergot pathogen into the rye host en masse. Wahlen had received "quite unpleasant and rude letters" threatening to make a big issue of the whole thing in the press. Concerns arose about a "danger of general contamination" of the country's rye stocks, including those destined for human consumption. The central point of criticism concerned the crediting of ergot production as having an "additional cultivation" status during the wartime cultivation battle. Furthermore, the angry letters, especially by seed breeders, suggested that it would be more expedient to restrict ergot breeding to a less-important region for grain cultivation and food production than the lowlands in the canton of Bern. "Finally, reference is made to the unpleasant and harmful influences of the inoculators and gatherers in various regions, who, according to the information received, cause disgruntlement in farming circles due to their origin and the wages paid to them," as one internal Sandoz document said.[11] Because of the labor-intensive inoculation process, Sandoz had to hire outsiders—most of them previously unemployed—and inmates of institutions for the poor and disabled.[12]

In the jointly determined cultivation program for 1942, it was noted by Wahlen and Sandoz that the latter should take better account of the higher altitudes, with the aim of concentrating ergot production in damp areas with heavy soil, and possibly also better involve farmers with large families in the highly elevated Entlebuch and Napf areas in Bern and Lucerne cantons.[13] Both in the inoculation and in the harvesting of the ergot, the respective topographical conditions required that numerous forms of production existed side by side. To support the local "notoriously poor peasant population with large families" by ergot production, a "semitechnical procedure," called "board vaccination," was invented. These were boards equipped with needles to inoculate the rye by hand. In the uneven mountainous terrain, the vaccination machine simply could not be used, and handheld pistol vaccination took too much time. With board inoculation as a semitechnical device, the disadvantage inherent in the uneven terrain was "largely compensated for."[14] As a result, there was a labor-intensive, peasant-style ergot culture in the mountainous regions relying on semitechnical procedures, and also an industrialized one in the lowlands.

As far as the ergot cultivation battle during the war was concerned, a compilation of reports by Sandoz recorded that the yield loss in rye production amounted to about 2.2 tons in 1939, 6 tons in 1940, and 8 tons in 1941. Due to the rise in the price of rye during the war, Sandoz felt compelled to increase the price of ergot, even though it was the only company that produced it on a large scale.[15] From 1943 on, the resistance of certain farming circles died down, and the relationship between Sandoz and the War Nutrition Office visibly improved.

LSD IN THE FIELD: BETTER LIVING THROUGH CHEMISTRY

In 1943, farmers were advised to use *Ceretan Trockenbeize* (ceretan dry dressing or stain), a chemical product that helped reduce the wintering of rye and to increase yields. And even if the fields fertilized with manure and slurry (a natural fertilizer) had given very good results, the use of mineral artificial fertilizers was now recommended.[16] While the ergot was experiencing its first surge of chemical inputs (and while the US chemical giant DuPont was creating one of the most succinct slogans in advertising history: "Better things for better living through chemistry"—or simply "Better living through chemistry"),[17] the psyche was also to open up to chemical processing methods. Hence, the chemical revolution in the field and the chemical revolution in the mind were intimately entangled; the pharmaceutical industry dealt with all aspects of human life.

For the immaterial effects of LSD to see the light of day, ever larger material flows were necessary. A passage from an early draft by Hofmann on the history of the discovery of LSD-25 is revealing in this regard. According to him, LSD-25 was discovered "by chance." In his view, it was "not pure coincidence," but some form of serendipity (i.e., "the occurrence of the event leading to the discovery [was] given a distinct chance").[18] Hence, Hofmann attributed his renewed interest on his intuition. But the success of Hofmann's synthesis of ergobasin, another alkaloid present in ergot that lead to the pharmaceutical product Methergin, had likely strengthened his position at Sandoz. In addition, and in view of the now flourishing ergot research, even his superior, Stoll, was likely not quite as suspicious of potentially lavishing too much ergot as research material as he had been in the late 1930s. Thus, the discovery relied on material factors, not only on intuition.

Solving the resource problems by industrializing ergot production had eventually paved the way for Hofmann's serendipitous discovery of LSD. But the substance produced effects that were neither easily classifiable nor easy to study. While ergot was growing in enormous amounts in the fields of the Swiss hinterland by 1943, Hofmann was in some sort of field as well. Less well known than his famous bicycle ride shortly after his first deliberate LSD self-experiment in April 1943 are three subsequent self-experiments during his military service in the small municipality of Claro in the canton of Ticino in the fall of the same year.

Perhaps due to his circumstances, Hofmann's original interpretations of LSD belonged to the register of war too: In his first series of self-experiments with LSD, he conceived of Pervitine, as he noted in his report to Stoll.[19] Pervitin was a methamphetamine miracle pill of the German Wehrmacht sometimes referred to as "National Socialism in pill form."[20] Hofmann, an admirer of the war-glorifying German writer Ernst Jünger and his 1920 novel *In Stahlgewittern* (storm of steel), believed that he had invented a new respiratory and circulatory stimulant, perhaps a Swiss version of Pervitin, with which Dr. Beerle, the doctor who had been called to help Hofmann on the occasion of his first deliberate self-experiment, had done his own work.[21]

The initial association of LSD with wartime drugs was only loosened when the substance entered yet another field—psychiatry. After his first self-experiment during his active military service (hence proverbially "in the field"), Hofmann suggested to Arthur Stoll that his son, Werner A. Stoll (1915–1995), who worked at Zurich's prestigious psychiatric research hospital Burghölzli (now the Psychiatric University Hospital at the University of Zurich), should investigate LSD clinically, "without waiting for further results of the animal test."[22] The elder Stoll expressed ethical concerns, writing that "a certain pharmacological and toxicological basis" must first be established for clinical investigations—"if one does not want to risk too much." "Responsibility towards the patients" on whom the preparations would have to be tested would require this.[23] Because of Stoll's concerns, Hofmann did two further self-experiments during his military service.[24] But it wasn't until the drug had been tested on a whole series of Sandoz employees in 1945 that Ernst Rothlin, the head of the Sandoz pharmacological laboratory, sent "20 vials of L. S. D. 25, together with 2 pipettes" to Werner Stoll for use at the Burghölzli psychiatric clinic.[25]

ERGOT AND THE CHEMICAL INPUTS IN AGRICULTURE

A new variety of rye called Kluser, bred by Sandoz to enhance ergot yields, was a distinctly "intensive variety," capable of converting much greater quantities of nutrients. Although Sandoz was familiar with the old farmer's saying "Manure is the better way to go," after the war, it recommended "top

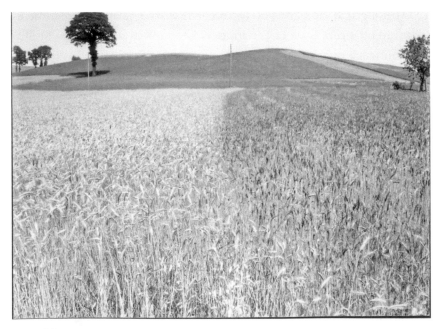

Figure 9.2
Ergot field, Emmental, 1954, with the right side inoculated. Reproduced with the permission of the Novartis archives, Basel. Source: FA Novartis, Sandoz: SA_FOT_3.5.049.

dressing" the rye. When the rye was about thirty centimeters high, it was to be fertilized with calcium nitrate, calcium cyanamide, or sulfuric acid ammonia.[26] This top-dressing process was to keep the rye green longer, which could result in one or two more harvests of ergot. Used as a trajectory to instruct farmers in the use of artificial fertilizers, which was already known but not done on a large scale in Swiss agriculture, ergot thus served as a gateway for agro-industrial knowledge to penetrate local knowledge and cycles. So far as plant nutrition was concerned, thinking in abstract analytical categories that dissolved the farm's own fertilizer into its individual nutrients led to the increased use of standardized artificial fertilizer.

Breeding of the new rye variety went hand in hand with experiments on its chemical treatment. In 1945, Swiss farmers received another important incentive to use chemical inputs into their fields. Since the ergot harvest that year had fallen short of expectations, "as a consolation and recognition for the effort expended," the agrochemical products Kupfer (meaning "copper") Sandoz, Extar, and Sandolin (all produced by Sandoz) were given to the farmers as a gift. The gifting of plant protection products such as Extar, a herbicide for cereal crops introduced in 1941, Sandolin, an insecticide introduced in 1942, and Copper Sandoz as a fungicide introduced in 1943, was done in the "hope of increasing yields through their application in the coming year."[27] Thus, in addition to the chemical adjuvants for extremely open, multiple cultivation under the sign of the cultivation battle, crop failures were important accelerators and catalysts for the increased use of chemical inputs to produce arable crops.

In addition to herbicides such as Weedone 402, experiments were also conducted at Sandoz with Stanormone 40, a phytohormone produced by the US-based DuPont. There were also trials with zinc fertilization, with the researchers exploring whether the alkaloid content could alter growth beyond yields. However, no difference was found between this and the control plant. Thus, no higher productivity could be achieved at the time by these sprays of the rye. Through breeding measures in combination with a certain push to include chemical inputs, "the practitioner could be provided with an increasingly more potent plant material." The correct handling of this more potent material was communicated to the farmers in particular via Sandoz's numerous area managers, who discussed weed control issues with the farmers. In addition, there were numerous presentations by Sandoz representatives. "Educational lectures" were organized for farmers, on topics such as "New research results in the control of soil pests (grubs and wireworms)."[28]

SEED BREEDING IN THE FIELD

By the 1950s, LSD had found a place in psychiatry, while ergot triggered fundamental changes in farmers' fields.[29] The ergot culture, as it came to be known, not only was a key element in the industrialization of agriculture and the introduction of mineral fertilizers and pesticides, but it also transformed the epistemic culture of plant breeding. Before World War II, seed breeding in Switzerland was a cooperative venture between universities, research institutes, seed-breeding associations, industries, and farming practitioners. But the breeding of the so-called Kluser Roggen Spezial (a specific new variety of Kluser rye that had been identified as a "more potent plant material") threatened to break down this collective, hybrid assembly of seed breeding. Kluser rye was bred by Sandoz (one of the predecessors of today's Syngenta/ChemChina strains) from the breeding variety Petkuser by means of so-called polyploidization. This work was completed on Sandoz's own farm in the Klus (in the village of Aesch, Basel-Landschaft). Sandoz bought the Klushof farm just after World War II, which had greenhouses to facilitate year-round research.

In 1949, "stem breeding of tetraploid rye" was initiated in the Klus to further enhance ergot productivity. By "consciously turning away from the classical system of grain breeding," Sandoz simplified rye breeding. The conventional procedure in grain breeding had consisted of pulling out individual plants after determining weaknesses, and examining them (in the present case: 50,000 individual plants) in the laboratory. For ergot grain, in contrast, it was now considered important that the "main act of selection" took place directly in the field. For this reason, in 1955, Sandoz researchers selected the canes for further breeding while they were still alive at their location, taking into account the following criteria: stability, late maturity, relative stem length, tillering, culm thickness, ear length, ear position, and glume closure. This method had the advantage that variations in the soil, as they are found in every field, could be taken into account more precisely. Through all these variables, the so-called elite plants finally had to remain viable in their specific environments.[30] These specific environments could be extremely diverse; for example, Sandoz had also tried to grow ergot in the Belgian Congo in the 1950s.[31]

Tetraploid forms—when an organism has four copies of each chromosome instead of two—were produced from several barley and especially rye varieties. In polyploidization, the chromosome set of a plant species is multiplied, and technically, the duplication of chromosomes produces tetraploid plants with four copies each. This happens either through a spontaneous, natural mutation or by trying to provoke it by irradiating the plant seeds. Unfortunately, how this mutation came about in the case of the Kluser Roggen Spezial is not known. Notwithstanding this unknown detail, beyond its life in the field and the laboratory, Kluser rye prepared the ground for a fundamental reorganization of the seed market in Switzerland.

Kluser rye's most revolutionary moment was not visible from the outside. Its explosive sociopolitical power came from the attempted inculcation of new property rights. On the order card for Kluser rye, the "Instructions on the Use of Kluser Roggen Special" explicitly stated that the ergot grower was obliged to use the seed exclusively for the cultivation of ergot for Sandoz. The company and the seed thus became inextricably linked, a model that later would become prevalent everywhere between agro-chemical firms and farmers. Furthermore, the farmer was prohibited from using Kluser rye for "seed purposes on his farm or to sell or otherwise disperse it to third parties." Sandoz aimed "to protect its rights in the event of a breach of the aforementioned obligations." The ergot farmer was informed via the order card that the fields planted with Kluser should not be located in the vicinity of fields planted with ordinary rye, especially when used for seed production. For its part, Sandoz declined responsibility for any consequences that might arise from Kluser spreading to neighboring fields.[32]

Sandoz and Hofmann were interested not only in native plants, but also exotic mushrooms. Thanks to LSD, and through the mediation of the French botanist Roger Heim (1900–1979), an eminent mycologist and director of the Museum National d'Histoire Naturelle (MNHN) in Paris,[33] *teonanacatl*, the "Flesh of the Gods," also entered the Sandoz laboratories. Since the director of Sandoz's Paris branch was Heim's good friend, the mushrooms cultivated in his laboratory were examined by Hofmann in a fresh, undried state. Therefore, the mushrooms were to be harvested on specific dates (namely, when someone traveled from Paris to Basel).

Meanwhile, the central material question that arose in the cultivation of Mexican mushrooms in the laboratories in Basel was that of the most suitable culture medium: manure. While the germination of spores for *Maltea agar* could be used as a culture medium to grow white, downy mycelium, cultivating these fruiting bodies turned out to be more complex (or, rather, more unusual) for the chemical industry. The instructions for preparing the best manure for fruiting mushroom bodies were at least as detailed as those for tillage and fertilization in ergot cultivation. The key condition was obtaining good-quality horse manure. Horse manure prepared for mushroom cultivation was used, but the following conditions had to be strictly observed:

> 1) It must be pure horse manure, without any admixture of cow manure, 2) There must be plenty of straw mixed with the horse manure, and 3) The manure must have undergone 4 to 5 fermentations together with the straw, with shoveling after each week, i.e., total fermentation [of] 4–5 weeks. The finished manure must now be washed thoroughly before use, 3–4 times in succession with a large volume of water until the wash water drains away completely colorless. The manure is squeezed out a little so that no water drips off when it is wrung out. For storage, the dung can be dried in this state, but it must then be soaked overnight before use.[34]

While *Stropharia mazatecorum* had already been cultivated in the laboratory in Paris, Heim now attempted to make Psilocybe grow under artificial conditions as one of the genera of this fungal family. As early as June 1957, the culture of *Psilocybe mexicana Heim* produced constant and good yields of fruiting bodies at Sandoz in Basel. In contrast, the culture of *P. zapatecorum Heim* was still unsatisfactory. But what particularly concerned Heim and Hofmann was the question of whether the mushrooms produced by these cultures had the same psychic effects as the mushrooms naturally grown in Mexico. A self-experiment carried out by Heim in the spring revealed that the same phenomena had occurred in an experiment in Mexico with the "naturally grown mushrooms"; hence, they believed that the mushroom produced in "artificial culture" also contained hallucinogenic substances.[35]

Because animal tests with the Mexican mushrooms had been disappointing, Hofmann felt "compelled" to work up the "leftover mushrooms" to carry out a test on himself. And indeed, for Hofmann, the mushrooms caused everything to take on "a Mexican character" when he ingested 2.4 grams of *Psilocybe mexicana* at his workplace. Hofmann tried to reproduce his impressions with these words: "Because I was fully aware that from the knowledge of the Mexican origin of these mushrooms I could now imagine Mexican sceneries, I consciously tried to see my environment as I normally knew it. However, all efforts of will to see things in their old familiar shapes and colors were unsuccessful. With my eyes open or with them closed, I saw only Indian motifs and colors." When this vision came to an end after about six hours, Hofmann felt the "re-entry into the familiar reality" like a "delightful return from a foreign world, experienced as quite real, to the old familiar homeland."[36] Sandoz's success in producing "Swiss psilocybin"[37] was celebrated by the director of the Sandoz pharmacological laboratory, Aurelio Cerletti (1918–1988), in similarly exoticizing terms: According to Cerletti (1959), the "small mushrooms and their inherent magic power could be snatched from the darkness of past centuries and from the spell of magical ideas."[38]

Thanks to Sandoz's laboratories and Heim, psilocybin existed in a wide variety of forms by the end of the 1950s. In addition to several naturally growing mushroom species containing psilocybin, there was psilocybin from artificially grown mushrooms in the laboratory and synthetically produced psilocybin in crystallized form. For some, the synthesis was hailed as definitive proof of the accuracy of the structural formula. However, one of the big questions was not yet answered in a satisfactory way regarding the psilocybin synthesis: Did the artificially produced, crystallized substance really have the same effects as the organically grown mushrooms? Heim suggested having the crystallized product taken by a Mexican *curandero* or *curandera*—perhaps best of all by María Sabina (1894?–1985) herself—to see whether she identified symptoms with those of the natural mushrooms. Upon learning that María Sabina had ingested Sandoz psilocybin pills in Huautla de Jiménez in 1959, Hofmann noted that "it was interesting to see how thrilled the Indians were in learning that we could provide them with pills. They were most eager to take them and though we had some real mushrooms, no one, on that night, cared for them."[39]

Fittingly, in 1962, not only did Albert Hofmann first come to the Sierra Mazateca region of Oaxaca in southern Mexico, but ergot-based drugs (Cafergot and Dihidroergotamina) produced in the Emmental Valley and in the Lucerne hinterland and manufactured in Basel made their way there via Sandoz de México. Sources even show that the antipsychotic chlorpromazine drug Largactil (which blocks the effects of LSD) was ordered by the governing medical authority in Huautla de Jiménez, Medico Jefe de la Sección de Salubridad,[40] while Indocybin (Sandoz's brand of psilocybin) was tested in Switzerland on patients who had been involved in ergot production.[41] It is remarkable that Swiss-produced ergot and other LSD allies had made their way to the Sierra Mazateca, while Mexican psilocybin arrived in Europe from the opposite direction, where it was transformed into a branded product.

EPILOGUE: "FLOWER POWER"? LSD, AGRIBUSINESS, AND BIOTECHNOLOGY

Ergot, or ergot rye, was fundamental to changes in material culture. It changed the view of living organisms, which were now regarded—like technical innovations—as patentable property and ultimately given very specific property rights. This process fundamentally changed the epistemic culture and practice of plant breeding. What was initially a collective, use-oriented endeavor became a private-sector, property-oriented industry, a central prerequisite for today's agribusiness. But the *Kluser Roggen Spezial* was also an important, very concrete gateway for the industrial modeling of agriculture. As an artificial rye variety, it homogenized the seed to such an extent that it could live only in association with the pathologization of plant breeding. In the farmers' fields, it survived in different biological, geographical, and meteorological conditions only because its surroundings were made reasonably uniform by relying on chemical inputs. More and more pesticides were necessary for it to thrive, and its nutrient balance could also be guaranteed only by standardized artificial, mineral fertilizers.

Ergot had extremely unforeseen and disparate effects. In addition to the mechanization and the increased use of chemical substances, it led to a reduction of diversity in agriculture, which now had to obey industrial rhythms and production methods. But ergot also led, surprisingly, to the expansion of natural substance chemistry. It was precisely this "technologizing of agriculture" that Albert Hofmann himself held partly responsible for the great demand for LSD.[42] Under the aegis of "flower power," ergot demonstrated the tremendous power of fungi and plants for synthetic chemistry. Hence, the idealization of the flower in that later movement already was present in Albert Hofmann's and Sandoz's practical work on ergot and the mushrooms. It led to a veritable boom of natural products research at Sandoz.[43] At the same time, ergot was an important fuel for Sandoz's entry into biotechnology, both in terms of plant breeding and the biotechnological production of large quantities of vaccines to inoculate rye, and later to produce lysergic acid in bioreactors. The new biotechnological possibilities meant that Sandoz began to withdraw more and more from farmers' fields before they stopped production completely in 1976.[44]

In view of the imponderables of people, plants, animals, machines, and vaccine strains, Sandoz was extremely pleased to gradually meet its demand for ergot alkaloids by fermentative means and synthetic reduction from 1968 onward. Due to the large-scale possibilities for the synthetic production of ergot alkaloids, naturally occurring ergot gradually disappeared from the fields in the mid-1970s. Farmers, for their part, increasingly became mere seed consumers, precisely via Sandoz's proprietary Kluser rye breed, and learned to adapt the new artificial varieties to unequal natural conditions with mineral fertilizers and chemical pesticides—some of them also produced by Sandoz. While LSD radically altered the psychological inner life, the cultivation, inoculation, and harvesting of ergot fundamentally plowed up numerous fields, as well as central aspects of capitalist material culture, such as traditional plant breeding, property rights on biological organisms, and agricultural means and methods of production. Hence, by focusing the collective effects of psychotropic substances, the agricultural history of LSD (and synthetic psilocybin) demonstrates how capitalist markets driven by a chemical revolution changed how we relate to plants, food, and psychoactivity.

NOTES

1. Jeannie Moser, *Psychotropen. Eine LSD-Biographie* (Konstanz, Germany: Konstanz University Press 2013), 194.

2. For more detail, see Beat Bächi, *LSD auf dem Land: Produktion und kollektive Wirkung psychotroper Stoffe* (Konstanz: Konstanz University Press 2020). All quotations from German are by the author.

3. The name "LSD-25" derives from the fact that it was the twenty-fifth substance in Hofmann's series of experiments on synthetic lysergic acid derivatives.

4. See Piero Camporesi, *Das Brot der Träume: Hunger und Halluzinationen im vorindustriellen Europa* (Frankfurt am Main, Germany: Campus, 1990); Dieter Hagenbach and Lucius Werthmüller, *Albert Hofmann und sein LSD* (Munich: AT Verlag, 2011); Hans Marti, "Von Mutterkornanbau, Wolfszähnen, Kornzapfen und Kribbelkrankheit," *Heimatkunde des Wiggertals* 43 (1985): 153–68, 157–159.

5. Robert Labhardt, "Mutterkorn und Calcium," in *Chemie und Pharma in Basel, Bd. 2: Wechselwirkungen einer Beziehung—Aspekte und Materialien,* ed. Georg Kreis and Beat von Wartburg (Basel, Switerland: Christoph Merian Verlag 2016), 122–133.

6. Hagenbach and Werthmüller, *Albert Hofmann und Sein LSD*, 56.

7. For example, ergot's characteristics as a national asset were quite similar to "purely Swiss Vitamin C," standing for self-sufficiency and independence from foreign raw materials during World War II. See Beat Bächi, *Vitamin C für alle! Pharmazeutische Produktion, Vermarktung und Gesundheitspolitik, 1933–1953* (Zurich: Chronos Verlag, 2009), 172–180.

8. Künstliche Züchtung von Mutterkorn, ca. 1939, FA Novartis, Sandoz, H 207.020, Sandoz A. G. Basel.

9. Brief von Traugott Wahlen, Sektionschef für landwirtschaftliche Produktion und Hauswirtschaft im Kriegsernährungsamt, an die Firma Sandoz A.G., Bern, Switerland, October 3, 1939, FA Novartis, Sandoz, H-202.019.

10. Dr. A. Brack, Mutterkorn-Feldversuche 1938, Bericht No. 35, Basel, Switerland, November 19, 1938, FA Novartis, Sandoz, H-207.028 (1938–1949), 2.

11. Brief des Kriegs-, Industrie- und Arbeitsamtes des Eidgenössischen Volkswirtschaftsdepartementes, Bern, Switerland, July 31, 1941, FA Novartis, Sandoz, H-202.018.

12. See also chapter 6 in this volume.

13. Briefe des Kriegs-, Industrie- und Arbeitsamtes, August 6, 1941 and September, 1941, FA Novartis, Sandoz, H-202.019. For a closer look at agriculture in Switzerland at this time. see Juri Auderset and Peter Moser, *Die Agrarfrage in der Industriegesellschaft. Wissenskulturen, Machtverhältnisse und natürliche Ressourcen in der agrarisch-industriellen Wissensgesellschaft (1850–1950)* (Vienna: Böhlau Verlag, 2018).

14. Brief von Stoll an Wahlen, August 1, 1942, FA Novartis, Sandoz, H-202.019.

15. Dr. A. Brack, Abschliessender Bericht über die künstliche Mutterkornzüchtung in der Schweiz 1940, Bericht No. 111, Basel, Switzerland, May 4, 1941, 11, FA Novartis, Sandoz, H-207.028 (1938–1949),

16. Sandoz A. G. Basel, Mutterkornzüchtung, 1943, FA Novartis, Sandoz H 207.020.

17. Nicolas Langlitz, *Neuropsychedelia: The Revival of Hallucinogen Research since the Decade of the Brain* (Berkeley: University of California Press, 2013).

18. Beilage zum Brief von Albert Hofmann an Ruedi Bircher, Sandoz Pharmaceuticals, New York, "Wie das Phantasticum LSD 25 entdeckt wurde," Basel, Switerland, December 12, 1952, 1 and 4f., Archiv IMG, N Hofmann 148: "LSD LA 111," Mappe 148.4.

19. Dr. med. Walter Schilling, Prakt. Arzt, Bottmingen, Bericht an Hr. Prof. Stoll, Beobachtungen bei Dr. A. Hofmann nach Einnahme von 0,25 mg des Diaethylamids der Lysergsäure am 19.4.43, 22. 4. 1943 (gez. Beerle), 1, Archiv IMG, N Hofmann 148.1: Berichte von Selbstversuchen mit d-Lysergsäure-diäthylamid-tartrat, 1943–1946.

20. Norman Ohler, "Nationalsozialismus in Pillenform: Der Aufstieg des Stimulanzmittels Pervitin im 'Dritten Reich'. Vom Einsatz des Medikaments als Element totaler Mobilmachung zum direkten Zugriff auf die Körper der Soldaten," in *Handbuch Drogen in sozial- und kulturwissenschaftlicher Perspektive*, ed. Robert Feustel, Henning Schmidt-Semisch, and Ulrich Bröckling (Wiesbaden, Germany: VS Verlag für Sozialwissenschaften, 2019), 71–79. See also Hans-Christian Dany, *Speed. Eine Gesellschaft auf Droge* (Hamburg: Nautilus, 2008). Nicolas Rasmussen, *On Speed: The Many Lives of Amphetamine* (New York: New York University Press 2009).

21. Berichte von Selbstversuchen mit d-Lysergsäure-diäthylamid-tartrat, 1943–1946: Dr. med. Walter Schilling, Prakt. Arzt, Bottmingen, Bericht an Hr. Prof. Stoll, Beobachtungen bei Dr. A. Hofmann nach Einnahme von 0,25 mg des Diaethylamids der Lysergsäure am 19.4.43, 22. 4. 1943 (gez. Beerle), 1, Archiv IMG, N Hofmann 148.1.

22. Brief von A. Hofmann (an Stoll), Im Felde, October 2, 1943, FA Novartis, Sandoz, H 105.022 (1940–1947).

23. Brief von Stoll an Hofmann, Basel, Switzerland, October 29, 1943, FA Novartis, Sandoz, H 105.022 (1940–1947).

24. Berichte von Selbstversuchen mit d-Lysergsäure-diäthylamid-tartrat, 1943–1946: Albert Hofmann an Herrn Prof. Stoll: Bericht über 3 Selbstversuche mit d-Lysergsäure-diäthylamid, 30.XII.1943, 1, Archiv IMG, N Hofmann 148.1.

25. Berichte von Selbstversuchen mit d-Lysergsäure-diäthylamid-tartrat, 1943–1946: Abschrift des Briefes von Dr. Werner Stoll, Assistent an der kantonalen Heilanstalt Burghölzli, an Prof. Dr. med. Ernst Rothlin, Leiter des pharmakologischen Laboratoriums der Sandoz A. G., Zürich, 7.5.1945, Archiv IMG, N Hofmann 148.10. See also Magaly Tornay, "Zugriffe auf das Ich. Psychoaktive Stoffe und Personenkonzepte in der Schweiz, 1945 bis 1980," (Tübingen, Germany: Mohr Siebeck, 2016), 143; and chapter 6 in this volume.

26. FA Novartis, Sandoz H-207.020, 1946.

27. FA Novartis, Sandoz H 207.020, Sandoz AG. An unsere Mutterkornzüchter, 1945.

28. FA Novartis, Sandoz, H 207.020, diverse Unterlagen. For applied entomology in Switzerland between 1874 and 1952, see Lukas Straumann, *Nützliche Schädlinge. Angewandte Entomologie, chemische Industrie und Landwirtschaftspolitik in der Schweiz 1874–1952* (Zurich: Chronos Verlag, 2005).

29. See also chapter 15 in this volume.

30. Herr Dr. H. Leemann, D. Gerber: Zusammenfassender Bericht über die im Jahre 1955 im Klushof durchgeführten Versuche, April 30, 1956, p. 8, FA Novartis, Sandoz, G 143.001.

31. For more detail, see Bächi, *LSD auf dem Land*, 113–19.

32. Bestellkarte für Kluser Roggen Spezial, 1955, FA Novartis, Sandoz, H-202.003.

33. See chapter 11 in this volume.

34. Dr. A. Brack, Psilocybe mexicana Heim. Besuch bei Prof. R. Heim, June 26 and 27, 1957, FA Novartis, Sandoz, H 207.019, 10.7.1957, 2–5.

35. Korrespondenz mit Prof. R. Heim Paris (1957–1972), Archiv IMG, N Hofmann 135.

36. Vortrag "Mexikanische Zauberpilze«gehalten vor Thurgauische Naturforschende Gesellschaft," Frauenfeld, April 25, 1961, 7–8, Archiv IMG, N Hofmann 151: Mappe 151.8.

37. See Nicolas Langlitz, *Neuropsychedelia*, 53–82.

38. Aurelio Cerletti, "Teonanacatl und Psilocybin," in *Deutsche Medizinische Wochenschrift*, Nr. 52, 84. Jg., 25. Dezember 1959, 2317–2321, here 2318.

39. Korrespondenz mit R. G. Wasson (1959–1986): Brief von Wasson an "Albert Hofmann," August 6, 1959, 2. Archiv IMG, N Hofmann 137.

40. Carlos Incháustegui Díaz (INI Centro Coordinador de la Sierra Mazateca, Huautla de Jiménez), to Antonio Salas Ortega, 1962, 4, Acervo / Fondo Documental "Dr. Alfonso Caso," Ex Convento de Santo Domingo Yanhuitlán, Mexiko: CCI Huautla de Jiménez, Dirección, Oficios enviados y recibidos.

41. See chapter 6 in this volume.

42. See Albert Hofmann, *LSD: Mein Sorgenkind* (Stuttgart: Klett-Cotta 1979), 63.

43. See Frank Petersen, "Naturstoffforschung bei Novartis Pharmaceuticals—ein historischer Überblick (Natural products research at Novartis Pharmaceuticals—a historical overview),"

in *Grenzgänge—Albert Hofmann zum 100. Geburtstag* (Exploring the frontiers—in celebration of Albert Hofmann's 100th birthday), ed. Günter Engel and Paul Herrling (Basel, Switerland: Schwabe Verlag, 2006), 28–73.

44. To give the reader an idea of the importance of the ergot campaign, it is worth mentioning here that Sandoz produced ergot in 1953 on 1,490 hectares, in 1963 on 940 hectares, and in 1970 on 826 hectares, among other instances.

BIBLIOGRAPHY

Primary Sources

Beilage zum Brief von Albert Hofmann an Ruedi Bircher, Sandoz Pharmaceuticals, New York, "Wie das Phantasticum LSD 25 entdeckt wurde," Basel, Switzerland, December 12, 1952, 1 and 4f., Archiv IMG.

Berichte von Selbstversuchen mit d-Lysergsäure-diäthylamid-tartrat, 1943–1946: Dr. med. Walter Schilling, Prakt. Arzt, Bottmingen, Bericht an Hr. Prof. Stoll, Beobachtungen bei Dr. A. Hofmann nach Einnahme von 0.25 mg des Diaethylamids der Lysergsäure am 19.4.43, 22. 4. 1943 (gez. Beerle), 1, Archiv IMG, N Hofmann 148.1.

Berichte von Selbstversuchen mit d-Lysergsäure-diäthylamid-tartrat, 1943–1946: Albert Hofmann an Herrn Prof. Stoll: Bericht über 3 Selbstversuche mit d-Lysergsäure-diäthylamid, 30.XII.1943, 1, Archiv IMG, N Hofmann 148.1.

Berichte von Selbstversuchen mit d-Lysergsäure-diäthylamid-tartrat, 1943–1946: Abschrift des Briefes von Dr. Werner Stoll, Assistent an der kantonalen Heilanstalt Burghölzli, an Prof. Dr. med. Ernst Rothlin, Leiter des pharmakologischen Laboratoriums der Sandoz A. G., Zürich, 7.5.1945, Archiv IMG, N Hofmann 148.10.

Bestellkarte für Kluser Roggen Spezial, 1955, FA Novartis, Sandoz, H-202.003.

Brief des Kriegs-, Industrie- und Arbeitsamtes des Eidgenössischen Volkswirtschaftsdepartementes, Bern, Switzerland, July 31, 1941, FA Novartis, Sandoz, H-202.018.

Briefe des Kriegs-, Industrie- und Arbeitsamtes, August 6, 1941 and September 6, 1941.

Brief von A. Hofmann (an Stoll), Im Felde, October 27, 1943, FA Novartis, Sandoz, H 105.022 (1940–1947).

Brief von Stoll an Hofmann, Basel, Switzerland, October 29, 1943, FA Novartis, Sandoz, H 105.022 (1940–1947).

Brief von Stoll an Wahlen, August 17, 1942, FA Novartis, Sandoz, H-202.019.

Brief von Traugott Wahlen, Sektionschef für landwirtschaftliche Produktion und Hauswirtschaft im Kriegsernährungsamt, an die Firma Sandoz A.G., Bern, Switzerland, October 3, 1939, FA Novartis, Sandoz, H-202.019.

Carlos Incháustegui Díaz (INI Centro Coordinador de la Sierra Mazateca, Huautla de Jiménez), to Antonio Salas Ortega, 1962, 4, Acervo/Fondo Documental "Dr. Alfonso Caso," Ex Convento de Santo Domingo Yanhuitlán, Mexiko: CCI Huautla de Jiménez, Dirección, Oficios enviados y recibidos.

Dr. A. Brack, Abschliessender Bericht über die künstliche Mutterkornzüchtung in der Schweiz 1940, Bericht No. 111, Basel, Switzerland, May 4, 1941, 11, FA Novartis, Sandoz, H-207.028 (1938–1949).

Dr. A. Brack, Mutterkorn-Feldversuche 1938, Bericht No. 35, Basel, Switzerland. November 19, 1938, FA Novartis, Sandoz, H-207.028 (1938–1949), 2.

Dr. A. Brack, Psilocybe mexicana Heim. Besuch bei Prof. R. Heim, June 26 and 27, 1957, FA Novartis, Sandoz, H 207.019, 10.7.1957, S. 2–5.

Dr. med. Walter Schilling, Prakt. Arzt, Bottmingen, Bericht an Hr. Prof. Stoll, Beobachtungen bei Dr. A. Hofmann nach Einnahme von 0,25 mg des Diaethylamids der Lysergsäure am 19.4.43, 22. 4. 1943 (gez. Beerle), 1, Archiv IMG, N Hofmann 148.1: Berichte von Selbstversuchen mit d-Lysergsäure-diäthylamid-tartrat, 1943–1946.

FA Novartis, Sandoz H 207.020, Sandoz AG. An unsere Mutterkornzüchter, 1945.

FA Novartis, Sandoz, H-202.019.

FA Novartis, Sandoz, H 207.020, diverse Unterlagen.

Herr Dr. H. Leemann, D. Gerber: Zusammenfassender Bericht über die im Jahre 1955 im Klushof durchgeführten Versuche, April 30, 1956, p. 8, FA Novartis, Sandoz, G 143.001.

Korrespondenz mit Prof. R. Heim Paris (1957–1972), Archiv IMG, N Hofmann 135.

Korrespondenz mit R. G. Wasson (1959–1986): Brief von Wasson an "Albert Hofmann," August 6, 1959, p. 2. Archiv IMG, N Hofmann 137.

Künstliche Züchtung von Mutterkorn, ca. 1939, FA Novartis, Sandoz, H 207.020, Sandoz A. G. Basel.

Sandoz A. G. Basel, Mutterkornzüchtung, 1943, FA Novartis, Sandoz H 207.020.

Vortrag "Mexikanische Zauberpilze«gehalten vor Thurgauische Naturforschende Gesellschaft," Frauenfeld, April 25, 1961, 7–8, Archiv IMG, N Hofmann 151: Mappe 151.8.

Secondary Sources

Auderset, Juri, and Peter Moser. *Die Agrarfrage in der Industriegesellschaft: Wissenskulturen, Machverhältnisse und natürliche Ressourcen in der agrarisch-industriellen Wissensgesellschaft (1850–1950).* Vienna: Böhlau Verlag, 2018.

Bächi, Beat. *LSD auf dem Land: Produktion und kollektive Wirkung psychotroper Stoffe.* Konstanz, Germany: Konstanz University Press 2020.

Bächi, Beat. *Vitamin C für alle! Pharmazeutische Produktion, Vermarktung und Gesundheitspolitik, 1933–1953.* Zurich: Chronos Verlag, 2009.

Camporesi, Piero. *Das Brot der Träume: Hunger und Halluzinationen im vorindustriellen Europa.* Frankfurt am Main, Germany: Campus, 1990.

Cerletti, A. "Teonanácatl und psilocybin." *DMW-Deutsche Medizinische Wochenschrift* 84, no. 52 (1959): 2317–2321.

Dany, Hans-Christian. *Speed. Eine Gesellschaft auf Droge.* Hamburg: Nautilus, 2008.

Hagenbach, Dieter, and Lucius Werthmüller. *Albert Hofmann und sein LSD.* Munich: AT Verlag, 2011.

Hofmann, Albert. *LSD: mein Sorgenkind.* Stuttgart: Klett-Cotta, 1979.

Labhardt, Robert. "Mutterkorn und Calcium." In *Chemie und Pharma in Basel, Bd. 2: Wechselwirkungen einer Beziehung—Aspekte und Materialien*, edited by Georg Kreis and Beat von Wartburg, 122–133. Basel, Switerland: Christoph Merian Verlag, 2016.

Langlitz, Nicolas. *Neuropsychedelia: The Revival of Hallucinogen Research since the Decade of the Brain.* Berkeley: University of California Press, 2013.

Marti, Hans. "Von Mutterkornanbau, Wolfszähnen, Kornzapfen und Kribbelkrankheit." *Heimatkunde des Wiggertals* 43 (1985): 153–168.

Moser, Jeannie. *Psychotropen. Eine LSD-Biographie.* Konstanz, Germany: Konstanz University Press, 2013.

Ohler, Norman. "Nationalsozialismus in Pillenform: Der Aufstieg des Stimulanzmittels Pervitin im 'Dritten Reich'. Vom Einsatz des Medikaments als Element totaler Mobilmachung zum direkten Zugriff auf die Körper der Soldaten." In *Handbuch Drogen in sozial- und kulturwissenschaftlicher Perspektive*, edited by Robert Feustel, Henning Schmidt-Semisch, and Ulrich Bröckling, 71–79. Wiesbaden, Germany: VS Verlag für Sozialwissenschaften, 2019.

Petersen, Frank "Naturstoffforschung bei Novartis Pharmaceuticals—ein historischer Überblick [Natural Products Research at Novartis Pharmaceuticals—A historical overview]." In *Grenzgänge—Albert Hofmann zum 100. Geburtstag* [Exploring the Frontiers—in Celebration of Albert Hofmann's 100th Birthday], edited by Günter Engel and Paul Herrling, 28–73. Basel, Switerland: Schwabe Verlag, 2006.

Rasmussen, Nicolas. *On Speed: The Many Lives of Amphetamine.* New York: New York University Press, 2009.

Straumann, Lukas. *Nützliche Schädlinge: Angewandte Entomologie, chemische Industrie und Landwirtschaftspolitik in der Schweiz 1874–1952*, vol. 9. Zurich: Chronos, 2005.

Tornay, Magaly. *Zugriffe auf das Ich: Psychoaktive Stoffe und Personenkonzepte in der Schweiz, 1945 bis 1980.* Tübingen: Mohr Siebeck, 2016.

10 THE FIRST APPLICATIONS OF LSD-25 IN SOUTH AMERICA (1954–1959)

Hernán Scholten and Gonzalo Salas

INTRODUCTION

The results of the first LSD-25 experiments administered to humans with the aim of investigating its effects on the psyche were published in 1947. Its author, the University of Zurich psychiatry professor Werner Stoll (1915–1995), was the son of Arthur Stoll (1887–1971), the director of Sandoz Laboratories in Basel, where Albert Hofmann first synthesized LSD in 1938. By virtue of the symptoms that accompanied its consumption, Stoll characterized LSD as a phantasticum, following the classification suggested in 1924 by the German chemist Louis Lewin to describe drugs such as cannabis and ayahuasca, which modify sensory perceptions, bring about hallucinations, and alter consciousness.[1] Given these properties, psychiatrists began to consider the possibility of using LSD as a research tool. Sandoz therefore made the new substance available under the name Delysid and recommended that psychiatrists self-administer the drug to gain an understanding of the subjective experiences of people suffering schizophrenia.[2]

In 1949, the German-born psychiatrist Max Rinkel (1894–1966) began spreading the word about LSD in the US. Gradually, it was no longer considered a phantasticum but rather a substance capable of producing temporary psychosis, a psychotomimetic.[3] Although it would eventually be applied in a variety of conditions (alcoholism, terminally ill patients, and even as a "cure" for homosexuality and frigidity), LSD was first used in research into psychosis, and later in the treatment of this condition. The substance was administered to healthy volunteers and used to provoke a transient psychotic state similar to schizophrenia, to allow researchers to study the disorder under experimental conditions.

In this context, and by virtue of renewed interest in this substance,[4] this chapter explores a forgotten tale in the history of LSD: its first applications in South America in the mid-1950s. These early encounters were carried out in a context similar to those in the US, which had itself assimilated a European psychiatric tradition. Indeed, LSD's potential for the experimental study of psychosis was a common feature of the first publications written by young psychiatrists dedicated to this substance in South America between 1954 and 1959.

LSD COMES TO SOUTH AMERICA: PSYCHIATRY AND EXPERIMENTAL PSYCHOSIS IN CHILE

Toward the mid-nineteenth century, psychiatry began to develop in young Latin American nations, growing out of institutions created during the colonial period. From the beginning, there was a wide circulation of theories, practices, and institutional models of European origin. During the first decades of the twentieth century, prominent regional figures such as Honorio Delgado (Perú), Gregorio Bermann (Argentina), and Juliano Moreira (Brazil) began amending the classical psychiatric literature reflected in the ideas of Pinel, Esquirol and Kraepelin, with the progressive impact of psychoanalytic theory.[5] At the same time, beginning in the 1920s, the mental hygiene movement initiated in the US by Clifford Beers was spreading, with broad support from the American psychiatric establishment.[6] By the end of World War II, this novel mental health paradigm was propagated throughout the region.[7] Further, until at least the middle of the twentieth century, South American psychiatrists took study trips to Europe and the US as an almost obligatory requirement for obtaining recognition and prestige within the field. In addition to strengthening their professional statuses, their activities show a clear openness to innovations coming from the main centers of scientific production.

In 1954, the first Spanish-language paper on psychedelics, "Psicosis experimentales con ácido lisérgico (Experimental Psychoses with Lysergic Acid)," appeared in the scholarly journal *Revista Chilena de Neuropsiquiatría*, signaling that LSD had arrived in the region. Its author, Agustín Téllez Meneses (1907–1977), was a physician-psychiatrist who took a job working in an asylum shortly after finishing his studies at the University of Chile. His LSD research exhibited a significant influence from contemporary German psychiatry and philosophy, which he had familiarized himself with while studying in Europe in the late 1930s on a Humboldt research grant.[8] It is therefore unsurprising that Téllez Meneses's experimental use of LSD relied heavily on German texts, particularly the work of Stoll and other European LSD researchers, including A. M. Becker, Roland Fischer, Felix Georgi, and Rolf Weber, and to a lesser extent the work of Rinkel.

Téllez Meneses's paper is a write-up of an oral presentation that he gave to a group of colleagues where he laid out an experimental framework based on experiments that he had carried out with Dr. Harda Fuchslocher Amthauer (1928–?) at the beginning of 1953.

His experimental framework included the hypothesis that "[p]sychotics and psychopaths are expected to be less sensitive to LSD-25 than normal subjects, and hallucinatory phenomena less frequent and less rich than in the latter. We would expect to see a triggering of the spontaneous hallucinations associated with the disease."[9] The twenty-five participants in the experiment were between fifteen and fifty-two years old, and all of them had been diagnosed with some form of psychosis (or "in the process of normalization,"[10] according to Téllez Meneses). Varying doses were administered, and a total of eleven checks were carried out, the first half an hour after ingestion and the last six days later.

Most of the paper was dedicated to a detailed description of his results, which were summarized in a final section that compared these Chile-based results to those from previous experiments carried out in Europe, ordered around ten central themes, such as optimal dose and symptom type. One factor that Téllez Meneses considered fundamental to explaining the differences between his results and those of the Europeans was in regard to the population chosen for the experiment: the majority of European experiments, including those of Stoll and Becker, were mainly carried out on subjects considered "normal," while Téllez Meneses had been administering LSD to subjects who had been diagnosed with a mental illness. This distinguishing feature allowed him to observe a double effect caused by the drug: reactivating and accentuating symptoms that were already present or developing, while simultaneously facilitating the appearance of new manifestations—a distinction that the patients themselves were able to make.

In Téllez Meneses's view, the results of this experiment challenged the European characterization of LSD as an "'eidetizant'[11] or producer of images . . . for us the most common symptoms manifest at the level of affective and psychomotor function."[12] He preferred to define the drug's action in terms of producing an "intoxicating, or psychotizing effect," as did his American colleagues, such as Rinkel and Sidney Cohen.

Moreover, noting that a feeling of relief was reported in some subjects after ingesting LSD, Téllez Meneses suggested that LSD had therapeutic potential, as had already been proposed as early as 1950 by Anthony Busch and Warren Johnson.[13] Without dwelling on the question further, he proposed to implement a therapeutic approach following the line of contemporary convulsive therapies, such as Metrazol (pentylenetetrazol) and electroconvulsive therapy (ECT), which had been in use since the 1930s.

The article concludes with various hypotheses regarding the neurophysiological mechanisms behind the effects produced by LSD, particularly its effects on the diencephalon and midbrain. These led Téllez Meneses to conclude that "the experimental psychosis produced [by LSD] could be a manifestation of diencephalosis," a short-lived psychiatric theory that referred to a physical disruption to normal functioning in this brain area, considered a possible effect of LSD by Werner Stoll in the late 1940s.[14]

Téllez Meneses does not appear to have continued his experiments, and later explorations in LSD research in Chile in the early 1960s were carried out in a different context altogether. Nevertheless, his early experiments resemble similar studies that were underway almost simultaneously in other countries in the region.

DISCONTINUED EXPERIMENTS WITH LSD IN ARGENTINA, BRAZIL, AND VENEZUELA

A year after Téllez Meneses's publication, several other articles exploring the effects of LSD appeared in Argentina, Brazil, and Venezuela. Although these papers have no direct connection to Téllez Meneses's work, the proliferation of such activities suggests that these substances were beginning to appeal a wider range of psychiatrists and researchers in Latin America.

In Argentina, the experimental use of LSD found its first expression in the work of Jorge Joaquín Saurí (1923–2003), a young psychiatrist with links to Catholicism and a patient of Céles Cárcamo, one of the founders of the Psycho-analytic Association of Argentina, established in 1942.[15] His article on the topic was written in collaboration with Amelia Cardoso de Onorato (1900–1965) and published in the journal *Acta psiquiátrica y psicológica de América Latina.*[16]

Like Téllez Meneses, they too probed the idea of using LSD to model psychosis and examined the hypothesis that ingesting LSD could bring about personality changes similar to hebephrenia (a term associated with chronic schizophrenia involving disordered thoughts, emotions, hallucinations, and behaviors). This working model of the drug's effects was corroborated by "most of the authors" whom they invited the reader to verify in the bibliography attached to the article. To this end, thanking the "kind collaboration of Sandoz," they conducted a study in which they analyzed drawings and paintings produced by a group of eight schizophrenics who took a dose of LSD on an empty stomach. [17]

Saurí and Cardoso de Onorato thus resumed a practice that had an extensive history in psychiatric practice, which was to have subjects engage in creative pursuits while under the drug's influence.[18] Indeed, Werner Stoll's landmark first paper on the psychological effects of LSD had included a sketch of substance-induced hallucination.[19] Along the same lines, the work of some Italian psychiatrists cited in the article, who had earlier showed an interest in LSD, are of particular interest.

This research led these Argentine authors to conclude that the reactions noted in their experimental subjects "failed on several occasions to correspond to the clinical framework employed,"[20] and the characteristics of the drawings allowed an appreciation of a "polarization of mood towards agitation and depression."[21]

Next, drawing on German sources, this inaugural study was especially inspired by the phenomenological-existential analysis proposed by Ludwig Binswanger (1881–1966), Jakob Wyrsch (1892–1980), and Eugene Minkowski (1885–1972)—three authors who incorporated the ideas of the philosophers Edmund Husserl and Martin Heidegger into their psychiatric practices. However, despite this international engagement, and much like the earlier work by Téllez Meneses, Saurí and Cardoso de Onorato's study seems to have been an isolated experiment that did not inspire follow-up studies, even though the "I." in its title suggests that a series of articles had been planned. Shortly after the publication of their study, however, the Argentinian doctor Alberto Tallaferro carried out his own research on experimental psychosis, leading to a more sustained set of studies that were included in the first book on the subject in Spanish, edited in 1956.[22]

Around the same time, Eustáchio Portella Nunes Filho (1929–2020), a young Brazilian doctor employed in the research division of the Institute of Psychiatry at the University of Brazil (today's Universidade Federal do Rio de Janeiro), published "Investigaçoes com a dietilamida do acido lisérgico" in the *Jornal Brasileiro de Psiquiatria*.[23] While Portella Nunes's bibliography for this work includes French and German authors, his influences were predominantly North American and continued to focus on psychoses, and the article provides a discussion of endogenous and exogenous psychoses. His experiments with LSD aimed at determining whether the drug could provoke or reactivate a specific type of psychosis. To test this hypothesis, he used a population of eight psychotic patients in remission (three hebephrenic schizophrenics, two catatonic schizophrenics, two manic-depressives, and one alcoholic with delirium tremens). Following previous tests with placebos, each subject was administered a 15-μg intravenous dose of Pervitin,[24] followed by a 1-gamma (μg) per kilogram dose of LSD (in one case, 2 gammas per kilogram) one week later. The effects produced by these two substances were then compared with the outcomes of preceding interventions in each subject, with the exception of the alcoholic. Portella Nunes concluded that Pervitin generated symptoms identical to those previously suffered by the subjects, while LSD produced a variety of effects: in the case of the schizophrenics (both hebephrenic and catatonic) it appeared to reactivate schizophrenic manifestations; in the case of the persons diagnosed with manic depression, it failed to elicit any pathological symptoms in one, while the other displayed schizophreniform symptoms. Neither substance provoked psychotic episodes in the patient who had suffered an episode of delirium tremens.

However, as with the other cases mentioned in this chapter, Portella Nunes seems to have discontinued experimenting with LSD, and a few years after this paper appeared, he turned to psychoanalysis and joined the Sociedade Psicanalítica do Rio de Janeiro—which was very common in Latin America at this time. As with the case of early LSD experiments in Chile, further studies using LSD did not appear in Brazil for another six years, and then they did so in a somewhat different context from the experiments carried out by Portella Nunes.[25]

For our final example of pioneering LSD work in South America, we turn to Venezuela, where a paper called "Experimental Psychiatry with L.S.D." was published in 1955 in the *Archivos Venezolanos de Psiquiatría y Neurología*. Although it was published as a coauthorship with Eduardo Quintero Muro (1913–?), the article was written by J. M. Hirsch (1907–1991), a Hungarian-born psychiatrist who arrived in Venezuela after fleeing growing anti-Semitism in Europe. He had studied medicine in Italy and been psychoanalyzed by a controversial Italian Franciscan friar, Father Agostino Gemelli (1878–1959), who was then rector of the Università Cattolica del Sacro Cuore in Milan. Hirsch's article is dedicated to Gemelli, referring to him as his "Master/Teacher in Experimental Psychology." Hirsch's first publications, which began emerging at in the early 1940s, show an interest in electroshock therapy,[26] which had been pioneered in the late 1930s in Rome and quickly spread throughout the continent. At the same time, Hirsch retained a significant interest in Freudian ideas. These Venezuelan researchers explained that they "wanted to experiment with L.S.D. because recent publications in scientific journals have caught our attention, and some newspapers are even writing about this drug."[27]

Despite the article's brevity—barely half a dozen pages—it was quite original in its review of the steps taken to have the substance delivered from the

Sandoz laboratory. It outlined LSD's distribution protocol, which in effect created opportunities for fellow researchers to solicit their own supplies. Following a request to have the drug delivered by mail, the authors received a warning written in French that described a few isolated accidents and listed various unforeseen or undesirable effects that could be caused by a drug that was still in the experimental phase: for example, apparently normal subjects could reveal a hidden or latent mental disorder under its influence. To conclude these warnings, there are two recommendations: to take care when administering the drug and carefully monitor the subjects to whom it was administered, and to publish the results of any experiments only in medical journals since publication in nonspecialized journals "cannot help but harm the interests of objective scientific research."[28] Sandoz finally agreed to supply the drug only after receiving a letter confirming that experimenters were aware of the warnings and would take full responsibility for acting in accordance with them.

Beyond this detailed account of the logistical hurdles to obtaining LSD, Hirsch's text gives a sparse description of his own self-experiment before spending the last two pages proposing a project—one lacking any explicit objective or hypothesis—in which the drug is administered to two subject groups (normal subjects and diagnosed psychotics), on whom various tests (e.g., neurological, electroencephalographic, Rorschach, and thematic apperception tests) would be carried out and whose self-assessments would be recorded.

It is not possible to confirm whether this experiment was in fact carried out, but a subsequent report by Hirsch does not seem to have been published anywhere, and his later publications contain no further reference to the use of LSD. Furthermore, LSD research by William Hidalgo Torres published a few years later confirm the suspicion that this initial experiment was not continued, and presumably it made no local impact within the field beyond perhaps helping researchers understand Sandoz's delivery protocols.[29]

THE ARRIVAL OF LSD IN PERU: A BUDDING RESEARCH TEAM

LSD in Peru serves as an important exception to the cases just described, displaying a distinctive feature that, until that time had not been found in other countries on the continent. Beginning in the mid-1950s, three young Peruvian psychiatrists carried out various experiments at Víctor Larco Herrera Hospital, a public psychiatric establishment in Lima, and sought to give broader visibility of LSD experiments in the country, which they pointed toward in their respective medical bachelor's theses (predoctoral), all completed in 1956.

The best-known of these psychiatrists was Javier Mariátegui Chiappe (1928–2008), the youngest son of the famous Latin American Marxist intellectual José Carlos Mariátegui (1894–1930). At the end of 1956, he published an extensive summary of his thesis in the *Revista de Neuro-psiquiatría*, based on research that he carried out under the direction of Enrique Encinas (1895–1971) in the experimental psychology lab of the pathological anatomy department at the Víctor Larco Herrera Hospital.[30] Mariátegui Chiappe placed his experiments within the framework of biochemical research into schizophrenia and hypothesized that there was a similarity between the action of LSD and psychiatric pathologies, a perspective that followed the approach proposed by Honorio Delgado (1892–1969).[31] Most of his paper was dedicated to a detailed presentation of the psychological changes observed in LSD-dosed subjects (arranged according to Delgado's classification), a description of physiological changes, a functional analysis of cognition (based on a method formulated by the German psychiatrist Konrad Zucker in 1935), and electroencephalographic studies. Although it did not stand out for its originality, this work gave visibility to a topic with no local precedents and opened the way for other studies.

In the same year, Manuel G. Zambrano (1922–2007) presented his own medical bachelor's thesis, titled "Phenomenology of Experimental Intoxication with LSD in Manic-Depressive Psychosis."[32] While his experiments involved subjects with manic depression (three men and one woman), his thesis shared a few theoretical references with Mariátegui Chiappe's work and the experimental setting was very similar to that used by his colleague. Zambrano confirmed the unusual appearance of new symptoms and noted similarities with results previously obtained using LSD on schizophrenics by international and local work teams.

A few months later, another of Mariátegui Chiappe and Zambrano's colleagues, Carlos Bambarén Vigil, published his own LSD study in the

Revista de Neuro-psiquiatría: "The Bender Test in Experimental Intoxication with LSD-25." The paper adapted a presentation that he gave at Sociedad de Psiquiatría, Neurología y Medicina Legal colloquium, in which he also summarized his bachelor's thesis, submitted the previous year, based on his involvement in experiments carried out by Mariátegui Chiappe and Zambrano. What set his work apart from that of his colleagues was the fact that he applied the Bender test[33] before and after the administration of LSD to twelve experimental subjects between the ages of twenty-six and sixty-four—five "normal," five schizophrenics, one manic-depressive, and one case of mixed psychosis. After describing his research protocols, Bambarén Vigil concluded that the difference between the two groups may reside in the fact that while normal subjects presented only motor disturbances, subjects diagnosed with some form of psychosis also experienced changes in perception, and this difference may be attributed to a "possible compromising of the intentional visual-motor act."[34] Thus, this young researcher introduced locally the application of psychological tests within the framework of the study of experimental psychoses.

During the same colloquium, Mariátegui Chiappe and Zambrano also presented some "preliminary aspects of a broader investigation that would be the subject of future articles"[35] and related the LSD experiments they had carried out with eleven subjects suffering endogenous psychoses (four manic-depressives and seven schizophrenics), as well as with two "normal" subjects and four "agitated schizophrenics" who were given d-lysergic acid ethylamide (LAE).

After a detailed account of the effects of the substances administered on the participants, there was a brief discussion among the attendees, which included Delgado himself. Amid the congratulations and specific clinical and theoretical questions, two respondents made statements that are of interest here.

The first was a comment made by the Peruvian psychiatrist Alfredo Saavedra Villalobos (1917–2014) regarding a problem that had emerged in many of the studies carried out with LSD up to that point: was there an ethical issue about administering such substances to patients whose symptoms were in remission or who were in the process of "normalization"? Saavedra

Villalobos went on to suggest that experiments using these drugs should not be carried out with these types of patients on ethical grounds, as it may exacerbate their condition.

The second was by the psychiatrist Pedro Aliaga Lindo, who made a striking remark concerning the "racial factor" in drug administration, asking if there were additional considerations "as individuals react differently depending on their race."[36] The authors responded by highlighting the need for more extensive research to assess this factor, and they observed that the effective doses appeared to depend somewhat on the regional environment, as those given in Peru were somewhat higher than those used in the US and Europe. They also referred to the aforementioned Argentine doctor Alberto Tallaferro's research, published the previous year, which shows that climate appears to have a certain influence on dosages.

Although unfortunately there have been no further mentions of research on the topic of race and LSD use in South America, their reference to Tallaferro's work leads us to another distinctive feature of these initial experiences with LSD in Peru, which sets it apart from studies published in other countries: these young Peruvian psychiatrists kept themselves informed and cited the LSD experiments carried out elsewhere in South America (namely, in Chile, Argentina, and Brazil).[37] However, although Zambrano and Mariátegui Chiappe published an article on the history of hallucinogenic drug use during colonial times the following year (1957), they did not continue their investigations with LSD—or if they did, they did not leave behind any evidence of such work.

FURTHER RESEARCH IN URUGUAY AND ECUADOR

A year after the experiences in Peru, the first publications on LSD use appeared in Uruguay and Ecuador, showing that interest in this substance continued to spread across the continent. Between 1957 and 1958, an extensive article published in the *Revista de Psiquiatría del Uruguay* under the title "Lysergic Psychosis" introduced LSD at a local level.[38] Its author, the Uruguayan scientist Juan Carlos Rey Tosar (1918–2008), was a prestigious figure in psychology in his country. By the mid-1950s, in addition to being one of the founders of the Uruguayan Psychoanalytic Association, he became a professor of psychiatry at the Faculty of Medicine (University of Uruguay). His wide and diverse output illustrates his interest in various clinical fields, and among them was narcoanalysis.[39] His paper on LSD, based on twenty experiments carried out with seven neurotic subjects, observed the psychological modifications produced by the drug: "sensory-perceptual alterations, modifications of time and space, of the body schema, hypomanic-type mood alterations, and symptoms of the schizophrenic type."[40]

One notable difference in his approach to using LSD concerned the choice of experimental subjects: although the title of his text mentions psychosis, Rey Tosar carried out his research with subjects who had been diagnosed as neurotic. This choice almost certainly arose from his interest in psychoanalysis, which can also be seen in the fact that he drew inspiration from research by Tallafero, who himself promoted the use of LSD in the treatment of obsessive neurosis.[41]

The use of LSD in the framework of experimental psychosis was also considered by other Uruguayan researchers, including Daniel Murguía (1910–2003) and Isidro Mas de Ayala (1899–1960), who took up Rey Tosar's ideas about the drug's effect on an element of the brainstem known as the "reticular formation."[42] Four years later, this topic was taken up again by the psychiatrists Ariel Duarte Troitiño and Franklin Bayley before disappearing definitively from the Uruguayan psychiatric literature.[43]

Finally, Ecuadorean research with LSD was instigated by Plutarco Naranjo Vargas (1921–2012), a doctor with strong socialist convictions, whose publications showed a wide diversity of interests, including botany, allergology (the study of allergies), and pharmacology. He held the position of public health minister under Rodrigo Borja Cevallos's government (1988–1992) and was elected president of the World Health Assembly—the decision-making body of the World Health Organization (WHO) and the highest international distinction in the field of medicine—from 1990–1991.

One distinctive feature of his work on LSD is that his publication of his research was not intended as a scientific publication, but rather was written for the magazine of the Ecuadorian House of Culture. It was there that he published his article, "Psychotomimetic Drugs," in 1957, and it was later published without modifications in *Archivos de Criminología, Neuro-Psiquiatría y Disciplinas Conexas* and the *Revista de la Confederación Médica Panamericana.*[44]

He began with a brief reflection on "psychotomimetic drugs," referring to them as a broad category of substances "capable of producing mental aberrations similar to those observed in psychosis."[45] Naranjo Vargas considered the term "hallucinogen" to be partial, and therefore incomplete; he preferred the term "psychedelic," presented at a meeting of the New York Academy of Sciences by the English psychiatrist Humphry Osmond that same year, which defined these drugs as "[s]ubstances that produce mental (thinking), perceptual, emotional, behavioral changes, and sometimes motor disturbances; changes that occur independently of each other or together."[46] Naranjo Vargas considered these drugs to be nonhabit forming, and he believed that the term excluded substances such as morphine and cocaine, as well as analgesics, anesthetics, and hypnotics.

With no claim to originality, he presented a summary comparing the psychotomimetic properties and other pharmacodynamic effects of harmine (an alkaloid now known to be a monoamine oxidase inhibitor) to LSD and mescaline using an experimental framework. The experimental subjects, in addition to other "human patients" (no further detail is given), included laboratory animals or some of their organs, which were studied at the Department of Pharmacology at the University of Utah in the US. Naranjo Vargas concluded that the three drugs would probably produce similar psychological changes and any differences would be mostly quantitative rather than qualitative. On the other hand, although these effects were generally categorized as experimental or model psychoses comparable to schizophrenia, Naranjo Vargas proposed that LSD produced a schizophrenic syndrome of the hebephrenic type, harmine a paranoid-type syndrome, and mescaline a catatonic-type syndrome with autistic tendencies.

To conclude his article, Naranjo Vargas highlighted the importance of psychotomimetic drugs "*not for their possible therapeutic applications*, but for their value as research tools."[47] However, although the publication of this article in three journals may indicate its author's enthusiasm for this topic, Naranjo Vargas did not continue his research, and his output on LSD was limited to this single text.

CONCLUSION

This chapter has set out to show the characteristics of the initial applications of LSD in psychiatric contexts in South America. In light of the first regional publications that appeared between 1954 and 1959, it is possible to detect some general features, as well as certain exceptions that also deserve to be considered.

First, for the most part, psychiatrists carried out isolated experiments that did not go on to continue this initial research—in fact, many of these experiments seem to be efforts to reproduce or verify the results of European or American researchers. Furthermore, each of these experiments was remarkably isolated from those being carried out by colleagues elsewhere in the region. Indeed, it is not clear that there was any meaningful network or direct influence among those writing and publishing LSD studies in Latin America at this time; the researchers for all the papers seem to have been relatively isolated in their own local context.

However, there are a few notable exceptions, as is clear from the experiments carried out in Peru. The work published by Javier Mariátegui Chiappe, Manuel Zambrano, and Carlos Bambarén Vigil between 1956 and 1957 show that something along the lines of a wider joint research project was carried out at the Víctor Larco Hospital. Here, despite their relative isolation, the Peruvian researchers were aware of developments in South America. In particular, the work of Mariátegui Chiappe and Zambrano (1957) exhibits a familiarity with LSD experiments that had previously been carried out by their colleagues in Chile, Brazil, and Argentina, some of which was used as sources of comparison and analysis in their own work. Although this cannot be used as a basis for any claims regarding the existence of a research network, or even of any interconnection between these early South American experiments carried, it allows us at least to observe an emerging set of regional references, as well as a certain desire to produce domestic work on the South American continent rather than merely assimilating the usual research monopoly emanating out of North America and Europe.[48]

In terms of LSD research in its broader global context, this early "South American model" of psychiatric research was abandoned shortly thereafter in light of the gradual abandonment of the toxic model of psychosis and the beginning of modern psychopharmacology that simultaneously emerged in the early 1950s.[49] It is well known that this does not imply that the use of LSD was abandoned within *psy* disciplines. As previously indicated, in the early 1960s, the substance began to be seen in a different light and to be used in a different field with different subjects. Indeed, as LSD became no longer widely viewed as a psychotomimetic, but rather as a hallucinogen, its use as an adjunct to psychotherapy—essentially for neurosis—became mainstream. In this sense, the Uruguayan psychiatrist Rey Tosar can be considered as a kind of "South American missing link": his publications toward the end of the 1950s show his passage from LSD's initial psychotomimetic experimental framework to its therapeutic application, a transition that none of his colleagues in the region appeared to have made.[50]

This application thus began a new chapter in the history of LSD, allowing its use to become widespread and making the substance famous beyond the restricted circle of *psy* professionals and institutions, even reaching certain local avant-garde movements.[51] In addition, some regional figures emerged, such as Alberto Fontana (Argentina) and Claudio Naranjo (Chile), who were able to connect their work with European and North American centers of scientific production until the early 1970s.

NOTES

1.   Albert Hofmann, *LSD: My Problem Child* (Oxford: Oxford University Press, 2013 [1979]).

2.   Robert F. Ulrich and Bernard M. Patten, "The Rise, Decline, and Fall of LSD," *Perspectives in Biology and Medicine* 34, no. 4 (1991): 561–78. https://doi.org/10.1353/pbm.1991.0062.

3.   Jay Stevens, *Storming Heaven: LSD and the American Dream* (New York: Grove Press, 1988). The history of LSD thus played out within a psychiatric tradition that had begun with the publication of the French psychiatrist Jacques-Joseph Moreau (1804–1884), who produced works on hashish and mental alienation. Michel Foucault pointed to the relevance of this author in the history of modern psychiatry in a lecture he gave on January 30, 1974; see Michel Foucault, *Psychiatric Power: Lectures at the Collège de France, 1973–1974* (Basingstoke, UK, and New York: Palgrave Macmillan, 2006).

4.   Juan José Fuentes et al., "Therapeutic Use of LSD in Psychiatry: A Systematic Review of Randomized-Controlled Clinical Trials," *Frontiers in Psychiatry* 10 (2020): 943.

5.   Mariano Plotkin and Mariano Ruperthuz, *Estimado doctor Freud, una historia cultural del psicoanálisis en América Latina* (Buenos Aires: Edhasa, 2017); Hernán Scholten and Fernando

Ferrari, *Los freudismos de Gregorio Bermann: Un recorrido sinuoso (1920–1962)* (Córdoba, Spain: Alethéia Clio, 2018).

6. Mathew Thomson, "Mental Hygiene as an International Movement," in *International Health Organisations and Movements, 1918–1939*, ed. Paul Weindling (Cambridge: Cambridge University Press, 1995), 283–304.

7. Alejandro Dagfal, "El pasaje de la higiene mental a la salud mental en la Argentina, 1920–1960: El caso de Enrique Pichon-Rivière," *Trashumante,* no. 5 (2015): 10–37.

8. Agustín Téllez, *Los Síntomas de la Esquizofrenia* (Santiago de Chile: Imprenta Universitaria, 1939); Agustín Téllez, *Aportes de la ciencia alemana a la psiquiatría moderna* (Santiago de Chile: Imprenta Universitaria, 1954).

9. Agustín Téllez, "Psicosis experimentales con ácido lisérgico," *Revista Chilena de Neuropsiquiatría,* no. 3 (1954): 289–391.

10. Téllez, "Psicosis expérimentales," 292.

11. This term, used by Tellez Meneses, was "eidetizante" in Spanish, and surely was inspired by the Greek *eidos* and/or the German *Ideen*. It can be found in some texts of Spanish-speaking philosophers inspired by German philosophers such as Edmund Husserl and other phenomenologists. We have not been able to locate the original German term or the equivalent in English.

12. Téllez, "Psicosis expérimentales," 298.

13. Anthony Busch and Warren Johnson, "L.S.D. 25 as an Aid in Psychotherapy; Preliminary Report of a New Drug," *Diseases of the Nervous System* 11, no. 8 (1950): 241–243.

14. Téllez "Psicosis expérimentales," 300.

15. Saurí's affinity with psychoanalysis is not surprising because, although Freudian doctrine began to spread regionally in the 1910s, by the mid-twentieth century, it had already been widely incorporated into Argentine culture. See Hugo Klappenbach et al., "Psychoanalysis in Argentina," *Oxford Research Encyclopedia of Psychology* (Oxford: Oxford University Press, 2021); Mariano Ben Plotkin, *Freud in the Pampas: The Emergence and Development of a Psychoanalytic Culture in Argentina* (Stanford, CA: Stanford University Press, 2002).

16. José Saurí and Amelia C. de Onorato, "Las esquizofrenias y la dietilamida del ácido d-lisérgico (LSD 25): I Variaciones del estado de ánimo," *Acta psiquiátrica y psicológica de América latina* 1, no. 5 (1955): 469–476.

17. Saurí and Onorato, "Las esquizofrenias," 469.

18. R. Stuart, "Modern Psychedelic Art's Origins as a Product of Clinical Experimentation," *Vernal Equinox,* no. 13 (2004): 12–22.

19. Werner A. Stoll, "Lysergsäure-Diäthylamid, ein Phantastikum aus der Mutterkorngruppe," *Schweiz. Arch. Neurol. u. Psychiat,* no. 60 (1947): 289.

20. Saurí and Onorato, "Las esquizofrenias," 469.

21. Saurí and Onorato, "Las esquizofrenias," 476.

22. Alberto Tallaferro, *Mescalina y LSD25* (Buenos Aires: Librería Jurídica Valerio Abeledo, 1956); Hernán Scholten, "Alberto Tallaferro y los usos experimentales de la LSD25 en Argentina (1954–1959)," *Sinopsis* 30, no. 59 (2017): 7–12.

23. Eustachio Portella Nunes, "Investigaçoes com a dietilamida do acido lisérgico," *Jornal Brasileiro de Psiquiatria* 4, no. 4 (1955): 407–418.

24. This was a brand of methamphetamine that became famous for its frequent use by German soldiers during World War II.

25. Paulo Guedes, "Experiencias com a dietilamina do ácido lisérgico (LSD25)," *Arquivos de Neuro-Psiquiatria* 19, no. 1 (1961): 28–34.

26. Concerning this period of his academic output, see Edward Shorter and David Healy, *Shock Therapy: A History of Electroconvulsive Treatment in Mental Illness* (London: Rutgers University Press, 2007).

27. J. M. Hirsch and Eduardo Quintero Muro, "Psiquiatría experimental con L.S.D.," *Archivos venezolanos de psiquiatría y neurología* no. 1 (1955): 24–29; 26.

28. Hirsch and Quintero Muro, "Psiquiatría experimental con L.S.D.," 27.

29. William Hidalgo Torres, "La dietilamida del ácido lisérgico," *Rev. Fac. Med.,* no. 3 (1957): 319–32; William Hidalgo Torres, "Estudio comparativo Psicofisiológico de la Mescalina, Dietilamida del ácido D-lisérgico y Psilocybina," *Acta médica venezolana,* no. 8 (1960): 56–62.

30. Javier Mariátegui, "Psicopatología de la intoxicación experimental con la LSD. Estudios en normales y en esquizofrénicos," *Revista de Neuro-psiquiatría* 19, no. 4 (1956): 474–517.

31. He was a prestigious Peruvian physician-psychiatrist, recognized throughout Latin America. Although he was an early regional disseminator of psychoanalysis and had fairly close contact with Sigmund Freud during the 1920s, soon afterward, he clearly distanced himself from the ideas of the Viennese doctor. See Plotkin and Ruperthuz, *Estimado doctor Freud,* 2017.

32. Manuel G. Zambrano, *Fenomenología de la intoxicación experimental con la LSD 25 en la psicosis maníacodepresiva* (Lima; Facultad de Medicina, Universidad Nacional Mayor de San Marcos, 1956).

33. Developed in 1938 by the child neuropsychiatrist Lauretta Bender, this is a psychological test used by mental health practitioners to assess visual-motor functioning, developmental disorders, and neurological impairments in adults and children aged three and older.

34. Carlos Bambaren Vigil, "La prueba de Bender en la intoxicación experimental con la LSD25," *Revista de Neuro-psiquiatría* 20, no. 4 (1957): 603.

35. Javier Mariátegui and Manuel Zambrano, "Psicosíndromes experimentales con los derivados del ácido lisérgico. Estudios preliminares con la LSD y la LAE," *Revista de Neuro-psiquiatría* 20, no. 4 (1957): 455.

36. Mariátegui and Zambrano, "Psicosíndromes experimentales con los derivados del ácido lisérgico," 469.

37. While Mariátegui Chiappe's text includes references to the articles by Téllez Meneses and Portella Nunes in its bibliography, Zambrano makes several references to the latter in his thesis. Finally, the article in collaboration with both authors includes references to the book by Argentine Alberto Tallaferro on *Mescaline y LSD-25* (1956).

38. Juan Carlos Rey, "Psicosis lisérgica," *Revista de Psiquiatría* 22, no. 131 (1957): 45–64; Rey, "Psicosis lisérgica," *Revista de Psiquiatría* 22, no. 132 (1957): 37–49; Rey, "Psicosis lisérgica," *Revista de Psiquiatría* 23, no. 133 (1958): 25–56.

39. Juan Carlos Rey, "Narcoanálisis," *Revista de Psiquiatría* 18, no. 105 (1953): 11–25.

40. Rey, "Psicosis lisérgica," *Revista de Psiquiatría* 23, no. 133 (1958): 25–56, 55.

41. Alberto Tallaferro, *Mescalina y LSD25*, 1956.

42. Isidro Más de Ayala, "Formación reticulada y alteraciones psiquiátricas," in *Anales de la Clínica Psiquiátrica: Curso de Perfeccionamiento II*, ed. Fortunato Ramírez (Montevideo, Uruguay: Rosgal, 1958), 153–60; Daniel L. Murguía, "Aportes modernos en terapéutico psiquiátrico," in *Anales de la Clínica Psiquiátrica: Curso de Perfeccionamiento I*, ed. Fortunato Ramírez (Montevideo, Uruguay: Rosgal, 1958), 177–204.

43. Ariel Duarte and Franklin Bayley, "Contribución al estudio del ácido lisérgico en clínica psiquiátrica," *Revista de Psiquiatría del Uruguay* 26, no. 1 (1961): 19–45.

44. Plutarco Naranjo Vargas, "Drogas psicotomiméticas: Estudio comparativo de la harmina, la dietilamida del ácido lisérgico (LSD-25) y la mescalina," *Revista de la Casa de la Cultura Ecuatoriana* 10, no. 19 (1957): 178–199; Naranjo Vargas, "Drogas psicotomiméticas: estudio comparativo de la harmina, la dietilamida del ácido lisérgico, LSD-25 y la mescalina," *Archivos de Criminología, Neuro-Psiquiatría y Disciplinas Conexas* 6, no. 23 (1958): 358–379; Naranjo Vargas, "Estudio comparativo de la Harmina, la Dietilamida del ácido lisérgico (LSD-25) y la Mescalina," *Revista de la Confederación médica panamericana* 6 (1959): 1–8.

45. Naranjo Vargas, "Drogas psicotomiméticas," 180.

46. Vargas, "Drogas psicotomiméticas," 181.

47. Vargas, "Drogas psicotomiméticas," 195 (emphasis added).

48. Anyway, the only relatively sustained program of study of LSD-25 as a psychotomimetic was carried out in Argentina by Alberto Tallaferro, who continued to publish his experiences until 1959. See Scholten, "Alberto Tallaferro y los usos experimentales de la LSD25 en Argentina (1954–1959)."

49. Alan Baumeister and Mike F Hawkins, "Continuity and Discontinuity in the Historical Development of Modern Psychopharmacology," *Journal of the History of the Neurosciences* 14, no. 3 (2005): 199–209; Joel T. Braslow and Stephen R. Marder, "History of Psychopharmacology," *Annual Review of Clinical Psychology* 15, no. 1 (2019): 25–50.

50. Juan Carlos Rey, "El esquema corporal en la psicosis lisérgica," in *Anales de la Clínica Psiquiátrica: Curso de Perfeccionamiento II*, ed. Fortunato Ramírez (Montevideo, Uruguay: Rosgal, 1959), 43–56; Juan Carlos Rey, "Desestructuración del esquema corporal y ácido lisérgico," *Revista uruguaya de psicoanálisis* 3, no. 4 (1960): 365–76.

51. In the case of Argentina, Luisa G. Álvarez de Toledo, the president of the local psychoanalytic association, openly promoted the use of LSD since 1957. However, at the beginning of the 1960s, the most orthodox sectors of this institution spurned the controversial substance, and two of its most renowned promoters were forced to resign.

BIBLIOGRAPHY

Baumeister, Alan, and Mike F. Hawkins. "Continuity and Discontinuity in the Historical Development of Modern Psychopharmacology." *Journal of the History of the Neurosciences* 14, no. 3 (2005): 199–209.

Braslow, Joel T., and Stephen R. Marder. "History of Psychopharmacology." *Annual Review of Clinical Psychology* 15, no. 1 (2019): 25–50.

Busch, Anthony, and Warren Johnson. "L.S.D. 25 as an Aid in Psychotherapy; Preliminary Report of a New Drug." *Diseases of the Nervous System* 11, no. 8 (1950): 241–243.

Dagfal, Alejandro. "El pasaje de la higiene mental a la salud mental en la Argentina, 1920–1960: El caso de Enrique Pichon-Rivière." *Trashumante*, no. 5 (2015): 10–37.

Duarte, Ariel, and Franklin Bayley. "Contribución al estudio del ácido lisérgico en clínica psiquiátrica." *Revista de Psiquiatría del Uruguay* 26, no. 1 (1961): 19–45.

Foucault, Michel. *Psychiatric Power: Lectures at the Collège de France, 1973–1974*. Basingstoke, UK, and New York: Palgrave Macmillan, 2006.

Fuentes, Juan José, Francina Fonseca, Matilde Elices, Magi Farré, and Marta Torrens. "Therapeutic Use of LSD in Psychiatry: A Systematic Review of Randomized-Controlled Clinical Trials." *Frontiers in Psychiatry* 10 (2020): 943.

Guedes, Paulo. "Experiencias com a dietilamina do ácido lisérgico (LSD25)." *Arquivos de Neuro-Psiquiatria* 19, no. 1 (1961): 28–34.

Hirsch, J. M., and Eduardo Quintero Muro. "Psiquiatría experimental con L.S.D." *Archivos venezolanos de psiquiatría y neurología* no. 1 (1955): 24–29.

Hofmann, Albert. *LSD: My Problem Child*. Oxford: Oxford University Press, 2013.

Klappenbach, Hugo, Antonio Gentile, Fernando Ferrari, and Hernan Scholten. "Psychoanalysis in Argentina." *Oxford Research Encyclopedia of Psychology*. 22 Jan. 2021; https://oxfordre.com/psychology/view/10.1093/acrefore/9780190236557.001.0001/acrefore-9780190236557-e-689.

Mariátegui, Javier and Manuel Zambrano. "Psicosíndromes experimentales con los derivados del ácido lisérgico. Estudios preliminares con la LSD y la LAE." *Revista de Neuro-psiquiatría* 20, no. 4 (1957): 451–474.

Mariátegui, Javier. "Psicopatología de la intoxicación experimental con la LSD. Estudios en normales y en esquizofrénicos." *Revista de Neuro-psiquiatría* 19, no. 4 (1956): 474–517.

Más de Ayala, "Isidro Formación reticulada y alteraciones psiquiátricas." In *Anales de la Clínica Psiquiátrica: Curso de Perfeccionamiento II*, edited by Fortunato Ramírez, 153–160. Montevideo, Uruguay: Rosgal, 1958.

Murguía, Daniel L. "Aportes modernos en terapéutico psiquiátrico." In *Anales de la Clínica Psiquiátrica: Curso de Perfeccionamiento I*, edited by Fortunato Ramírez, 177–204. Montevideo, Uruguay: Rosgal, 1958.

Nunes, Eustachio Portella. "Investigaçoes com a dietilamida do acido lisérgico." *Jornal Brasileiro de Psiquiatria* 4, no. 4 (1955): 407–418.

Plotkin, Mariano Ben. *Freud in the Pampas: The emergence and Development of a Psychoanalytic Culture in Argentina*. Stanford, CA: Stanford University Press, 2002.

Plotkin, Mariano, and Mariano Ruperthuz. *Estimado doctor Freud, una historia cultural del psicoanálisis en América Latina*. Buenos Aires: Edhasa, 2017.

Rey, Juan Carlos. "Desestructuración del esquema corporal y ácido lisérgico." *Revista uruguaya de psicoanálisis* 3, no. 4 (1960): 365–476.

Rey, Juan Carlos. "El esquema corporal en la psicosis lisérgica." In *Anales de la Clínica Psiquiátrica: Curso de Perfeccionamiento II*, edited by Fortunato Ramírez, 43–56. Montevideo, Uruguay: Rosgal, 1959.

Rey, Juan Carlos. "Narcoanálisis." *Revista de Psiquiatría* 18, no. 105 (1953): 11–25.

Rey, Juan Carlos. "Psicosis lisérgica." *Revista de Psiquiatría* 22, no. 131 (1957): 45–64.

Rey, Juan Carlos. "Psicosis lisérgica." *Revista de Psiquiatría* 22, no. 132 (1957): 37–49.

Rey, Juan Carlos. "Psicosis lisérgica." *Revista de Psiquiatría* 23, no. 133 (1958): 25–56.

Saurí, José, and Amelia C. de Onorato. "Las esquizofrenias y la dietilamida del ácido d-lisérgico (LSD 25): I Variaciones del estado de ánimo." *Acta psiquiátrica y psicológica de América latina* 1, no. 5 (1955): 469–476.

Scholten, Hernán. "Alberto Tallaferro y los usos experimentales de la LSD25 en Argentina (1954–1959)." *Sinopsis* 30, no. 59 (2017): 7–12.

Scholten, Hernán, and Fernando Ferrari. *Los freudismos de Gregorio Bermann: Un recorrido sinuoso (1920–1962)*. Córdoba, Argentina: Alethéia Clio, 2018.

Shorter, Edward, and David Healy. *Shock Therapy: A History of Electroconvulsive Treatment in Mental Illness*. London: Rutgers University Press, 2007.

Stevens, Jay. *Storming Heaven: LSD and the American Dream*. New York: Grove Press, 1988.

Stoll, Werner A. "Lysergsäure-Diäthylamid, ein Phantastikum aus der Mutterkorngruppe." *Schweiz. Arch. Neurol. u. Psychiat.* no. 60 (1947): 279–323.

Stuart, R. "Modern Psychedelic Art's Origins as a Product of Clinical Experimentation." *Vernal Equinox*, no. 13 (2004): 12–22.

Tallaferro, Alberto. *Mescalina y LSD25*. Buenos Aires: Librería Jurídica Valerio Abeledo, 1956.

Téllez, Agustin. *Aportes de la ciencia alemana a la psiquiatría moderna*. Santiago de Chile: Imprenta Universitaria, 1954.

Téllez, Agustín. "Psicosis experimentales con ácido lisérgico." *Revista Chilena de Neuro-psiquiatría*, no. 3 (1954): 289–391.

Téllez, Agustín. *Los Síntomas de la Esquizofrenia*. Santiago de Chile: Imprenta Universitaria, 1939.

Thomson, Mathew. "Mental Hygiene as an International Movement." In *International Health Organisations and Movements, 1918–1939*, edited by Paul Weindling, 283–304. Cambridge: Cambridge University Press, 1995.

Torres, William Hidalgo. "La dietilamida del ácido lisérgico." *Rev. Fac. Med.*, no. 3 (1957): 319–332.

Torres, William Hidalgo. "Estudio comparativo Psicofisiológico de la Mescalina, Dietilamida del ácido D-lisérgico y Psilocybina." *Acta médica venezolana*, no. 8 (1960): 56–62.

Ulrich, Robert F., and Bernard M. Patten. "The Rise, Decline, and Fall of LSD." *Perspectives in Biology and Medicine* 34, no. 4 (1991): 561–578. https://doi.org/10.1353/pbm.1991.0062.

Vargas, Naranjo. "Drogas psicotomiméticas: Estudio comparativo de la harmina, la dietilamida del ácido lisérgico, LSD-25 y la mescalina." *Archivos de Criminología, Neuro-Psiquiatría y Disciplinas Conexas* 6, no. 23 (1958): 358–379.

Vargas, Naranjo. "Estudio comparativo de la Harmina, la Dietilamida del ácido lisergicolisérgico (LSD-25) y la Mescalina." *Revista de la Confederación médica panamericana* 6 (1959): 1–8.

Vargas, Plutarco Naranjo. "Drogas psicotomiméticas: Estudio comparativo de la harmina, la dietilamida del ácido lisérgico (LSD-25) y la mescalina." *Revista de la Casa de la Cultura Ecuatoriana* 10, no. 19 (1957): 178–199.

Vigil, Carlos Bambaren. "La prueba de Bender en la intoxicación experimental con la LSD25." *Revista de Neuro-psiquiatría* 20, no. 4 (1957): 508–607.

Zambrano, Manuel G. *Fenomenología de la intoxicación experimental con la LSD 25 en la psicosis maníacodepresiva*. Lima: Facultad de Medicina, Universidad Nacional Mayor de San Marcos, 1956.

11 "I AM A SCIENTIST!" ROGER HEIM'S INTERDISCIPLINARY AND TRANSNATIONAL RESEARCH ON HALLUCINOGENIC MUSHROOMS (AND THE PROBLEM OF DIVINATION)

Vincent Verroust

Roger Heim (1900–1979) was a French biologist and a professor of mycology at the *Muséum National d'Histoire Naturelle* (MNHN) in Paris. He directed this old and prestigious academic institution, following in the footsteps of famous biologists like Georges-Louis Leclerc, Comte de Buffon, and Georges Cuvier. During the 1950s, at a time when his brilliant career was already underway, his research took a new turn when he became actively involved in the discovery of Mexican hallucinogenic mushrooms among Western researchers.

In doing so, he helped pave the way for groundbreaking research in the modern psychedelic history. Of course, archeological evidence indicates that Amerindians had known hallucinogenic mushrooms in ill-known practices deep into pre-Columbian times,[1] but Western scientific investigations are recent, notwithstanding some references in sixteenth-century Spanish manuscripts[2] and in some ethnographic observations published in Europe in the 1920s and 1930s. The famous Harvard ethnobotanist Richard Evans Schultes (1915–2001) had also collected samples in 1938 and 1939.[3] In any event, records that reveal the intentional use of psilocybin mushrooms in Europe do not appear until the second half of the twentieth century; what traces of interest were shown in this topic before this time were isolated to a handful of erudite scientists with a limited audience.[4] On the other hand, there is evidence of psilocybin mushrooms in nineteenth- and early-twentieth-century European medical literature[5] that describes cases of involuntary intoxication and shows that nobody understood their psychoactive effects.

The year 1953 marks the critical starting point for contemporary scientific investigations into Mexican mushrooms through the work of Robert Gordon Wasson (1898–1986) and Valentina Pavlovna Wasson (1901–1958), a banker and a pediatrician, respectively. Both of them were passionate about mushrooms. While their story is usually depicted as independent scholars forging a new path, their friendship and collaboration with Heim is little known. Heim's correspondence, housed at the MNHN, reveals that Gordon Wasson and Roger Heim became friends in the late 1940s via correspondence and met in person in Paris in the spring of 1950. Subsequently, the two traveled around France in 1952, including one trip with Valentina, as they were preparing their seminal monograph *Mushrooms, Russia and History*, which was published in 1957 in two splendid volumes.[6] In fact, Heim diligently copyedited their book, and their close friendship and intellectual affinity is also reflected in their dedications in their respective works.[7] Beginning in 1956, Heim joined the Wassons on several expeditions to visit various Indigenous peoples in Mexico in an attempt to find traces of mushroom consumption.

Following this early work discovering the existence and uses of hallucinogenic mushrooms, Heim went on to collaborate with Albert Hofmann, the anthropologist Guy Stresser-Péan (1913–2009) and the psychiatrist Jean Delay (1907–1987). From the 1950s onward, his career took an unexpected turn, building bridges with the humanities, medicine, and visual arts. Heim's work thus deserves to be analyzed along interdisciplinary and transnational lines. Recent historical scholarship reveals how the psychopharmacological study of serotoninergic hallucinogens spilled out of the lab and into groundbreaking collaborations. This is apparent in Milana Aronov's work of on LSD as a source of creativity[8] and Erika Dyck's history of the influence of LSD on architecture in psychiatric hospitals.[9]

The global history of psychedelics calls into question the specific nature of the psychic effects triggered by the serotoninergic hallucinogens, which can vary quite dramatically according to the context and from one user to another. By way of hypothesis, intimate experiences with psychedelics within the scientific realm have led to specific knowledge, such as the end of the psychotomimetic paradigm and Humphry Osmond's coining of the word "psychedelic," which helped move toward a therapeutic understanding of LSD and mescaline in psychiatry.[10] The Czech pharmacologist Stephen Szára likewise defended the heuristic value of personal familiarity with psychedelics, as did the Italian theoretical physicist Carlo Rovelli, who pointed to the influence of his LSD experiences on his scientific work.[11]

Roger Heim's career is a case in point. I wish to focus on one particular episode: his appraisal of their use in divination. In conjunction with his appreciation for their psychic effects, and according to the anthropological, psychiatric, and experimental perspectives that emerged through his collaborations, Heim developed an interest in the practice of divination, and in so doing, he operated on the scientific fringe. I wish to show that although he attempted to incorporate allusions to extrasensory perception into his own research, which is evidenced by the archives and hinted at in his interdisciplinary understanding of hallucinogenic mushrooms, it caused him a great deal of unease. How did he negotiate between his interest in paranormal phenomena and the rigorously rational imperatives of Western science? From this perspective, it is illuminating to dwell on the research happening in France in the 1950s and 1960s and how it is related to scientism and rationalism.

ROGER HEIM'S ACADEMIC TRAINING

Beginning in his youth, Heim was fascinated by the natural sciences, and as early as 1920, he spent time at the MNHN's cryptogam (botanical organisms that reproduce by spores, without flowers or seeds) laboratory. However, his father made it clear that he would only settle for his son getting an engineering degree, and that same year Heim entered the *École Centrale*, one of the country's oldest and most prestigious institutions (*grandes écoles*), as well as an elite school where he received advanced training in applied industrial science. He received his engineering degree in 1923 before immediately returning to his initial passion and completing his degree in natural science in 1924. He did his military service at the MNHN's organic chemistry laboratory, and later in the biochemistry laboratory of *L'institut Pasteur* in Paris, while simultaneously training in mycology. He defended his dissertation

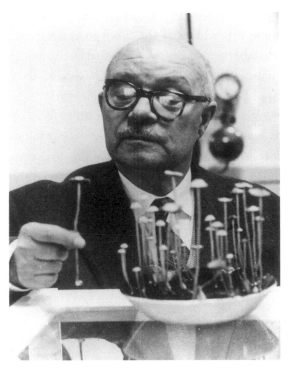

Figure 11.1
Roger Heim with a culture of *Psilocybe mexicana* at the cryptogamy laboratory of the MNHN in Paris, c. 1958. Reproduced with the permission of the MNHN.

on the *Inocybe* genus of fungi in 1931, reflecting his developing interest in mushroom classification, tropical mycology, and phytopathology. Soon, he made a name for himself by publishing high-impact papers on the topic. After World War II,[12] he joined the *Académie des Sciences* in 1946, after which he began conducting fieldwork around the globe before taking assuming the position of director of the MNHN in 1951. Over the course of his career, he was the recipient of several academic distinctions and honorary degrees.

Heim's training reveals that his main area of interest was the biology of organisms, based on a naturalistic approach to the living world. What this survey of Heim's education and career overlooks is his general interest in psychology (and parapsychology in particular), which came to the fore only after his first contact with hallucinogenic mushrooms.[13] There is no indication that Heim was interested in paranormal phenomena when he began collaborating with the Wassons—neither in his publications, nor in his personal papers, nor in any other archival source. Given his rigorous scientific training, it is quite likely that he would have had, at least initially, an unfavorable opinion of the issue. Indeed, theories based on metapsychic phenomena, such as animal magnetism and somnambulism, had already been discredited by French science and medicine in the eighteenth century. While research on psychic phenomena in France was temporarily part of the field of psychology during the last two decades of the nineteenth century, the so-called occult sciences were far afield from the perspectives of most scientists, were too busy defending their positivistic methodologies.[14] Hence, scientific research into paranormal phenomena in France quickly waned at the turn of the century and was abandoned permanently just before World War II.[15] When Heim was a student, these phenomena had thus been banished to the domain of occultists and spiritualists, as well as the *Institut Métapsychique International*, created in 1919, which was not part of academia.

When the fifty-something Heim first heard about Mexican psychotropic mushrooms, he was the respected director of the MNHN and brilliant biologist, known around the world for his exemplary, naturalistic fieldwork. This placed him in a very prominent and public position, and given the intellectual context of the time, it is hard to imagine him taking up the study of paranormal phenomena.

THE DISCOVERY OF MUSHROOM-BASED AMERINDIAN DIVINATORY PRACTICES

In 1953, the Wassons began their ethnographic fieldwork in Mexico and collected four types of samples that they shipped to the MNHN for analysis and classification. It was through them that Heim learned about the use of hallucinogenic mushrooms in divination. In 1956, he acknowledged this aspect of mushroom use at the French *Académie des Sciences* in a note stating that these mushrooms were indeed "divinatory."[16]

The Wassons first witnessed a mushroom *velada* in the Mazatec village of Huautla de Jimenez in northern Oaxaca, Mexico in August 1953. To justify their request for such a ceremony and to be able to observe it as ethnographers, they asked the *curandero* Aurelio Carreras for some news about their son Peter, who had stayed in the US. They believed that he was in Boston, where he worked, but under the influence, Aurelio told them that he was in New York, that he was in a bad way, and that the army was going to send him to Germany. He also predicted that a family member would be afflicted by a serious condition later that year.

The Wassons had no trouble admitting that they doubted Aurelio's divinatory powers, most notably because Peter was exempted from the draft. Upon returning to the US, they were surprised to learn that their son was indeed in New York (and not Boston) at the time that Aurelio made his prediction. Peter told them that he was heartbroken, which led to a major emotional crisis, which caused him to join the army. He was to be shipped off to Japan, but after receiving basic combat training, he was stationed in Germany. A few months later, to everyone's shock, a young cousin of Gordon Wasson died of a heart attack. Aurelio's account had come to pass. In *Mushrooms, Russia and History*, where this story appears, the Wassons remained uncertain about what they had experienced: "We record, as in duty we are bound to do, but without further comment, these strange sequelae to our Huautla visit."[17] The comment without further elaboration suggests that the Wassons were aware of their reputations and remained cautious. After all, they were trying to introduce a new field of study—ethnomycology—and were intent on legitimizing this new field in academia.

Nothing indicates that Gordon Wasson and Heim discussed this divinatory event in their correspondence, but it is possible that they talked about it during their joint expedition in July and August 1956.[18] Heim too had undergone a bemushroomed prediction, via the soon-to-be famous *curandera* María Sabina, which he acknowledged on French television in 1966.[19] Appearing on the show *Entrée libre*, Heim said: "Wasson and myself have experienced, quite by chance, the predictions of María Sabina . . . and I have to say that she made predictions for both of us, and we had no reason to believe them, and they both turned out to be accurate." In 1970, Heim briefly discussed this again at a meeting organized by Sandoz,[20] during a debate on "social chemical substances," where participants discussed the reasons for some Indigenous peoples to use the intoxicating mushrooms—in this case for divination. Heim had this to say:

> So—and this a scientist talking to you—I have to say that I've been impressed by the divinatory meaning of the predictions made by the shaman as she was under the influence of the mushroom. I would just like to tell you that, to my friend Wasson and to myself, the *curandera* María Sabina, in Mexico, in a small Mazatec village, after ingesting the mushrooms, predicted two events that both of us could never have guessed. . . . During this extraordinary experience that we witnessed, María told us with precision: 'OK, in Paris, this is about to happen which concerns you, and for you, there is this other thing in New York.' It was a double prediction that was really unthinkable for both of us. I say this to you because it turned out to be accurate and she told us that a lot of Mexicans were coming over to consult with her hoping that she will answer some of their questions.

Unfortunately, Heim does not provide the details about these predictions. In *Les champignons hallucinogènes du Mexique* (1958), he makes no mention of it, but in the conclusion, he adds:

> María Sabina's rituals would only be distinguished in detail from the formulas of many other ceremonies where exorcism is integral, where occultism is absolute, if an essentially objective, tangible, and controllable element had not long been introduced into these esoteric practices (unless they had spurred them): the exacting power of certain hallucinogenic mushrooms.[21]

His word choices are worth dwelling on: "occultism," "exorcism," and "esoteric," which Heim uses to refer to Mazatec "ceremonies," are certainly clumsy. To be sure, these words are drawn from the nineteenth-century realms of mediums and spiritualism rather than from anthropology—the comparative scientific study of different peoples—which had experienced academic renewal in the 1930s and 1940s and which accepted magic and science as both integral to many human societies and distinguished between notions of magic and superstition.[22] His choice of these words in this context indicates that Heim had made inroads into the world of magic. At the same time, his statement reflects the strong influence of the twentieth-century positivist and scientist traditions.

In the excerpt quoted here, it is noteworthy that Heim underscored the effects of psilocybin on the psyche, which scientists were beginning to study in this context. He added that "it is striking that the divinatory characteristics of the totem are indeed based on the *true* hallucinatory effects of the teonanácatl, perfectly distinguished, precisely experienced by the Indians." Heim emphasized the adjective "true." Was this a hypallage? Was he implicitly suggesting "true divinatory characteristics" being inherent in the mushroom through this figure of speech? This hypothesis does not seem far-fetched. Another hint suggests that it was during his first trip to Huautla that Heim experienced María Sabina's prophetic abilities, as this excerpt indicates: "All these different kinds of staging, like many others, could have been the result of total occultism or a partially subconscious form of self-suggestion. That is not the case. That some of the facts turned out to be real was a decisive and powerfully convincing factor, revealing that the Indian sorcerers were sincere actors in part." [23]

What were those facts? Heim does not say. On the one hand, the French translation of the Wassons' 1953 fieldwork appears in the text, as does Aurelio Carreras's prediction about Peter and their ill family member. On the other hand, it is the only mention of a successful prediction provided in the book that was verified by the scientists' personal experiences. Moreover, Heim mentions "facts," plural. In light of a spoken anecdote related much later, first on television and then in the journal *Entretiens de Rueil*, it seems that during his first visit, María Sabina offered Heim a prediction that turned out to be true. He found this troubling, for it was inconceivable to Heim, the rationalist, that the predictions of a native soothsayer could shake his certainties. If Heim had no trouble recognizing the accuracy of the ecological knowledge of the Indigenous people he met in his many travels around the world, as well as the effectiveness of their medicines,[24] it was a real surprise to him that María Sabina forced him to question his own logic.

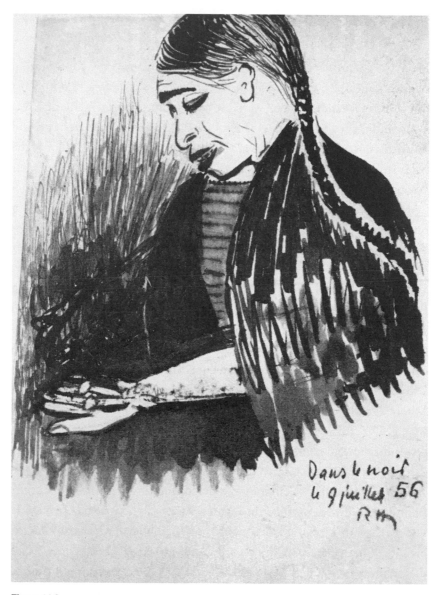

Figure 11.2
Sketch of María Sabina by Roger Heim on July 9, 1956. Reproduced with the permission of the
Société des amis du Muséum national d'Histoire naturelle.

ACADEMIC DISTANCE IN THE FIRST WRITINGS
ON MEXICAN MUSHROOMS

Heim's and Gordon Wasson's letters offer a window into their collaboration on their joint study, *Les champignons hallucinogènes du Mexique* (1958). Wasson wrote the sections dealing with historical sources, ethnographic observations, and archeological data, many of which were translated from his and Valentina's *Mushrooms, Russia, and History*. Heim, as the main author of the volume, described the collected species and took charge of the study of their taxonomic, embryological, and cultivational features. The chapter written by Heim in this study is an exhaustive account of his mycological research on those species, with a few basic incursions into the realm of ethnobiology.

Heim also cowrote chapters, with Albert Hofmann and other scientists at Sandoz, on the pharmacology of psilocybin, as well as the drug's effects on the psyche, which begins with an account of his self-experimentations in Paris and Mexico. Here, he described the visual phenomena, physiological symptoms, mood changes, "joyous clairvoyance of the mind," and "exceptional well-being" that he experienced the day after the sessions.[25] He also discussed reports by other mushroom experimenters like the Wassons', but also the mescaline experiences of Aldous Huxley, the neurologist Silas Weir Mitchell, and the poet Henri Michaux, as well as Hofmann's experiments with LSD.

Indigenous discourses on the effects of the mushrooms did not appear in this psychopharmacological study, framed by Western subjective experiences and ways of knowing. Heim omitted describing his impressions about the feelings of knowledge gained through revelations, which he had previously associated with Mexican practices, about which he had previously written in a note on divinatory mushrooms at the *Académie des Sciences* in 1956. In the 1958 volume, this analysis of the "first experiences resulting from the ingestion of Mexican agaric hallucinogens" was followed by a psychophysiological and clinical study of psilocybin conducted by a team of psychiatrists at the Sainte-Anne Hospital in Paris. Here, these French psychiatrists described psilocybin's somatic, psychic, and electroencephalographic effects on normal subjects and mental patients. Of course, there were no mentions of clairvoyance. The physicians, for their part, describe "delirious constructions" and "reminiscences," observed "relatively often," which "made for one the most interesting aspects of the mechanisms of psilocybin."[26]

Speculation notwithstanding, it remains interesting to note that under the mushroom's effects, Indigenous Mexicans sought to become aware of the future, while European subjects tended to experience a recollection of memories. Even so, Wasson had explicitly referred to the divinatory power of the mushrooms in his account of his first Mazatec ritual. Heim also appears to acknowledge this feature of the mushroom in wandering innuendoes in the last pages of his conclusion. Even if representing just a tiny portion of the book, the topic of the divinatory power of mushrooms was impossible to ignore.

A MORE OPEN FORM OF CORRESPONDENCE

In the spring of 1959, Heim received an invitation from the American journalist Martin Ebon, on behalf of the Parapsychology Foundation, to participate in the international conference on parapsychology scheduled for the next year in Saint-Paul-de-Vence entitled "Pharmacology and Parapsychology." Heim could not make it, but he wrote to Hofmann soon afterward to see whether he might consider attending. Hofmann replied by asking if the Parapsychology Foundation was "a seriously scientific society." This organization, which Hofmann seemed to perceive as pseudoscientific, would certainly have threatened their reputations if they had responded favorably to the invitation.

Indeed, parapsychology was still considered a controversial and quite unstable discipline at the time of this exchange. In the US, Joseph Rhine (1895–1980) and his wife, Louisa Rhine, both at Duke University, pioneered the use of quantitative methods for the study of extrasensory perception (ESP) and became staunch defenders of the field from the 1930s onward. Joseph Rhine also founded the Parapsychological Association in 1957, and in New York City, the Irish spiritualist and medium Eileen J. Garrett had created the Parapsychology Foundation, which organized the Vence Congress, a few years earlier. Garrett also worked toward the legitimization of parapsychology as an academic discipline, especially by lending herself to numerous laboratory experiments as a subject.

In the 1960s, Heim corresponded with Roberto Cavanna, an Italian biochemist from the Instituto Superiore di Sanita in Rome, whose letters were often accompanied by a few sentences from his fellow countryman Emilio Servadio. The latter, who received his PhD in legal theory from the University of Genoa, was the founder of the Italian Psychoanalytic Society and the Italian Society of Parapsychology. In their letters, Cavanna and Servadio expressed interest in parapsychology, in conjunction with the mushroom experiences. The first letter, dated March 31, was an invitation to discuss the topic over dinner while the two Italians traveled through Paris on their way to New York, having accepted an invitation to visit from the Parapsychology Foundation (with "no mushrooms on the menu!" they specified). They also suggested that Heim invite the Sainte-Anne Hospital–based psychiatrist Jean Delay to lunch. Heim responded favorably by dispatching a note to Delay, where he mentioned the arrival of the two Italians and noted their link with the Parapsychology Foundation, although Heim himself could not attend.

Heim did not seem embarrassed to broach the subject of parapsychology with Delay. Apparently, Cavanna and Servadio were very eager to have a face-to-face exchange with Heim and were disappointed to miss him; they also tried to meet him on their return journey. A July 11, 1960, letter from Heim to Cavanna indicates that they had finally met, with Heim expressing his "great pleasure" at their acquaintance and adding that it "will be very pleasant to continue our contacts around hallucinogenic mushrooms and the problems of Psychopharmacy [sic]."

Heim added that he considered an article published by Servadio that June in the Italian periodical *La Stampa* was "the best report that has been made regarding the discovery of Mexican hallucinogenic mushrooms and psilocybin." This article, which ends by referring to María Sabina's ability to "read minds," came to this conclusion: "Illusion or truth? We can only say . . . that alongside psychological research and psychiatric studies on psilocybin, other studies are underway regarding its possible, and so-far only hypothesized, ability to 'trigger' extra-sensory perceptions."[27] Thus, if Heim was indeed troubled by a startling prediction of María Sabina, it is quite understandable that he approved of this conclusion. In any event, it seems very likely that these mysterious divinatory phenomena were the topic of the discussions during Heim's meeting with the Italians, given their focus on the potential of psilocybin in experimental parapsychology.

The 1960 correspondence between Cavanna and Heim also reveals that Garrett, a close associate to Aldous Huxley and Humphry Osmond,[28] carried out experiments under the effects of eight milligrams of psilocybin by the sublingual route, which occurred on July 19 in Nice, in the presence of Cavanna and Servadio. During this session, however, Garrett allegedly spoke about Roger Heim and his life on several occasions, although she did not know anything about him—a form divination, in short. Cavanna quickly sent Heim the transcript of the experience "to examine it together." But Heim watered down his enthusiasm by replying that he had read it "with interest," but as far as he was concerned, "the observations of Mrs. Garrett seemed very approximate and imprecise." He added: "However, there is no doubt that this report deserves attention."

Heim's correspondence with Cavanna and Servadio also includes an undated document they had sent him for feedback, entitled "Headlines of a Preliminary Investigation on Human Volunteers (Two 'Sensitives' and Two 'Normal') in Order to Study the Possible Occurrence of ESP Phenomena under the Influence of Psychopharmaca." In a letter dated March 12, 1962, Cavanna expressed his interest in sending Heim this draft protocol designed to test the possibility of psilocybin-induced ESP. This was likely a preliminary reflection that would later form the basis of Cavanna and Servadio's book *ESP Experiments with LSD-25 and Psilocybin: A Methodological Approach*, published in 1964 by the Parapsychology Foundation.[29]

In this book, the two Italian authors clearly expressed their gratitude to Heim. Other psychedelic scientists were thanked as well, including the Canadian psychiatrist Abram Hoffer, Albert Hofmann and the pharmacologist Ernst Rothlin from Sandoz Laboratories in Switzerland, the Italian philosopher Francesco Sirugo, the German psychologist Inge Strauch, the American psychologist Robert Sommer, "the late Aldous Huxley," and, finally Eileen Garrett herself.[30] From the perspective of the global history of psychedelics, reference to these figures is interesting because it documents the intellectual exchanges and aspects of this research. These acknowledgments can be understood as part of an attempt to legitimize parapsychology and as proof of correspondence and collaboration with respected authorities. Around that time, research into ESP and psychedelics were already underway in North America,[31] such as seen in the work of Stanley Krippner, who published studies on the electroencephalography of ESP in 1969.[32] The 1960s were indeed a decisive time for parapsychology. After much effort, the Parapsychological Association became affiliated with the American Association for the Advancement of Science in 1969, thus consolidating a precarious legitimacy in the face of a large number of detractors.

Another letter that stands out in Heim's massive trove of correspondence confirmed his conviction that divinatory power is real. He was responding to a letter that he had received after a report on Mexican mushrooms appeared in the Christmas 1965 issue of the prominent women's magazine *Marie France*. A female reader asked him if María Sabina could read minds, to which Heim took the trouble of answering "that one cannot speak exactly of transmission of thought but of a sense of inexplicable forecast . . . a sense of divination." His responding letter concludes somewhat apologetically: "I have to give up a rigorous explanation but, although I am a scientist, even I have to admit my interest in this observation."[33]

Here, a marked tension can be seen between Heim's scientific status and the recognition of inexplicable and seemingly unexplainable facts. This left little room to admit his interest in parapsychology. How could he not have feared for his reputation—he, who directed the *Muséum national d'Histoire naturelle* and who sat at the *Académie des sciences*? France, which had seen the development of the occult sciences at the turn of the eighteenth century, as well as debates regarding its legitimacy, did not lead to formalization of the controversial discipline.[34]

A VERY SPECIAL CASE AMONG THE VOLUNTEERS OF FILMED MUSHROOM EXPERIENCES

Given the importance of the discovery of the divinatory mushrooms of Mexico for Heim, he soon considered making a documentary film on the subject. He teamed up with the videographer and physician Pierre Thévenard as the project's scientific advisor. In 1963, this materialized in a film called *Les champignons hallucinogènes du Mexique*, which from the outset has remained somewhat secretive, having been screened on only a very few occasions.[35] The film deals with archaeological, historical, ethnographic, biological and, of course, psychological aspects of the mushroom experience.

Beginning back in 1959, Heim and Thévenard had filmed the reactions of four volunteers who agreed to ingest mushrooms cultivated at the MNHN, in an attempt to investigate the psychological dimension of the experience. The diversity of the reactions underlined the deeply subjective character of the experiences and their relation to "the psychic individuality of the experimenter." They filmed follow-up interviews four years later to measure any long-lasting consequences. One of the volunteers, Miss Michaux (her first name is not known), an advertising designer, experienced two mushroom experiments. During the second, she expressed a desire to draw, in response to which Heim observed noticeable changes in her artistic style, which became more refined. Four years from this experience, Heim asked her a follow-up question: "Miss, I would like to ask you if, after your experiments with the hallucinogenic mushrooms . . . are you changed? Are you now different from the prior Miss Michaux?" Here, Heim was interested in any personality changes that may have been caused by the drug. A little later in the interview, it became apparent that the changes in the designer's artistic style had persisted, though Heim was much more interested in any global changes that may have happened to her. When he hesitantly mentioned, in an unclear formulation, "the acquisition of a possibility of analysis," she immediately answered:

> I absolutely have the impression of having acquired a new lucidity, which was unknown to me before and which allows me to let myself be guided when I have an important decision to make. Moreover, I sometimes have some intuitions, which are quite surprising, I can give you an example. The other day, I called my mother, at her place, the phone was ringing, she did not answer. It was puzzling. And when I hung up, I was immediately positive that she was in a particular place. A place moreover she rarely ever went to. I called that place, and I spoke to her on the phone! To her amazement and mine too!

It is striking that such an unusual anecdote appeared in the documentary. Heim seemed to balk at the possibility of using the word divination, preferring the more cautious and abstract phrase "possibility of analysis." He remarked as follows:

> This is really most interesting. Because, it seems to me that we can compare these impressions which you have now, with those which, in a way, ordered, among the *curanderos* and the *curanderas* of Mexico, the shamans, that sort of . . . well, of religion, during which questions were put to them, night sessions where . . . the clients came by and said: 'well here someone has stolen my mule, where can it be and who stole it?' And I was able to see for myself during the sessions that I underwent, several nights with María Sabina and other *curanderas*, the rather astonishing value of some of their predictions!

Heim then asked Michaux about the possibility of applying "this kind of instinct of premonition" to "a better knowledge of faces." She replied that she "really has the feeling of having acquired a power" that allowed her, when she "sees someone, to guess what his temperament is, what his character is." After this short back-and-forth, the documentary focused on the drawings made by Miss Michaux after her second experience.

These filmed experiences were recounted in Heim's second volume on hallucinogenic fungi, *Nouvelles investigations sur les champignons hallucinogènes*, published in 1967.[36] The section devoted to Michaux first reflects on imagery, with reproductions of her drawings. She refers to "the mark left in her" by the mushrooms, long after her experiences: "My power of prediction has been exacerbated, a sort of intuitive vision of certain facts has imposed itself; I have acquired a predictive lucidity of certain realities that I would have previously been unable to suspect." Heim concluded the passage about Michaux's experience by asking a question, followed by a remarkable apophasis:

> Power of transmission of thought? Aptitude for divination? We will not go down that road, nor will we refer to in detail the observations that made her suddenly pick up the phone, for example, because she was seized with the certainty that her mother was in a precise place, where she rarely went to, but where she was indeed, quite surprised to get this call. . . . [37]

Heim mentioned this astonishing anecdote while perhaps distancing himself from a personal interest in such an unusual phenomenon, as evidenced by his use of a trailing off ellipsis. On the book's last page, he returned to the issue: "In fact, although the spiritualism of the 19th century—and earlier manifestations of course—does not resist explanation through an objective psychophysiology, it does not follow that some of the older parapsychological data, specific to paranormal phenomena, do not deserve to be reexamined and interpreted under a different light."[38]

CONCLUSION

Roger Heim agreed that it was legitimate that science should dismiss "spiritualism," but he nevertheless pleaded for a reexamination of "paranormal phenomena." In his 1966 television appearance, he explained María Sabina's predictions accordingly:

> These men and women, exposed like mediums to the effects of these mushrooms, had a kind of foreknowledge, it seems, I dare not pronounce the word divination, because *I am a scientist*! [emphasis added] But foreknowledge, foresight, in response to certain questions put to them . . . These women, accustomed to being in an ecstatic state under the influence of the mushroom, have an imagination which overflows, in a way, a sort of subconscious which reappears, a contact with the visitor which is exacerbated, and which leads to revelations which do seem quite extraordinary sometimes. . . . I won't go any further in my conclusions. But I still consider that this sense . . . multiplied . . . exacerbated . . . of the power of analysis and even going beyond through irrational and subconscious elements, cannot be absolutely eliminated a priori. That is a fact.[39]

"I am a scientist!" he added, once again emphasizing the tension between his academic position and his acknowledgment of the existence of divinatory phenomena. On several occasions during the interview, Heim visibly felt compelled to acknowledge the unbelievable, courageously underscoring the limits of his rationality, tested by his own lived experience.

The fact that he revealed the accuracy of María Sabina's predictions only orally, and that they were only later transcribed in this televised interview, certainly revealed his reluctance to bring up the subject to his peers: for example, he never broached the topic in his presentations at the *Académie des Sciences*. But in 1964, during a phytochemistry conference in Nouméa, in the former French colony of New Caledonia—a distant location to be sure!—he made the following statement about the "provinces of knowledge" attainable through the study of psilocybin: "One of them corresponds to psychopathology and psychiatric therapy. . . . The other belongs to a dual sector that scientists are perhaps wrong to brand as contemptible or at least far removed from the limits of objective sciences: that of parapsychology and of divination."[40]

He ended his talk by mentioning the possibility of understanding the effects of drugs like psilocybin as a way to "make inroads into the most intimate mechanisms of our perceptions and reflections"; that is, as a tool of scientific exploration. This brief defense of parapsychology can also be found in a 1969 column that he published in a supplement of the *Revue de mycologie*.[41]

The topic of divinatory power accessed through the ingestion of mushrooms represents only a very small element of the titanic research that Heim devoted to hallucinogenic mushrooms. However, even though he proved to be elusive or cautious in his publications, he did not ignore the subject altogether—a testimony to his intellectual integrity. Faced with his own and others' bemushroomed encounters with divination, Heim seems to have responded to the "rationalist commitment" defined by the French philosopher Gaston Bachelard, a commitment that involves fighting dogmatism by accepting the unknown, and according to which reason can be specified only in its relation to the reality it encounters.[42] Heim was indeed a scientist.

NOTES

1. See Valentina P. Wasson and R. Gordon Wasson, *Mushrooms, Russia and History* (New York: Pantheon Books, 1957); and R. Gordon Wasson, *The Wondrous Mushroom: Mycolatry in Mesoamerica*, Ethno-Mycological Studies 7 (New York: McGraw-Hill, 1980).

2. For a review of the sources and the analysis of the Western reception of the peyote cactus and psilocybin mushrooms, see Samir Boumediene, *La colonisation du savoir, Une histoire des plantes médicinales du «Nouveau Monde» (1492–1750)*, Vaulx-en-Velin, les Editions des mondes à faire, 2016.

3. Richard Evans Schultes, "The Identification of Teonacátl, a Narcotic Basidiomycete of the Aztecs," *Botanical Museum Leaflets of Harvard* 7, no. 3, (February 21, 1939): 37–54, and "Teonacátl: The Narcotic Mushroom of the Aztecs," *American Anthropologist* 42 (1940): 429–443.

4. See, for example, B. P. Reko, "De los Nombres Botanicos Aztecos," *El Mexico Antiguo* 1, no. 5 (February 1919):113–117; W. E. Safford, "Narcotic Plants and Stimulants of the Ancient Americans," *Annual Report of the Smithsonian Institution,* Washington, DC, 1916, 387; C. G. Santesson, "Einige Mexikanische Rauschdrogen," *Archiv für Botanik* 29A, no. 12 (1939): 1–9.

5. See, for example, *London Medical and Physical Journal.* John Souter, 1816. 451; A. E. Verrill, "A Recent Case of Mushroom Intoxication," *Science* 40, no. 1029 (September 18, 1914): 408–410.

6. Wasson and Wasson, *Mushrooms, Russia and History.*

7. There a great deal of praise for Roger Heim in the preface of *Mushrooms, Russia and History.* R. Gordon Wasson's *The Wondrous Mushroom,* published in 1980, is incidentally dedicated to his "loyal collaborator" and his "valiant friend," who is described further as a "beloved friend." Heim, for his part, states in the preface of *Les champignons hallucinogènes du Mexique* (1958) that it had been a "great pleasure . . . for several years . . . to have been able to share ideas and documents with Mr. and Ms. Wasson" regarding "the folkloric aspect manifest in the relations between mushrooms and primitive populations."

8. Milana Aronov, "(Micro-) 'Psychedelic' Experiences: From the 1960s Creativity at the Work-place to the 21st Century Neuro-Newspeak," *Ethnologie française* 49, no. 4 (2019): 701–718.

9. Erika Dyck. "Spaced-out in Saskatchewan: Modernism, Anti-Psychiatry, and Deinstitution-alization, 1950–1968," *Bulletin of the History of Medicine* 84, no. 4 (2010): 640–666.

10. Erika Dyck, *Psychedelic Psychiatry—LSD from Clinic to Campus,* Baltimore: Johns Hopkins University Press, 2008.

11. See Stephen Szára, "Are Hallucinogens Psychoheuristic?" *NIDA Research Monograph* 146 (1994): 33–51; Carlo Rovelli and Sophie Lem, *Écrits vagabonds* (Paris: Flammarion, 2019).

12. It is worth mentioning that Roger Heim was part of the French Resistance and that he was betrayed and deported to Buchenwald, and subsequently to Mauthausen and Gusen. In the concentration camps, he carried on his scientific reflections and gave conferences to his fellow inmates. He was saved by the US Army on May 6, 1945, in a state of extreme fatigue.

13. Although Heim self-experimented with fly agaric in 1923, which indicates a brief interest in psychopharmacology. See Roger Heim, "Analyse de quelques expériences personnelles produites par l'ingestion des Agarics hallucinogènes du Mexique," in *Comptes rendus heb-domadaires des séances de l'Académie des sciences,* Gauthier-Villars., Paris, Académie des Sci-ences, 245 (1957): 597–603.

14. See Peter Schötter, "Scientisme, sur l'histoire d'un concept difficile," *Revue de synthèse,* no. 134 (2013): 89–113.

15. Marmin Nicolas, "Métapsychique et psychologie en France (1880–1940)," *Revue d'Histoire des Sciences Humaines* 4, no. 1 (2001): 145–171.

16. Roger Heim, "Ethnomycologie—les champignons divinatoires utilisés dans les rites des Indiens Mazatèques, recueillis au cours de leur premier voyage au Mexique, en 1953, par Mme Valentina Pavlovna Wasson et M. R. Gordon Wasson," *Comptes-Rendus Des Séances de l'Académie Des Sciences* t. 242 (February): 965–68.

17. Wasson and Wasson, *Mushrooms, Russia and History*. The fact that Peter traveled to Germany rather than Japan is mentioned in the French translation of this excerpt published in *Les champignons hallucinogènes du Mexique* the following year.

18. Heim went to Mexico three times to study hallucinogenic mushrooms—1956, 1959, and 1961.

19. Jean Lallier, "Champignons et hallucinations," Entrée libre, Office national de radiodiffusion télévision française, 1966.

20. Collectif, *Entretiens De Rueil / Les Cahiers Sandoz—Ivresse chimique et crise de civilisation*, Rueil-Malmaison, Laboratoire Sandoz, 1970.

21. Roger Heim, and R. Gordon Wasson, *Les Champignons Hallucinogènes du Mexique: Études Ethnologiques, Taxinomiques, Biologiques, Physiologiques et Chimiques*, 7, VI. Archives Du Muséum National d'histoire Naturelle (Paris: Muséum national d'Histoire naturelle, 1958), 317.

22. Although the paradigm understanding the succession of magic, religion, and science was no longer dominant in anthropology in the first half of the twentieth century, the condemnation of magic as superstition remained the dominant framework for the interpretation of a number of anthropologists, ranging from Edward Tylor to Lucien Lévy-Bruhl. At the end of the 1940s, Claude Levi-Strauss took part in a renewal of the analysis of magic through his own brand of structuralism, which made it possible to consider the shamanic complex on the one hand and the symbolic efficacy of magic on the other. See, for instance, Claude Lévi-Strauss, "Le sorcier et sa magie," *Les Temps Modernes* 4, no. 41 (March 1949), 385–406. Finally, it should be noted that while Lévi-Strauss and Heim had the opportunity to meet at the Académie des Sciences, nothing indicates that they were aware of their respective work in the early 1950s.

23. Roger Heim, and R. Gordon Wasson, *Les Champignons Hallucinogènes du Mexique: Études Ethnologiques, Taxinomiques, Biologiques, Physiologiques et Chimiques*, 7, VI. Archives Du Muséum National d'histoire Naturelle (Paris: Muséum national d'Histoire naturelle, 1958), 318.

24. Roger Heim, *Un naturaliste autour du monde* (Paris: Editions Albin Michel, 1955). See, for example, "Malagasy medicine is as good as ours, by its results. It is made of observations, experiments, traditions and arts, like ours," 130.

25. Roger Heim, and R. Gordon Wasson, *Les Champignons Hallucinogènes du Mexique: Études Ethnologiques, Taxinomiques, Biologiques, Physiologiques et Chimiques*, 7, VI. Archives Du Muséum National d'histoire Naturelle (Paris: Muséum national d'Histoire naturelle, 1958), 275.

26. Heim and Wasson, *Les Champignons Hallucinogènes du Mexique*, 305.

27. Press clipping in box number 5 of the Roger Heim archive at the Bibliothèque centrale du Muséum national d'Histoire naturelle.

28. Cynthia Carson Bisbee et al., *Psychedelic Prophets: The Letters of Aldous Huxley and Humphry Osmond* (Montreal, Kingston, London, and Chicago: McGill-Queen's University Press, 2018).

29. Roberto Cavanna and Emilio Servadio, *ESP Experiments with LSD-25 and Psilocybin: A Methodological Approach* (Parapsychology Foundation, 2010).

30. The list is in alphabetical order right up to Huxley, who died as the book was published. This is not a reflection of the importance of Huxley's involvement in the research project on Italian parapsychologists, but it does confirm that he was involved, likely through oral discussions during their meetings.

31. For a review of the parapsychological scholarship on the effects of hallucinogens, see David Luke, *Otherworlds: Psychedelics and Exceptional Human Experience* (London: Muswell Hill Press, 2017).

32. See, for instance, S. Krippner, and M. Ullman, "Telepathic Perception in the Dream State: Confirmatory Study Using EEG-EOG Techniques," *Perceptual and Motor Skills*, 29, no. 3 (1969), 29, 915–918. In his book *Song of the Siren: A Parapsychological Odyssey*, Krippner mentions a key event that sparked his interest in parapsychology: a personal episode of clairvoyance during a psychedelic session hosted by Timothy Leary. See S. Krippner, *Song of the Siren: A Parapsychological Odyssey* (New York: Harper & Row, 1975).

33. Correspondence of Roger Heim, January 1966, box number 5 of the Heim archive, Bibliothèque centrale du Muséum national d'Histoire naturelle, Paris, France

34. Bertrand Méheust, *Somnambulisme et Médiumnité, tome 2: Le choc des sciences psychiques* (Le Plessis-Robinson, France: Les Empêcheurs de penser en rond, 2003).

35. I had the privilege of attending a screening of this film during the Paris mushroom exhibition on October 14, 1999. I found it in the audiovisual section of the MNHN in October 2017—and they were unaware that they had a copy—in the form of two Betacam tapes, which I had digitized.

36. Roger Heim, *Nouvelles investigations sur les champignons hallucinogènes, Archives du Muséum national d'Histoire naturelle, 7ème série* 9 (1967).

37. Roger Heim, *Nouvelles investigations*, 207.

38. Roger Heim, *Nouvelles investigations*, 218.

39. Lallier, "Champignons et hallucinations." Author's translation.

40. Roger Heim, "Histoire de la découverte des champignons hallucinogènes du Mexique," Noumea, Editions du Centre national de la recherche scientifique. Author's translation.

41. Roger Heim, "Réflexions sur le pouvoir des champignons hallucinogènes," *Revue de mycologie* 33, no. 4 (1969), 322. Author's translation.

42. See Gaston Bachelard, *Le nouvel esprit scientifique* (Paris: PUF (1934) 1960), 10.

BIBLIOGRAPHY

Primary Sources

Heim, Roger. *Analyse de quelques expériences personnelles produites par l'ingestion des Agarics hallucinogènes du Mexique*. Paris: Gauthier-Villars, Académie des Sciences, 1957.

Heim, Roger. "Les champignons divinatoires utilises dans les rites des Indiens Mazateques, recueillis au cours de leur premier voyage au Mexique, en 1953, par Mme Wasson, Valentina Pavlovna et Wasson, Mr Gordon." *Comptes Rendus Hebdomadaires des Seances de l'Academie des Sciences* 242, no. 8 (1956): 965–968.

Heim, Roger. *Histoire de la découverte des champignons hallucinogènes du Mexique*. Noumea, Editions du Centre national de la recherche scientifique, 1966.

Heim, Roger. *Un naturaliste autour du monde*. Paris: Editions Albin Michel, 1955.

Heim, Roger. "Nouvelles investigations sur les champignons hallucinogènes." *Archives du Muséum national d'Histoire naturelle, 7ème série* 9 (1967): 1–218.

Heim, Roger. "Réflexions sur le pouvoir des champignons hallucinogènes." *Revue de mycologie* 33, no.4 (1969).

Heim, Roger, and R. Gordon Wasson. "Les champignons hallucinogènes du Mexique-Etudes ethnologiques, taxinomiques, biologiques, physiologiques et chimiques." *Archives du Muséum national d'Histoire naturelle, 7ème série* 6 (1958): 1–445.

Roger Heim archive. Correspondence of Roger Heim, boxes 1 to 5. *Bibliothèque centrale du Muséum national d'Histoire naturelle*, Paris, France.

Thévenard, Pierre, dir. 1964. *Les champignons hallucinogènes du Mexique*. Film. Documentaire scientifique. Fondation Singer-Polignac.

Wasson, Valentina Pavlovna, and R. Gordon Wasson. *Mushrooms: Russia and History*. New York: Pantheon Books, 1957.

Secondary Sources

Aronov, Milana. "(Micro-) 'Psychedelic' Experiences: From the 1960s Creativity at the Workplace to the 21st Century Neuro-Newspeak." *Ethnologie française* 49, no. 4 (2019): 701–718.

Bachelard, Gaston. "Le nouvel esprit scientifique." Librairie F. Alcan, Paris, 1934.

Bisbee, Cynthia, Paul Bisbee, Erika Dyck, Patrick Farrell, James Sexton and James Spisak, eds. *Psychedelic Prophets: The Letters of Aldous Huxley and Humphry Osmond*. Kingston (Ontario) and Montreal (Quebec): McGill-Queen's University Press, 2018.

Boumediene, Samir. *La colonisation du savoir. Une histoire des plantes médicinales du «Nouveau Monde» (1492–1750)*. Vaulx-en-Velin, *Éditions des Mondes à faire*. 2016.

Cavanna, Roberto, and Emilio Servadio. *ESP Experiments with LSD 25 and Psilocybin: A Methodological Approach*, no. 5. Parapsychology Foundation, New York, 1964.

Collectif, 1970, Entretiens De Rueil / Les Cahiers Sandoz—Ivresse chimique et crise de civilisation, Rueil-Malmaison, France, Laboratoire Sandoz.

Dyck, Erika. *Psychedelic Psychiatry: LSD from Clinic to Campus.* Baltimore: Johns Hopkins University Press, 2008.

Dyck, Erika. "Spaced-out in Saskatchewan: Modernism, Anti-Psychiatry, and Deinstitutionalization, 1950–1968." *Bulletin of the History of Medicine* 84, no. 4 (2010): 640–666.

Krippner, Stanley. *Song of the Siren: A Parapsychological Odyssey.* Harper & Row, New York, 1977.

Krippner, Stanley, and Montague Ullman. "Telepathic Perception in the Dream State: Confirmatory Study Using EEG-EOG Monitoring Techniques." *Perceptual and Motor Skills* 29, no. 3 (1969): 915–918.

Lallier, Jean. 1966. "Champignons et hallucinations." Entrée libre. Office national de radiodiffusion télévision française.

Lévi-Strauss, Claude. *Le sorcier et sa magie.* Imprimerie Chantenay, Paris, 1949.

Luke, David. *Otherworlds: Psychedelics and Exceptional Human Experience.* London: Aeon Books, 2019.

Marmin, Nicolas. "Métapsychique et psychologie en France (1880–1940)." *Revue d'Histoire des Sciences Humaines* 1 (2001): 145–171.

Méheust, Bertrand. *Somnambulisme et Médiumnité, tome 2: Le choc des sciences psychiques.* Le Plessis-Robinson, France: Les Empêcheurs de penser en rond, 2003.

Reko, Blas Pablo. *De los nombres botánicos aztecas.* H. Beyer, Mexico, 1919.

Rovelli, Carlo, and Sophie Lem. *Écrits vagabonds.* Paris: Flammarion, 2019.

Safford, William Edwin. *Narcotic Plants and Stimulants of the Ancient Americans.* Annual Report of the Smithsonian Institution, Washington D C, 1916, 387.

Santesson, C. G. "Einige Mexikanische Rauschdrogen." *Archiv für Botanik* 29, no. 12 (1939): 1–9.

Schöttler, Peter. "Scientisme sur L'histoire D'un Concept Difficile." *Revue de synthèse* 134, no. 1 (2013): 89–113.

Schultes, Richard Evans. "The Identification of Teonacátl, a Narcotic Basidiomycete of the Aztecs." *Botanical Museum Leaflets of Harvard* 7, no. 3 (February 1939): 37–54.

Schultes, Richard Evans. "Teonanácatl: The Narcotic Mushroom of the Aztecs." *American Anthropologist* 42, no. 3 (1940): 429–443.

Szára, Stephen. "Are Hallucinogens Psychoheuristic?" *NIDA Research Monograph* 146 (1994): 33–51.

Verrill, A. E. "A Recent Case of Mushroom Intoxication." *Science* 40, no. 1029 (September 18, 1914): 408–410.

Wasson, Robert Gordon. *The Wondrous Mushroom: Mycolatry in Mesoamerica.* New York: McGraw-Hill, 1980.

12 BEATITUDE, DREAD, AND MOTHER-BLAMING: THE ORIGINS OF CLINICAL THEOLOGY, FROM INDIA TO ENGLAND AND CANADA

Andrew Jones

INTRODUCTION

Psychiatrists in the 1950s and 1960s who used LSD as an adjunct to psychotherapy were facing the challenge of interpreting the mystical-like experiences that the drug often produced. For several groups, the experiences of unity, bliss, and transcendence generated by LSD were the key to its therapeutic potential. For others, the purported mystical dimension of the LSD experience awkwardly blurred the boundary between rigorous scientific investigation and spirituality.

This chapter explores how the challenge of drug-induced mystical experience was navigated in a Christian context by examining the international collaboration between two medical missionaries who came to see LSD as a valuable psychiatric tool. Florence Nichols (1913–1987), a Canadian psychiatrist, and Frank Lake (1914–1982), a British physician, met in the late 1940s while working at the Christian Medical College in the city of Vellore, in southern India. Nichols traveled to Vellore in 1946 to establish a psychiatric unit at the college. Lake, whose background was in parasitology, took a position as the college's medical superintendent in 1948. After witnessing Nichols's dedicated Christian approach to psychiatry, Lake became more interested in treating the mind and began his own psychiatric training after returning to England in 1950.

In England, Lake encountered LSD while working with the British psychiatrist Ronald Sandison at Powick Hospital. Sandison was using the drug in psychotherapy to help access the unconscious processes of his patients.

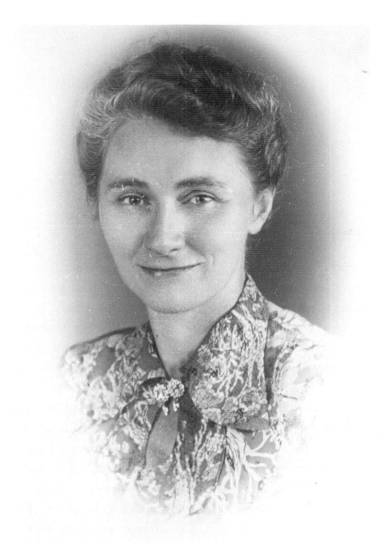

Figure 12.1
Dr. Florence Nichols, 1951. Courtesy of the General Synod Archives, Anglican Church of Canada.

Watching patients relive trauma under the influence of LSD convinced Lake of the validity of psychodynamic psychiatry and the therapeutic potential of this drug. In the late 1950s, he introduced it to Nichols and guided her through her own LSD experience. After reliving episodes from her infancy, she was immediately convinced of the value of LSD, and she incorporated it into her psychiatric practice in Vellore.

After Nichols left India in 1959, she visited Lake in England, where they continued to practice LSD therapy. There, Nichols helped Lake develop "clinical theology," a pedagogical discipline aimed at educating clergy members about mental illness. Clinical theology responded to a real need among Christian clergy. While psychotherapy was becoming more socially acceptable in Europe and North America in the 1960s, many people still relied on church leaders to ease their mental distress. In serious cases, clergy members felt unequipped to handle the psychological problems that arose during pastoral encounters. The aim of clinical theology, therefore, was to provide tools to help clergy recognize and address the deeper roots of mental disorders among the laity.

To this end, Lake and Nichols conducted seminars illustrating the theory and practice of their Christian approach to psychiatric treatment. Interest in clinical theology grew. By 1963, Lake and his colleagues had organized over 100 training programs across England and established the Clinical Theology Association. In 1966, Lake published a massive textbook for clinical theology, containing many descriptions of his observations of LSD therapy that supported his claims about the roots and nature of mental distress.

Nichols played a vital role in clinical theology's development and dissemination. While the discipline's origins remain primarily associated with Lake, who is now regarded as a pioneer in the British pastoral counseling movement, almost nothing is known about Nichols or her impact on him and his work.[1] This is surprising and disappointing, as the earliest roots of clinical theology are found in her psychiatric work in Vellore, which in fact prompted Lake to take up psychiatry himself. Furthermore, in addition to helping him work out the theoretical basis of clinical theology while working together in England, she personally introduced the discipline to Canada in the early 1960s.

Lake's approach to psychiatry was heavily influenced by the object-relations school of psychoanalytic thought associated with the pioneering psychoanalyst Melanie Klein and others that gained traction in postwar Britain. In contrast to Freud's emphasis on the child's gratification of libidinal instincts, proponents of object-relations theory stressed the primacy of the infant's need to establish relationships with surrounding objects, particularly the mother. Object-relations theorists held that a loving mother-infant relationship was crucial for each individual's proper psychological development.[2]

Examining clinical theology therefore provides an interesting opportunity to consider how maternal-deprivation or mother-blaming psychoanalytic hypotheses interacted with LSD in this period. The object-relations approach was one of several psychiatric theories that reflected the prevalent focus on the role of the mother in postwar psychiatry. As mothers increasingly entered the workforce, psychiatrists and policymakers worried about the impact that their absence would have on child development and family structure. Drawing on studies suggesting that prolonged periods of maternal deprivation led to negative outcomes later in life, many psychiatrists highlighted the importance of mother-infant attachments and thus placed the burden of ensuring mental health on mothers.[3]

This widespread concern about maternal deprivation shaped how Lake and Nichols explained LSD experiences. The science and technology studies scholar Ido Hartogsohn has pointed out the complex relationship between scientific frameworks and the LSD experience. Not only do scientific theories provide lenses through which actors interpret the psychedelic experience, but they also contribute to the cultural set and setting that affects the nature of the experience.[4] In Lake's case, the object-relations framework influenced how he and his patients understood and reacted to LSD. He continually found that by inhibiting repression, the drug allowed his patients to reexperience the trauma of maternal neglect from early infancy. For Lake, these experiences provided empirical evidence for the object-relation school's claims about the importance of mother-infant relationships in the first months of life.

However, in addition to this psychoanalytic framework, Lake superimposed a theological-existential framework onto the mother-infant relationship. In his view, the mother acted as "God's vice-regent" for the infant, who lacked a differentiated sense of self, let alone a concept of God.[5] From the infant's perspective, the mother took on God's role as the ultimate source of "being and well-being," and her loving "countenance" channeled the necessary ontological resources for the infant's adequate personal and spiritual development. When deprived of these resources (i.e., when the mother was unloving or absent for prolonged periods), the infant was confronted with the loss of being and intense existential anguish.[6] These experiences of maternal deprivation, Lake concluded, distorted the individual's subsequent relationship with and attitude toward God.

Lake's view of positive and negative LSD reactions then was determined by this combination of theology, existentialism, and object-relations theory. His patients' negative reactions were visceral recollections of the preverbal experience of dread in the face of maternal neglect, which threatened their infant self's sense of being and well-being. Positive or spiritual reactions that involved sensations of bliss, unity, and transcendence were recollections of beatific union with maternal warmth and love in the earliest months of life, before the infant had developed a differentiated sense of itself from others. In this way, Lake expanded the mother-blaming framework to account for the effects of a drug.

Fully uncovering and entering these buried experiences of existential anguish were the primary goals of LSD therapy for Lake. Positive experiences of "mystical union" with the source of being merely served to help provide patients with the courage to face terrifying infantile experiences of ontological dread. By fully reexperiencing and consciously integrating this deep sense of infantile distress, patients could relinquish the impact that it had on their mental lives and on their understanding of God. In contrast, then, to the North American psychedelic psychiatrists, whose primary aim was to generate positive, transcendent experiences, LSD therapy for Lake was about facing dread, and he used prayer, Christian sacraments, and biblical passages to prepare his patients for this unsettling encounter.

Since she was a child, Florence Nichols dreamed of becoming a missionary. Knowing that her parents did not approve of this path, she quietly pursued medicine with the hope that one day, this would allow her to follow her dream. She earned her bachelor of arts from the University of Toronto in 1934 and her medical degree in 1937. During a surgical internship, Nichols realized that she was more concerned with her patients' mental lives than their bodily woes, so she decided to pursue psychiatry. After earning a diploma in psychiatry in 1941, she worked at the Ontario Hospital in Toronto until she finally mustered the courage to apply to the Missionary Society of the Church of England. By 1946, she was on her way to India to become, in her words, "the first woman missionary psychiatrist."[7]

Nichols was assigned to work at Vellore's Christian Medical College. However, physicians there did not view psychiatry as a priority, and at first they were not sure what to do with her. Psychiatric resources were only beginning to expand in postcolonial India, and missionary projects had neglected mental health.[8] The college lacked funding and space for psychiatric patients, and Nichols was forced to use a cramped nurse's pantry as her office. She treated fellow missionaries as well as locals, while struggling to learn Indian languages. As its only psychiatrist, Nichols encountered a range of conditions, from mild cases of neuroses to severe forms of depression or schizophrenia. While she saw no conflict between Christian faith and psychiatry, she refused to view all mental ailments in exclusively spiritual terms, and she also focused on emotional or biological causes. This perspective allowed her to employ a variety of treatments, from Christian prayer, psychoanalysis, and family therapy to electroconvulsive and insulin coma treatments. Nichols was willing to use any method that she thought would work, at times having a translator help her conduct barbiturate-assisted talk therapy or taking her patients mountain climbing as a form of occupational therapy.[9]

By the late 1940s, Nichols had gained a reputation in India as an effective psychiatrist. Her work convinced local and missionary physicians of the value of her profession. In 1948, Lake was appointed the Christian Medical College's medical superintendent, and tasked with helping Nichols set up a psychiatry department. Lake's medical training was in parasitology and tropical medicine, but after arriving in Vellore, he was impressed by the significant transformations that he saw in Nichols's patients.[10] Missionaries who visited Nichols as "psychological wrecks" became "spiritually renewed." One Indian Christian pastor even described psychotherapy with Nichols as "a profound spiritual experience."[11] In another example, in July 1949, a young Christian minister came to the medical college with a variety of physical complaints. He was brought to Nichols after a medical examination failed to reveal any organic problems. Nichols found the minister to be full of despair; he felt that he had wasted his life and God would not forgive him for that. Nichols connected his understanding of God to events in his childhood that predisposed him toward feelings of guilt. She prayed with him and emphasized God's love and compassion. After a few similar visits, the minister had the ecstatic realization that "God is love" and became "drunk with joy." He attributed this realization to his sessions with Nichols, who helped him transform his attitude toward God.[12]

Nichols discussed these kinds of cases with Lake, who became increasingly excited about her Christian approach to psychiatry. In 1950, Lake returned to England and pursued psychiatric training, spending six years working at Scalebor Park Hospital in Yorkshire. By 1958, he had won a diploma in psychological medicine from the University of Leeds. According to Lake, however, his "real education in psychodynamics" began when he first encountered LSD. In 1954, Lake's supervisor assigned him to a team investigating the new drug as a treatment for alcoholism. After working with Ronald Sandison, who was then pioneering the therapeutic use of LSD in Britain at Powick Hospital in Worcestershire, Lake incorporated LSD into his own practice and exclusively focused on it for the following two years.[13]

Lake's work with LSD made genuine for him "the world of Freudian interpretation," and it guided his psychiatric education. He was shocked by the number of his patients who reported reliving their first months of infancy, or even their own birth trauma, while under LSD. Although initially skeptical, he began taking these reports seriously as he found independent evidence from doctors and parents that corroborated his patients' descriptions. He continued using the drug as an adjunct to psychotherapy throughout the 1950s and 1960s.[14]

Nichols also left Vellore in 1950 to continue her training in psychoanalysis at the University of Pennsylvania in Philadelphia. In 1955, she returned to Vellore to finish building a department of psychiatry at the Christian Medical College. By this time, the college had secured funding for psychiatry, and she worked with the superintendent to plan her ideal psychiatric unit. The Mental Health Center opened in June 1958 and was officially inaugurated by the vice president of India, Sarvepalli Radhakrishnan.[15]

Lake and Nichols had kept in touch during these years apart. In the late 1950s, he guided her through her first LSD experience. Nichols relived the preverbal experience of "extreme physical pain and terror" after being left outside in the Canadian winter as an infant.[16] Her mother later confirmed that this event did in fact happen when she was four months old. According to Nichols, this experience taught her more about the roots of her psychological problems in 4 hours than she had learned in 700 hours of analytical training.[17]

Nichols began using LSD to help some of her private patients in Vellore, which led to some controversy. In March 1959 the administrative staff at the Christian Medical College were concerned that she was using the drug indiscriminately. According to one staff member's report, Nichols allowed a male patient, Peter Cooper, and his family to move into her private residence. While this decision reflected her focus on family therapy, it soon blurred the doctor-patient boundary, as she and Cooper had been giving each other LSD on a weekly basis for a few months. In addition, while her department was still understaffed, Nichols had allowed Cooper to practice psychotherapy with some of her other patients. At the time of the report, Nichols had just received news that her mother was suffering a depressive episode, and she returned to Canada. The administrative staff recommended that she should not return to Vellore as the head of the Mental Health Center.[18] With a heavy heart, Nichols wondered whether she would ever again work in India.

LSD AND MATERNAL DEPRIVATION: CLINICAL THEOLOGY IN ENGLAND

In 1960, Nichols visited Lake in England for six months. While there, she continued to practice LSD therapy, and she helped Lake articulate the "theoretical basis" of what they had started calling "clinical theology."[19] Clinical theology was fundamentally an educational program that equipped clergy with the resources to recognize and handle the psychological difficulties that emerged in pastoral encounters.

Starting in 1958, Lake began conducting seminars that introduced clergy to the world of psychiatry. The three-hour seminars took place twelve times a year during a multiyear program. In the seminars, participants reviewed diagrams and engaged in role-playing activities that illustrated the relationship between specific personality types and experiences in early infancy. They discussed tools for easing psychological distress, such as attentive listening, compassionate dialogue, and authentic countenance expressed through eye contact and facial expressions. The seminars also involved sharing groups, which enhanced self-awareness by having participants recount their deepest psychological pain and discomfort with each other.[20]

In the early 1960s, church leaders supported these clinical theology seminars, and they quickly spread across England. In 1962, the Clinical Theology Association was established, and by 1966, over 2,000 clergy members had participated in two years of seminars.[21] These meetings were so prominent that even notable figures, such as the Scottish psychiatrist R. D. Laing and the British psychologist Harry Guntrip, had attended.[22] Lake published a 1,282-page textbook titled *Clinical Theology: A Theological and Psychiatric Basis to Clinical Pastoral Care* in 1966. Drawing on thousands of hours of observations during LSD therapy, the book served as a practical and theoretical guide for those interested in a Christian approach to psychiatry.

Watching patients undergo the LSD experience had a major impact on Lake's understanding of psychiatry and theology. He continually stressed that these observations confirmed the views of object-relations theorists who claimed that ego development is primarily shaped by early-infantile interpersonal relationships. Lake's view of object-relations theory was most informed by the formulations of the Scottish psychiatrist Ronald Fairbairn. While Melanie Klein, a pioneer in object-relations theory, retained Freud's view that development is driven by a libido centered on "pleasure-seeking" behavior, Fairbairn argued instead that from birth, the libido is "object-seeking"; the infant is driven to establish an adequate relationship with the mother.[23]

Fairbairn stressed that a mother's love and emotional support were central to proper ego development, especially in early infancy. He distinguished between two stages of development that took place within the first year of life. During the first stage, "infantile dependence," the mother-infant relationship was one of "primary identification": the infant has no sense of differentiation from its mother as a separate object. Fairbairn's second stage, "mature dependence," was characterized by the infant's growing awareness of itself as separate from other objects.[24] Fairbairn theorized that experiences of maternal neglect were particularly damaging during the first stage since they would cause an infant to associate pain with object-seeking. These painful experiences, which the infant's underdeveloped ego could not bear, would be repressed or dissociated from conscious awareness.[25]

Lake added an existential-theological dimension to this psychoanalytic framework. For him, the first nine months of life were crucial not only for the development of the ego, but also for the development of "personal and spiritual being." He referred to this period as "the womb of the Spirit"; just as the mother provides physical sustenance to the infant during gestation, the mother also needs to supply spiritual and ontological resources to the infant in the first months after birth.[26] In this period, which roughly corresponded to Fairbairn's stage of infantile dependence, the infant identifies with the mother and lacks a differentiated sense of self. In Lake's terms, the "baby has no capacity for separate personal existence. It can conceive of itself as 'in Being,' or Alive, only by identification with the Mother's Being and Person. The dichotomy which later distinguishes the boundaries between the baby's 'I' and the Mother's 'Thou', is not possible at this stage."[27]

During what Lake called the "womb of the Spirit," the mother provides the infant with the "genesis of being" and the "sustenance of being," which are both necessary for the infant to develop an adequate sense of personal existence and selfhood. Continuing the womb metaphor, Lake stated that the infant's sensory experience of the mother acts as an "umbilical cord" that connects to the mother's spiritual and ontological resources. He placed particular emphasis on the importance of the infant's visual experience of the mother's face, stressing that it is the "light of her countenance" that transmits God's resources of being and well-being to the infant.[28]

Maternal deprivation, therefore, detached the infant from these ontological resources, creating experiences of existential or ontological anxiety. To highlight this point, Lake drew on the work of Laing, who suggested that the "child who cries when its mother disappears from the room is threatened with the disappearance of his own being, since for him also percipi = esse [perception equals being]. It is only in the mother's presence that he is able to fully live and move and have his being."[29] Lake found that this existential perspective explained the experiences of patients who reported reliving their infancies under LSD. His patients often reported preverbal sensations of "unendurable loneliness," nothingness, and nonbeing, which were usually accompanied by extreme terror and dread. For example, one patient, while "writhing, groaning and moaning," stated that "I was absolutely lost . . . there was no one, no one, no one there. No one to give me life . . . In the centre—nothing—no meaning . . . I am not life but death, there is nobody . . . I was past longing for anything, it was all pain and misery and death."[30]

To connect these experiences of maternal deprivation to specific psychological reaction patterns, Lake drew on the Russian physiologist Ivan Pavlov's notion of "transmarginal stressing." Pavlov found that dogs who had been exposed to extreme stress suddenly switched from a trusting relationship with him to an aversive one. Lake's LSD observations suggested to him that this drastic switch occurred in infancy when a certain margin of suffering was crossed in response to experiences of maternal deprivation. If an infant had been left alone in anguish for too long, the longing to reconnect with the mother would turn into an aversion toward her. Lake described the experience of crossing this margin of suffering as "the most sharply split-off and deeply repressed core of wretchedness and affliction."[31] Infants who approached this margin, but did not cross it, developed hysterical reaction patterns; their neurosis centered on securing relationships. Infants who crossed this margin, who became averse to relationships and consequentially identified with nonbeing, developed schizoid personalities.

Since Lake viewed the mother as a stand-in for God in the first months of infancy, he emphasized that the mother-infant relationship also determined the individual's subsequent understanding of God. Experiences in early infancy shaped how individuals reacted to their "dependence on source persons."[32] From Lake's Christian perspective, the ultimate source of being and well-being that humans depended on was God. Therefore, a mother's unloving facial expression or countenance could result in distorted images of God as unloving or vengeful. In the worst case, experiences of dread and nonbeing in the mother's prolonged absence could lead to an unwillingness to have any relationship at all with God and the denial of God's existence.[33]

While Lake's patients often had terrifying experiences during LSD sessions, they also often had "monistic mystical experiences" of identification with the source of being. Lake himself had this kind of reaction when he took LSD; he described it as an experience of "identification with the sources of life itself, without boundaries to the ego, without limitation or frustration."[34] He was clear, though, that the drug did not cause these experiences of beatitude or blessedness, just as it did not cause the negative experiences of dread. Instead, he suggested, LSD merely inhibited repression and allowed the individual to regress to these buried, preverbal experiences.[35] Negative reactions to LSD were regressions to painful experiences of maternal neglect, and positive reactions were regressions to the state of loving union that existed with the mother in the womb or in the "early months of sheer maternal beneficence," before any separation or trauma had occurred.[36] For infants who had not gone through significant stress during their first year, who "entered into a glorious inheritance of mother love," these positive experiences were the dominant LSD reaction. For them, "there is evoked into consciousness by LSD an experience of transcendent joy with no hint at all of separation."[37]

However, generating positive reactions to LSD was not Lake's main therapeutic goal. According to him, LSD was useful because it allowed one to face the terrifying experiences of dread and integrate them into consciousness.[38] Lake criticized the tendency in psychiatry, and in pastoral care, to temporarily bandage psychological ailments with sedatives or superficial spiritual advice.[39] Healing for Lake was not about restoring proper defenses or normalcy within the status quo. Rather, he stressed the need to fully experience and enter into the unconscious infantile experiences of pain that shaped personality.[40]

Facing the deepest experiences of infantile dread under LSD required preparation and the presence of a trained and trusted therapist or pastor. For Christian patients, Lake established peace before the session by using prayer, Holy Communion, and Scripture.[41] He claimed that clinical theologians were ideally suited for helping patients face dread. Psychiatry could not address existential anxiety, but spiritualty could. It was thus, in the existential nature of anxiety, that Lake saw a cohesion between religion and psychiatry; Christian ontological resources—an "inflow of being and well-being" from God—were necessary to address the threat of nonbeing, and clinical theologians could provide these resources in interpersonal relationships through supportive countenance and compassionate listening.[42]

Although reliving positive experiences of blessedness under LSD was not the main aim of therapy, Lake believed that these blissful experiences could provide patients with the courage to face dread. Lake's focus on courage came from the German-American theologian Paul Tillich's book *The Courage to Be*. Tillich argued that individuals can derive courage from the source of their being, God, to face the existential anxiety surrounding nonbeing.[43] Lake felt that this courage to overcome nonbeing was instilled into the infant through repeated experiences of maternal beneficence.[44] Reliving experiences of maternal love, then, could help patients develop the courage to feel dread during their LSD sessions.[45] When these positive experiences were combined with the supportive resources of a trusted guide, the patient was in the optimal position to tackle the deepest regions of their own mental pain.

Lake warned, though, that the persistent desire to relive ecstatic experiences of mystical union from early infancy was a sign of a schizoid or alienated personality. Christian spirituality, he claimed, was about having a personal relationship with God in Christ. Experiences of monistic union or of oneness removed the personal element: as Lake said, "The Christian goal ultimately heightens personality, it does not annihilate it." He stressed that Christians commune with God through "active goals in the world," through relationships with others, and through the church. While Christians often regressed to "monistic experiences" during LSD therapy, "these are always secondary and inessential factors, a bonus of joy."[46] For Lake, individuals or religions that placed monistic experiences of oneness at the foundation of their spirituality were caught in a reaction pattern to infantile trauma and were not pursuing genuine spiritual connections.

Perhaps unsurprisingly, Lake's *Clinical Theology* textbook received mixed reviews. While some found it helpful for understanding their emotional lives, others questioned whether Lake had successfully integrated theology and psychiatry.[47] Several critics noted that it was obscure or felt that Lake's use of LSD was controversial.[48] Nevertheless, the discipline spread throughout the 1960s. Lake began conducting clinical theology seminars for missionaries with the intent of bringing the discipline to other countries,[49] and when she returned from England, Nichols brought clinical theology to Canada.

"NO CASE IS HOPELESS WITH LSD": SPREADING ENTHUSIASM IN CANADA

After arriving back in Toronto in 1960, Nichols worked at the Ontario Hospital, a public psychiatric institute, and the Bell Clinic, a private hospital that centered on treating addiction. She continued practising LSD therapy and conducting clinical theology seminars.

Much of her LSD work took place at the Bell Clinic. Founded by the Canadian physician R. Gordon Bell in 1954, the clinic offered inpatient and outpatient services to men and women suffering from alcohol addiction. Treatment for alcoholism was increasingly recognized as a medical need at this time, but as Bell later wrote, many Canadian physicians still considered it to be "a controversial area of health care." Bell's motivation, then, was to provide a space for patients whose most pressing issues related to drinking.[50] Between 1961 and 1963, Nichols used LSD to treat around 100 patients at the clinic. She found that the "large majority" had become sober or at least improved, including patients who had struggled with alcohol addiction for twenty years.[51]

Nichols's position as a psychiatrist using LSD in Canada in the early 1960s embroiled her in debates surrounding the Canadian government's decision to restrict access to the drug. Prompted by the thalidomide tragedy, which centered around an insufficiently tested morning sickness drug that caused thousands of birth defects in the late 1950s, the government became increasingly concerned about the unknown side effects of experimental drugs. In 1962, the Food and Drug Directorate introduced a bill that would heavily restrict physicians' access to LSD.[52] Many psychiatrists, and even a group of clergy members, protested the bill in Canadian news media. After the bill was announced, Nichols told one reporter that "my alcoholic patients phoned from all over the country in panic . . . They said, 'this is our lifeline.' It would be dreadful if LSD were removed."[53]

At this time, Nichols was not shy about expressing her enthusiasm about LSD to reporters. She appeared on a Canadian television program that documented a woman's experience of LSD therapy at Toronto Western Hospital. She described her own experience with the drug and explained how it helped patients reach back to the earliest roots of their emotional disturbances.[54] "No case is hopeless with LSD," she told a reporter in 1963, adding, "It brings not only awareness but also revelation, insight, reintegration and a lessening of anxiety."[55]

However, Nichols's use of LSD was not without controversy. In 1961, she participated in an experimental program at the Prison for Women in Kingston, Ontario. Initiated by the Canadian psychologist Mark Eveson, the program involved giving LSD to twenty-three prisoners to help uncover emotional trauma that he thought caused criminal behavior.[56] Recognizing that Nichols had several years of experience with the drug, Eveson invited her to train the prison staff in its therapeutic use. In February of that year, Nichols travelled to Kingston and demonstrated her therapeutic technique by giving LSD to one of the inmantes from the prison at a nearby psychotherapy clinic. The inmate, Christine Bauman, was a German immigrant who was incarcerated for fraud. Bauman had volunteered for the study, but she later claimed that it was a devastating experience. According to Bauman, Nichols presented LSD "as something very pleasant" and had given her a total of 450 μg in one day, along with an injection of Ritalin.[57] "I kept wanting someone to help me," she later said, "but people kept lighting lights, playing music, giving me things to drink and asking how it was." Seven years later, Bauman was arrested for stealing a sweater, but she was acquitted, as her defense argued that the LSD experiment had a long-term negative impact on her personality.[58]

After years of working with experimental psychiatric techniques, though, Nichols was no stranger to unsuccessful cases, and she continued to integrate psychedelics into her Christian approach to psychiatry. As soon as she arrived back in Canada in 1960, Nichols began organizing a network of clinical theology seminars throughout Ontario. As it had in England, this approach appealed to Canadian church leaders, who were trying to incorporate clinical training into their pastoral work. The social transformations of the 1960s created a "decade of ferment" for Canadian churches, which were eager to revive their image to appeal to new generations.[59] Building bridges with the world of psychiatry was one way to do this. Starting in 1961, Nichols organized monthly seminars with clergy in churches and psychiatric clinics. Soon the seminars caught the interest of the Canadian Mental Health Association, who began sponsoring them. By 1965, the seminars took place in seven locations across southern Ontario, with about fifty clergy members attending monthly.

During the seminars, through discussion and role-play, Nichols illustrated various psychiatric disorders and explained to audiences that experiences of maternal deprivation can distort one's image of God later in life. One example, which she shared with a reporter in 1965, was of a pessimistic patient who felt that God would not allow him to maintain his relationship with his wife. Nichols had him use psilocybin to help him recover experiences from infancy. While under the drug, he relived an early experience of abandonment, which was later confirmed by his family.[60]

In 1968, Nichols left for Singapore to continue teaching psychiatry to clergy members. As concern grew in Canada about uncontrolled recreational use of LSD in the late 1960s, the Bell Clinic discontinued its use with patients.[61] LSD was made illegal in Canada in 1968, while Nichols was in Singapore. When she heard this news, she became concerned. She had an office in a clergyman's basement in Toronto, where she kept a supply of LSD.

She was worried that the minister could get in trouble if it were discovered, so she called her sister-in-law and asked her to go over and throw it out.[62]

CONCLUSION

Lake also stopped using LSD around 1970, once it became difficult to access legal supplies. He then explored a number of alternative therapeutic approaches to help patients access repressed trauma from infancy and birth, including primal therapy, a method based on verbally and physically acting out emotional pain, and Reichian breathwork, which used breathing techniques to promote a state of relaxation. Based on these approaches, he developed the concept of the "Maternal-Foetal Distress Syndrome," according to which the roots of psychiatric disorders reached back, beyond infancy or birth, to the first trimester of pregnancy.[63] By the late 1970s, he began engaging with the work of the psychedelic pioneer Stanislov Grof and incorporated Grof's notion of perinatal matrices into his discussions of birth trauma.[64] After his death in 1982, the Clinical Theology Association continued as the Bridge Pastoral Foundation.

Nichols moved to British Columbia in the 1970s and began treating sex offenders at a maximum-security prison until she retired in 1983. With her conviction that positive relationships could transform personalities, she continued to develop close connections with her patients, often inviting them to her home for social events, as she had in India and Ontario.[65]

The story of clinical theology provides an example of how LSD interacted with psychoanalytic psychiatry in the mid-twentieth century. Before discussions of neurotransmitters became dominant, the psychoanalytic framework provided the lens through which most psychiatrists understood LSD. In Lake's case, object-relations theory, with its emphasis on mother-blaming, served as the particular psychoanalytic approach that shaped his interpretation of LSD experiences. The emphasis on mother-blaming extended into explanations of the effects of a drug; Lake understood the blissful or spiritual experiences so often occasioned by LSD as reexperiences of maternal beneficence, and "bad trips," or negative reactions, as reexperiences of dread in the face of maternal deprivation.

The object-relations framework also influenced Lake's and Nichols's understanding of the goal of LSD therapy. For them, LSD therapy was not about inducing positive or transcendent experiences. Instead, it was about reliving dread. Only by fully reentering the pain and suffering of maternal deprivation in infancy could patients relinquish the hold that these experiences had on their lives. While Lake's emphasis on pain certainly had theological underpinnings, it also reflected a psychoanalytic approach to LSD psychotherapy, in which negative experiences were a sign that the drug was doing its job by overcoming repression. As psychedelic therapy reemerges in the era of neuroscience, the question of the therapeutic value of negative experiences is seen through a new lens.[66]

In the case of Lake and Nichols, LSD therapy traveled through postcolonial contexts and across three continents. Beginning after their meeting in India, they continued to influence each other's approaches to psychiatry, resulting in clinical theology, a discipline that was heavily informed by their own and their patients' experiences with LSD. In their missionary spirit, Lake and Nichols brought the discipline to England and Canada in an attempt to further spread their message of Christian psychiatry.

NOTES

I would like to thank Jill Campbell-Miller and Christopher Harding for sharing their research on Florence Nichols with me. I would also like to thank Laurel Parson from the General Synod Archives of The Anglican Church of Canada for sending me copies of Nichols's papers, and Chris Elcock for helpful and encouraging comments.

1.   Christopher Harding has written about Nichols's work in Vellore but does not explore her interactions with Lake. See Christopher Harding, "The Emergence of 'Christian Psychiatry' in Post-Independence India," *Edinburgh Papers in South Asian Studies*, 24 (2011). Even in Lake's biography, Nichols is mentioned only briefly, on one page, and her name is misspelled to boot. See John Peters, *Frank Lake: The Man and His Work* (London: Darton, Longman & Todd 1989), 47.

2.   Judith M. Hughes, *Reshaping the Psychoanalytic Domain: The Work of Melanie Klein, W. R. D. Fairbairn, and D. W. Winnicott* (Berkeley: University of California Press, 1989).

3.   See Marga Vicedo, "The Social Nature of the Mother's Tie to Her Child: John Bowlby's Theory of Attachment in Post-War America," *British Journal for the History of Science* 44, no. 3 (2011): 401–426; and Bican Polat, "Mental Hygiene, Psychoanalysis, and Interwar Psychology: The Making of the Maternal Deprivation Hypothesis," *Isis* 112, no. 2 (2021): 266–290.

4. Ido Hartogoshn, *The American Trip: Set, Setting, and the Psychedelic Experience in the Twentieth Century* (Cambridge, MA: MIT Press, 2020).

5. Frank Lake, *Clinical Theology: A Theological and Psychiatric Basis to Clinical Pastoral Care* (London: Darton, Longman & Todd, 1966), 184.

6. Lake, *Clinical Theology*, 140.

7. Florence Nichols, "Chapter I Alternate, p. 1, Memoirs of a Missionary Doctor in India, 1984–1986," n.d., Florence Nichols Fonds, M2019–06 Box 1 File 1, Anglican Church of Canada/General Synod Archives (hereafter cited as Memoirs, ACC/GSA).

8. Harding, "The Emergence of 'Christian Psychiatry'" 5.

9. Nichols, "Chapter IX, 6–8," n.d., Memoirs, ACC/GSA.

10. Lake, *Clinical Theology*, xix.

11. Nichols, "Chapter IX, 26," n.d., Memoirs, ACC/GSA.

12. Nichols, "Chapter VII, 6–12," n.d., Memoirs, ACC/GSA.

13. Lake, *Clinical Theology*, xix.

14. Lake, *Clinical Theology*, xix–xx.

15. Anju Kuruvilla, "Dr. Florence Nichols," *Indian Journal of Psychiatry* 52, no. 6 (2010): 146.

16. Lake, *Clinical Theology*, 184.

17. Frank Lake, "Discussion," in *Proceedings of the Quarterly Meeting of the Royal Medico-Psychological Association on Hallucinogenic Drugs and their Therapeutic Use*, ed. Richard Crocket, R. A. Sandison, and Alexander Walk (London: H. K. Lewis, 1963), 151.

18. Harding, "The Emergence of 'Christian Psychiatry'," 13–14.

19. Lake, *Clinical Theology*, xii.

20. Sylvia Lake, "Forward," in Peters, *Frank Lake*, viii.

21. Lake, *Clinical Theology*, 32.

22. Lake, *Clinical Theology*, xi.

23. Hughes, *Reshaping the Psychoanalytic Domain*, 95–96.

24. Hughes, *Reshaping the Psychoanalytic Domain*, 99.

25. Hughes, *Reshaping the Psychoanalytic Domain*, 104.

26. Lake, *Clinical Theology*, 140.

27. Lake, *Clinical Theology*, Fold-out Chart 1.

28. Lake, *Clinical Theology*, Fold-out Chart 1.

29. R. D. Laing, *The Divided Self: An Existential Study in Sanity and Madness* (London: Tavistock Publications, 1960), 118.

30. Lake, *Clinical Theology*, 682–683.

31. Lake, *Clinical Theology*, xxi.

32. Lake, *Clinical Theology*, 242.

33. Lake, *Clinical Theology*, 179–180.

34. Lake, *Clinical Theology*, xxii.

35. Lake, *Clinical Theology*, 478; See also Frank Lake, appendix to *A Christian Therapy for a Neurotic World*, by Eric N. Ducker (New York: Taplinger Publishing Co., 1961), 216–217.

36. Lake, *Clinical Theology*, 802.

37. Lake, *Clinical Theology*, 791.

38. Lake, *Clinical Theology*, 881.

39. Lake, *Clinical Theology*, xxii–xxiii.

40. Lake, *Clinical Theology*, 1137.

41. Lake, *Clinical Theology*, 660.

42. Lake, *Clinical Theology*, 15.

43. Paul Tillich, *The Courage to Be* (London: Nesbitt, 1953).

44. Lake, *Clinical Theology*, 627.

45. Lake, "Discussion," 150–151.

46. Lake, *Clinical Theology*, 738.

47. Peters, *Frank Lake*, 20–21.

48. Peters, *Frank Lake*, 59.

49. Peters, *Frank Lake*, 21.

50. R. Gordon Bell, *A Special Calling: My Life in Addiction Treatment and Care* (Toronto: Stoddard Publishing, 1989), 157–160.

51. Jeanine Locke, "The Drug That Brings the Alcoholic Face to Face with Himself," *Star Weekly Magazine*, February 16, 1963.

52. "Drug Acclaimed by Researchers May Be Banned," *The Globe and Mail*, October 20, 1962. For more on these regulations, see Erika Dyck, "Just Say Know: Criminalizing LSD and the Politics of Psychedelic Expertise, 1961–8," in *Social, Legal, and Historical Perspectives on the Regulation of Drugs in Canada*, ed. Edgar-André Montigny (Toronto: University of Toronto Press, 2011), 169–196.

53. Blaik Kirby, "Doctors Protest Most to Ban 'Alcoholics' Drug," *Toronto Star*, December 5, 1962.

54. Alan Edmonds, "TV Sequel: Drug Row Spreads to Clergy," *Toronto Star*, December 14, 1962.

55. Locke, "The Drug That Brings the Alcoholic."

56. Mark Eveson, "Research with Female Drug Addicts at the Prison for Women," *Canadian Journal of Corrections* 21, no. 6 (1963): 25–27. The project also involved experiments on Indigenous women. For more on LSD experiments in the Kingston Prison for Women, see Dorothy Proctor and Fred Rosen, *Chameleon: The Lives of Dorothy Proctor* (New Jersey: New Horizon Press, 1994).

57. Nichols likely learned the practice of combining stimulants with LSD while working with Lake in England. Lake initially found that methedrine could enhance LSD's ability to help patients overcome defenses and experience infantile dread. However, he eventually discontinued this practice, as he felt that methedrine distorted the experience of dread by making it more palatable. See Lake, *Clinical Theology*, 682.

58. Shiela Gormerly, "LSD-Defence Women Wins Her Freedom," *Toronto Telegram*, January 17, 1968.

59. Phillip Gardner, "A Holy or a Broken Hallelujah: The United Church of Canada in the 1960s Decade of Ferment" (PhD thesis, University of Toronto, 2018).

60. Janice Tyrwhitt, "Psychiatry and the Pulpit," *Montreal Gazette*, June 12, 1965.

61. John Marshall, "Quiet Campaign Pushes Potential Good of LSD," *The Globe and Mail*, October 4, 1976. For more on the LSD controversy in Canada in the late 1960s, see Marcel Martel, "Setting Boundaries: LSD Use and Glue Sniffing in Ontario in the 1960s," in *Social, Legal, and Historical Perspectives on the Regulation of Drugs in Canada*, ed. Edgar-André Montigny (Toronto: University of Toronto Press, 2011), 197–218.

62. Margaret Janack (Nichols's sister-in-law), interview with Jill Campbell-Miller, August 2018. I am grateful to Jill Campbell-Miller for granting me permission to use this excerpt from the interview.

63. Frank Lake, *Tight Corners in Pastoral Counselling* (London: Darton, Longman and Todd, 1981), xi.

64. Lake's story has some interesting parallels with the work of Stanislov Grof. During the 1950s and 1960s, they both found that LSD allows patients to relive birth trauma, and when LSD became restricted, they both switched to alternative methods to help patients access these experiences. It is unclear when they first met, but in 1977, Lake attended a workshop led by Grof. See Alix Pirani, "Frank Lake 1915–1982," *Self & Society* 10, no. 4 (1982): 209; and Frank Lake, "The Significance of Perinatal Experience," *Self & Society* 6, no. 7 (1978): 224–232.

65. Florence Nichols, "Chapter IV, Life with Father and Mother as told by Barney Poodle," 1988, box 1, folder 2, Florence Nichols Fonds, M2019–06, Anglican Church of Canada/General Synod Archives.

66. For more on interpreting bad trips, see Erika Dyck and Chris Elcock, "Reframing Bummer Trips: Scientific and Cultural Explanations to Adverse Reactions to Psychedelic Drug Use," *Social History of Alcohol and Drugs* 34, no. 2 (2020): 271–296.

BIBLIOGRAPHY

Primary Sources

"Drug Acclaimed by Researchers May Be Banned." *The Globe and Mail*, October 20, 1962.

Edmonds, Alan. "TV Sequel: Drug Row Spreads to Clergy." *Toronto Star*, December 14, 1962.

Gormerly, Sheila. "LSD-Defence Women Wins Her Freedom." *Toronto Telegram*, January 17, 1968.

Kirby, Blaik. "Doctors Protest Most to Ban 'Alcoholics' Drug." *Toronto Star*, December 5, 1962.

Lake, Frank. *Clinical Theology: A Theological and Psychiatric Basis to Clinical Pastoral Care* (London: Darton, Longman & Todd, 1966)

Locke, Jeanine. "The Drug That Brings the Alcoholic Face to Face with Himself." *Star Weekly Magazine*, February 16, 1963.

Marshall, John. "Quiet Campaign Pushes Potential Good of LSD." *The Globe and Mail*, October 4, 1976.

Nichols, Florence. "Chapter I Alternate, Memoirs of a Missionary Doctor in India, 1984–1986," n.d., Florence Nichols Fonds, M2019–06 Box 1 File 1, Anglican Church of Canada/General Synod Archives (hereafter cited as Memoirs, ACC/GSA).

Nichols, Florence. "Chapter IV, Life with Father and Mother as told by Barney Poodle," 1988, box 1, folder 2, Florence Nichols Fonds, M2019–06, Anglican Church of Canada/General Synod Archives.

Nichols, Florence. "Chapter IX, 26," n.d., Memoirs, ACC/GSA.

Nichols, Florence. "Chapter IX, 8," n.d., Memoirs, ACC/GSA.

Nichols, Florence. "Chapter VII, 6–12," n.d., Memoirs, ACC/GSA.

Tyrwhitt, Janice. "Psychiatry and the Pulpit." *Montreal Gazette*, June 12, 1965.

Secondary Sources

Bell, R. Gordon. *A Special Calling: My Life in Addiction Treatment and Care*. Toronto: Stoddard Publishing, 1989.

Dyck, Erika. "Just Say Know: Criminalizing LSD and the Politics of Psychedelic Expertise, 1961–1968." In *Social, Legal, and Historical Perspectives on the Regulation of Drugs in Canada*, edited by Edgar-André Montigny, 169–196. Toronto: University of Toronto Press, 2011.

Dyck, Erika, and Chris Elcock. "Reframing Bummer Trips: Scientific and Cultural Explanations to Adverse Reactions to Psychedelic Drug Use." *Social History of Alcohol and Drugs* 34, no. 2 (2020): 271–296.

Eveson, Mark. "Research with Female Drug Addicts at the Prison for Women." *Canadian Journal of Corrections* 21, no. 6 (1963): 25–27.

Gardner, Phillip. "A Holy or a Broken Hallelujah: The United Church of Canada in the 1960s Decade of Ferment." PhD thesis, University of Toronto, 2018.

Harding, Christopher. "The Emergence of 'Christian Psychiatry' in Post-Independence India." *Edinburgh Papers in South Asian Studies*, 24 (2011): 1–16

Hartogoshn, Ido. *The American Trip: Set, Setting, and the Psychedelic Experience in the Twentieth Century*. Cambridge, MA: MIT Press, 2020.

Hughes, Judith M. *Reshaping the Psychoanalytic Domain: The Work of Melanie Klein, W. R. D. Fairbairn, and D. W. Winnicott*. Berkeley: University of California Press, 1989.

Kuruvilla, Anju. "Dr. Florence Nichols." *Indian Journal of Psychiatry* 52, no. 6 (2010): 145–146.

Laing, R. D. *The Divided Self: An Existential Study in Sanity and Madness*. London: Tavistock Publications, 1960.

Lake, Frank. *A Christian Therapy for a Neurotic World*. New York: Taplinger Publishing, 1961.

Lake, Frank. *Clinical Theology: A Theological and Psychiatric Basis to Clinical Pastoral Care*. London: Darton, Longman & Todd, 1966.

Lake, Frank. "Discussion." In *Proceedings of the Quarterly Meeting of the Royal Medico-Psychological Association on Hallucinogenic Drugs and Their Therapeutic Use*, edited by Richard Crocket, R. A. Sandison, and Alexander Walk, 146–57. London: H. K. Lewis, 1963.

Lake, Frank. "The Significance of Perinatal Experience." *Self & Society* 6, no. 7 (1978): 224–232.

Lake, Frank. *Tight Corners in Pastoral Counselling*. London: Darton, Longman and Todd, 1981.

Lake, Sylvia. *Foreword to Frank Lake: The Man and His Work*, by John Peters, vii–x. London: Darton, Longman & Todd, 1989.

Martel, Marcel. "Setting Boundaries: LSD Use and Glue Sniffing in Ontario in the 1960s." In *Social, Legal, and Historical Perspectives on the Regulation of Drugs in Canada*, edited by Edgar André Montigny, 197–218. Toronto: University of Toronto Press, 2011.

Peters, John. *Frank Lake: The Man and His Work*. London: Darton, Longman & Todd, 1989.

Pirani, Alix. "Frank Lake 1915–1982." *Self & Society* 10, no. 4 (1982): 209–211.

Polat, Bican. "Mental Hygiene, Psychoanalysis, and Interwar Psychology: The Making of the Maternal Deprivation Hypothesis." *Isis* 112, no. 2 (2021): 266–290.

Proctor, Dorothy, and Fred Rosen. *Chameleon: The Lives of Dorothy Proctor*. Far Hills, NJ: New Horizon Press, 1994.

Tillich, Paul. *The Courage to Be*. London: Nesbitt, 1953.

Vicedo, Marga. "The Social Nature of the Mother's Tie to Her Child: John Bowlby's Theory of Attachment in Post-War America." *British Journal for the History of Science* 44, no. 3 (2011): 401–426.

13 PSYCHEDELICS, POLITICAL RADICALISM, AND TRANSNATIONAL ACID-ANARCHISM IN THE 1970s

Hallam Roffey

In 1970, an anarchist commune was established in a three-bedroom, terraced house on Havelock Square in the Broomhall suburb of the northern city of Sheffield, England. The commune, "a hotbed of radical debate," established several enduring principles, including the door never being locked and nobody ever being turned away.[1] Living arrangements, including the bedrooms, were communal. In the fall of that year, a young anarchist named Dave Lee moved into the commune and remained there for about two years. Lee has recalled how the anarchists at Havelock Square "did not see their role as selling papers, or building an organization aimed at insurrection"—they could see from the vantage point of the 1970s that insurrections, even leftist ones, did not necessarily result in a better society—rather, what they were doing "was about everyday relationships, breaking the patterns of bourgeois society to underpin a new kind of social movement."[2]

What made this commune significant in the history of British psychedelia was the integral place of LSD within it, and what the drug meant to this brand of anarchism more broadly. Indeed, Lee remembers that "many people in the anarchist milieu took LSD, which was very easy to acquire. In fact, it would be fair to say that much of our social scene floated on a small lake of LSD. And the people I am talking about were not the pop-mystics that psychedelic culture has become associated with; there was less an emphasis on achieving 'enlightenment' and more on living true to ourselves." For Lee and his fellow anarchists, LSD not only infused them with a "militant anti-materialism," it was crucial in their emphasis on "total cultural transformation, via transformation of everyday life," and they especially valued features of youth subculture that Lee thought might now be derided as "hippy values."[3]

It is certainly true that "hippy values"—the utopian and communitarian "peace and love" ethos of the 1960s counterculture—and the explosive psychedelia of the same era have, since their inception, been endlessly disparaged and reduced to recognizable tropes, characterized as bourgeois, escapist, undisciplined, antisocial, and preoccupied with lifestyle choice and exhibitionism.[4] The result has been an overriding of the truly radical, politically threatening potential of the counterculture's use of psychedelic drugs during the 1960s and 1970s, which masked a great deal of serious, politically engaged content that requires salvaging in the historiography. Cynicism reigns among those historians who continue to reduce the counterculture and psychedelic culture of the mid-to-late twentieth century to their "commodified components."[5]

However, there are signs of growing interest in what the political theorist Jeremy Gilbert termed "acid socialism," inspiring the cultural theorist Mark Fisher's "acid communism."[6] This is summarized by the philosopher Emma Stamm as representing "the idea that psychologically profound experiences—including the use of psychedelic drugs—should be used to galvanize anticapitalist movements."[7] Both Fisher and Gilbert have explored the notion that to imagine alternatives to capitalism, we must explore the limits of consciousness, and the countercultures of the 1960s and later might provide valuable insights to the left in this project.[8] The premise is that experiences of ego dissolution, unity, and connectedness, to which psychedelics are one route, can be useful to the radical left when properly programmed (notwithstanding the concurrent challenge from a "psychedelic right").[9]

To be sure, there have always been significant tensions in Britain between the counterculture and other parts of the political left. As the historian Willie Thompson has observed, from the 1960s on, the counterculture offered an "alternative version of and path to utopia" than the revolutionary far-left, and the counterculture seldom appeared in the radical left press of the late 1960s. In part, this is because revolutionary socialists of all stripes were essentially rationalists (all being fundamentally Marxist), and therefore the counterculture's own rejection of rationality, frequently catalyzed by psychedelics, was generally anathema.[10]

As this chapter argues, attempts to infuse psychedelics and psychedelic philosophy into radical leftist politics is no new endeavor, and it seeks to refute any notion that psychedelics have transcended politics by examining their use in politically radical contexts in Britain and Ireland in the 1970s. The 1960s has tended to dominate the history of psychedelics, and the focus here on the 1970s shows that while any psychedelic heyday may have passed by this period, key actors and organizations continued to use these substances to radical ends. In addition, it is the counterculture of the mid-1960s period that receives the most attention in historiographical studies of psychedelics rather than other radical movements; this chapter partly reorients this existing focus. This exploration centers around one key individual in the history of what is here called "acid-anarchism": the Irishman Bill "Ubi" Dwyer (1933–2001), who offers a fascinating conduit into the complex relationship between psychedelics, anarchism, the radical left, and the counterculture of 1970s Britain.

BILL DWYER AND PSYCHEDELIC ANARCHISM

Bill Dwyer was born in 1933 in County Kildare, Ireland. In the mid-1950s, he emigrated to New Zealand, where he was first introduced to anarchism, and he became active in politics. In his book *Rabble Rousers*, the historian Toby Boraman has described how in Wellington and Auckland, Dwyer was a regular speaker at political gatherings, and his "lyrical" Irish voice made him a popular orator, well regarded for his sociability and generosity.[11] In 1966, Dwyer moved to Sydney, Australia, where he sold LSD to finance anarchist projects and propaganda (selling around 1,000 tabs a week by mid-1968).[12] Dwyer noticed that it was mainly "heads," referring to people who used acid and other drugs, who visited Sydney's anarchist hangout The Cellar, which he described as an "embryonic anarcho-hippie sub-culture," and he felt it was in fact these people who were "most likely to find the anarchist message true to their aspirations." Bringing in around 500 pounds a week from collective drug sales, all money at The Cellar was spent communally and "in advancement of our principles." While there, Dwyer observed how people would "willingly work together as a co-operative," and there had been "a cohesive spirit of mutual aid, trust and affection which provided sound foundations for the community."[13] He took these lessons with him and would later apply them to his own brand of acid-anarchism.

However, according to Boraman, many Sydney anarchists deemed him as something of a joke and were suspect of his apparent enthusiasm for the place of LSD in anarchist movements. In fact, at this stage, Dwyer did not think that there was necessarily any direct connection between LSD and the creation of an anarchist society—"the only direct connection as far as I was concerned was my use of the latter to raise funds for the former"—but he did believe that acid was a "symbol of the rejection of the status quo"; in any case, his view on the role of LSD in anarchist projects was soon to shift considerably.[14]

An "action-hungry," committed radical, Dwyer came to believe passionately in "the possibility of an anarchist revolution."[15] In his 1968 pamphlet *Anarchy Now!* Dwyer appealed for "an unceasing battle against authority . . . every individual must repudiate the claim of anyone else to rule and exploit him (or her)."[16] While he was classically anarchist, to the extent that he considered capitalism, the state, the church, and the army to all be public enemies, and he viewed anarchism principally as a working-class movement, unlike other 1960s anarchists, Dwyer saw few differences between "competing" strands of anarchism and recognized revolutionary potential among multiple sections of society, including students and "hippies," the latter of which, following his experiences at The Cellar, he thought were "basically anarchists."[17]

In 1968, Dwyer was arrested for dealing LSD and imprisoned for eighteen months before being deported back to Ireland in 1969, after which he moved to London to work as a civil servant in the Stationary Office as he continued his activism. He became involved in anarchist, squatting, and countercultural scenes, as well as with the anarchist publishing house Freedom Press, writing a regular column—"This World"—for their weekly newspaper, *Freedom*. He changed his name to Bill Ubique Dwyer (short for "Ubiquitous") but was widely known as "Ubi." In 1970, Dwyer attended the third and final Isle of Wight Festival, where, as with Woodstock in the US the year before, various anarchist groups pulled down the barriers surrounding the festival site and declared the event "free." For Dwyer, this was an example of true anarchism in action, and he became enthusiastic about the subversive potential of free music festivals. He was best known as a principal founder of the Windsor Free Festival, following an inspirational acid trip in London's Windsor Great Park. The first iteration of the festival in 1972 was the forerunner for the whole "free festival" movement of the 1970s.[18]

Anarchism in the 1960s and 1970s was, as it always has been, a broad-church philosophy. But a reliable commitment to libertarianism meant that from the peak of "flower power," despite differing views on drugs, anarchists almost invariably defended the right of the individual to consume whatever they wanted to; there was rarely dissent on this specific point within anarchist literature.[19] Rather, the key internal tension was whether psychedelic drug use—and drug use more broadly—was desirable within radical movements or not, and the extent to which those within them should actively discourage their comrades and others from using drugs. Ido Hartogsohn has highlighted the common notion that psychedelics had an "inherent tendency to destabilize the powers-that-be by inducing a radical rebelliousness that rejected cultural norms and challenged any authority or ideology."[20] Some anarchists subscribed to this view while others rejected it wholesale.

This debate had played out in October 1966 in one of the earlier references to psychedelics in *Anarchy* magazine. In one letter, a reader from Blackburn argued that if anarchists "really wish to achieve something approaching an enlightened society," then "advocacy propaganda for psychedelic drugs is an important prerequisite," with the letter writer viewing particular mind-altering substances as being "chemical short-cuts" to achieve useful personal and social insights.[21] The same kind of language was being used contemporaneously by those interested in the more spiritual and mystical dimensions and possibilities of psychedelics, but here it was being inserted into a new—and more explicitly political—context.[22] The writer's aspiration was to promote an expansion of collective consciousness so that radicals free themselves of "hereditary conditioning, tribal inhibition and taboo," a version of the concept of "deconditioning" or "deschooling," which was prominent in popular psychology at this time and has been explored by the historian David Farber.[23]

Accompanying this letter in print, however, was another from "J. Jack," who argued that the "principal objective" of libertarians should indeed be the liberation of the mind but—in a reversal of the acid-logic of the previous letter writer—asserted that "tangible results" in this field would be achieved only with an "increasingly clear view of reality."[24] For this reader, this necessitated the development of the strength to experience reality "without the dubious crutches of analgesics, be they drink, drug, dogma or irresponsible escapism." Representing a more sober radicalism, the author thought that not only would permitting "the irresponsibility of a few adolescent inadequates" alienate the very people they should be aiming to attract, but that drugs would only serve to increase the user's "dependence on the existing social system." These were the broad contours of a debate that played out only very rarely in anarchist magazines over the next several years. *Anarchy* appeared every month throughout the mid-to-late 1960s, and *Freedom* every week, and yet there were only a handful of references to psychedelic drugs, most of which are not particularly insightful. Psychedelics started to receive more serious coverage, even if still in very small doses, only from the start of the 1970s, aligning with the passing of the 1971 Misuse of Drugs Act, which prohibited their possession.

After the head rush of the 1960s and its association with the "Summer of Love," and the turn to more direct confrontation with authority in Europe and the US during 1968, the early 1970s in Britain saw a cooler cultural climate, the result of the Organisation of Petroleum-Exporting Countries (OPEC) oil crisis, domestic economic turmoil, successive states of emergency, national strikes, race riots, and a new and more aggressive form of politics. The beginning of the decade saw the start of a bombing campaign by the Angry Brigade in 1970, polarizing factions within the counterculture. There was a general image of a society fraying at the seams, establishing Britain as the "sick man of Europe" and making notions of dropping out and pursuing drug-enhanced experiences appear considerably riskier.[25] The 1970 Isle of Wight festival signaled this changing mood as some of the positive youthful energy that had emerged around 1967 began to ebb away. However, psychedelics continued to be employed in radical contexts and countercultural values endured in the form of underground magazines, communes, community projects, activism, and head shops. The ideologists and idealists who envisioned a more profound social role for psychedelics did not disappear altogether.

In May 1970, a symposium on LSD took place at the US embassy in Dublin, Ireland. It was attended by a wide range of interested parties: academics, teachers, social workers, drug squad detectives, and a few priests. According to Dwyer, who was invited to the conference to speak and who wrote about his visit for *Freedom* and *Anarchy*, there were several "heads" there, but they had all been hurriedly stewarded toward the back of the hall.[26] The symposium reflects how far Dwyer's views on the radical potential of psychedelics had moved by this stage. Dwyer's assessment of the event was that, for a meeting about LSD, it was "pretty dull." More sensationally, a suited Dwyer revived the audience by announcing at the start of the talk that he had been on around 250 LSD trips in total and had never had any of the catastrophic experiences that other speakers at the event had warned about. Dwyer claimed that there was "little to no knowledge or information at this assembly," but in its place, there was "plenty of prejudice." He told the audience that LSD was, in fact, "the greatest gift from nature to mankind in the twentieth century."[27] His speech even resulted in one of the priests later coming up to him to tell him that he wanted to try acid. Unfortunately for the priest, LSD became illegal in Ireland shortly after the conferehnce.[28]

A year later in 1971, apparently inspired by the Dublin meeting, Dwyer organized his own open and free Acid Symposium, to take place on April 28 in Conway Hall, the prestigious home of the British humanism and free-thought movements.[29] Posters appeared around London's Red Lion Square, announcing that the event was to be sponsored by *Anarchy* magazine and would be an opportunity to "get a HEAD LIBERATION FRONT moving!" Afterward, Dwyer organized an inaugural meeting for the newly formed Head Liberation Front, which he promoted in *Freedom* and various other underground magazines.[30] The new movement was founded on a stated set of principles and objectives, including "the development of communes and co-operatives" and "enlightenment of public opinion on the subject of psychedelic drugs." It would also work toward the "furtherance of research into the social use of LSD and allied psychedelics" and the development of "knowledge into LSD as a truth revealer relating to the individual personality."[31]

That same month, the third issue of the new series of *Anarchy* was published. Dwyer's attempts to advocate for at least a consideration of the place of drugs within anarchist movements had reaped dividends, and the issue was designated "The Acid Issue," dedicated to an exploration of the place of LSD and other psychedelics in the struggle for radical liberation and revolution.[32] Taken as a whole, this issue was much more carefully balanced than *Oz* magazine's own "Acid Issue" the year before, which had included pieces that did little more than enthusiastically promote the use of psychedelic drugs for personal and spiritual development.[33] In *Anarchy*'s Acid Issue, alongside a report on the Dublin symposium, Dwyer contributed a seven-page article called "Feed the Head," in which he contemplated the connection between LSD and freedom.[34] Attempting to couch his argument more precisely in anarchist vocabularies and objectives, Dwyer suggested that the two "primary fundamentals" of a free society were the rejection of authority and the espousal of a society organized *without* authority. He argued that these corresponded with the central themes of hippie culture—the rejection of rat-race materialism and a desire for mutual aid and communitarianism.

Dwyer reminded the readers of *Anarchy* that everyone was born conditioned to authority, amounting to "a society, at essence, of slaves." However, he did not believe the cause was hopeless; for him, it was "self-discovery and an awareness of one's own dignity, sovereignty and sacredness" that held the key. It was in this objective that Dwyer claimed that LSD was a powerful catalyst: "I maintain that LSD is of enormous assistance in liberating the mind, in learning respect for yourself (and, therefore, of others)." He still did not deny that all this could be done *without* psychedelic assistance, but he did feel certain that LSD was a "powerful spur to truth and sensitivity, an awakener of the inner man."[35] Again, this provides some measure of the ideological distance that Dwyer had traveled since he left Sydney.

The issue included challenges to Dwyer's perspective by several pieces from anarchists who rejected the kinds of claims that Dwyer was making for LSD. In one article, the anarchists Chris Broad, Alison Cattell, David Godin, Graham Moss, and Roger Willis cast serious doubt on the revolutionary aspects of the embryonic acid-left, finding that the whole scene only *appeared* revolutionary because of the very fact that it was based on an illegality.[36] "LSD users," they posited, "reject the authority that denies them acid, but do not appear to reject authoritarianism . . . LSD and revolution? We are not convinced. LSD and evolution? A contradiction in terms."

In another article, "A New Consciousness & Its Polemics," John O'Conner wrote somewhat disparagingly about the incursion of psychedelics and psychedelic philosophy into anarchist spaces. O'Conner acknowledged that one characteristic of what he termed "acid fairyland," which revolutionaries seemed to find encouraging, was the "noticeable sensitivity to any form of authority among its inhabitants . . . I imagine, and some value acid for this insight, that it reproduces the extreme sensitivity of a child at the stage when park-keepers, schoolmasters and parents are mysteriously in league with each other." In this, O'Conner echoed some of Dwyer's own points. However, O'Connor also argued that while the psychedelic experience might create a "nice person" with no interest in controlling others, that person would be vulnerable to manipulation by those who did seek power over others—"the state might one day need as many groovy citizens as can be indoctrinated into being satisfied with the pleasures of just existing."[37]

In another piece, the anarchist writer and cartoonist Donald Rooum contended that acid's "protagonists" suggest that the chemical "reveals a world inside your head as marvelous as the world outside. But of course there is nothing inside your head except your brain . . . which functions by trillions of delicate chemical exchanges."[38] Presenting a hardcore materialist response to Dwyer's own ideas about the relationship between acid and freedom, Rooum thought that all LSD provided was "freedom from the ability to control your thoughts, freedom from common sense." For him, anarchism and acid had "nothing in common," and while he did not claim that they were not mutually exclusive, he did think that they were "mutually irrelevant . . . like anarchism and ingrowing toenails." *Anarchy's* Acid Issue ultimately left the debate around psychedelics and anarchism wide open.

PSYCHEDELICS, POST-SCARCITY, AND LIFESTYLE RADICALISM

Community and communal lifestyles were central to Dwyer's philosophy and worldview, and he assigned a key place to psychedelics in facilitating these radical forms of living and being. From 1970 to 1972, Dwyer ran the "Island Commune" on Merrion Road in Dublin. He called this "an experiment in communal living" that "provided an opportunity of meeting girls and boys who actually lived on hippy farming communities in the US."[39] There were important links between Dwyer's lifestyle radicalism, his anarchism, and his approach to psychedelics. The communal lifestyle advocated by Dwyer and his associates in this period was part of a broader project to challenge and subvert bourgeois norms and traditional Western-capitalist social structures and hierarchies.[40]

Similarly, the anarchism at the Havelock Square commune in Sheffield was explicitly based, according to Dave Lee, on an interpretation of the American anarchist Murray Bookchin's (1921–2006) essay collection *Post-Scarcity Anarchism* (1971), a response to ideas that were widely circulating about the white heat of technological advancement ushering in a milieu of automation, computerization, increased leisure time, and ultimately self-actualization rather than workplace alienation.[41] The goal at the commune and others like it was wholesale cultural change rather than a direct assault on the political or economic order, and it was believed that psychedelics could facilitate this kind of cultural shift.

Post-scarcity thinking along the lines that Bookchin envisioned had been circulating for some time prior to his own work. By 1967 and the Summer of Love, *Anarchy* had been occasionally featuring articles on this theme—for instance, in August, when a contributor imagined a future where "the machines would work for man. Free communities would stand, in effect, at the end of a cybernated industrial assembly line with baskets to cart the goods home."[42] This notion had underpinned the counterculture's emphasis on play and childhood, often greatly enhanced through the use of psychedelic drugs, which was (and is) incorrectly taken as the antithesis of political, or a reflection of middle-class, hedonistic indifference. From this view, the British underground and its use of psychedelics amounted to little more than the consumption of commercially marketable goods and ultra-exclusive fun, not radical cultural politics. Much of the British "new left," for instance, saw this turn to play and childhood not merely as apolitical but frivolous, exposing these tensions between the more libertarian sections of the counterculture and the more serious materialist politics of the "new" and "radical" left. The historian and feminist Sheila Rowbotham (1943–), for example, has reflected on the fact that she was never able to be part of the underground in the mid-1960s because of its "abnegation of any attempt to change the external world."[43] Apparent lack of strategy, organization, or grander plan also prompted the orthodox Marxist David Widgery (1947–1992) to write in the August 1967 issue of *Oz* that "at the moment hippies in England represent about as powerful a challenge to the power of the state as the people who put foreign coins in their gas meters."[44]

However, while many within the counterculture may have themselves explicitly rejected political engagement because they saw the problem as being a common culture on top of which the state was erected, this was a radical stance in itself. In his prominent countercultural text *An Essay on Liberation* (1969), the philosopher and sociologist Herbert Marcuse (1898–1979) argued that "the 'trip' involves the dissolution of the ego shaped by established society . . . the revolution must at the same time be a revolution in perception which will accompany the material and intellectual reconstruction of society."[45] Therefore, the pervasive 1960s theme of "play" and the present-oriented "Be here now" ethics of the counterculture gave a real challenge to the status quo insofar as it attempted to be the antithesis of a prevailing work ethic and tried to point to possible alternatives.[46] This should be read not as apathy or impotence, but rather an active attempt to fashion something different.[47] This idea of subversion through changing the way that one lived and acted in the world was augmented by theories of postscarcity and absorbed by those on the radical and anarchist left, such as Dwyer, who took these ideas and the place of psychedelics within them seriously.

Communes were one site where psychedelics often helped enact these alternative modes of living (and often ruined them too). The Island Commune and Havelock Square were not the only communes buoyed by a reliable supply of psychedelic drugs in the early 1970s. When the journalist William De'Ath (1937–2020) wrote his anthropological "Notes from the English Underground" for the magazine *The Listener* in 1970, he observed that there were about forty communes in Britain, which were growing in number and strength.[48] LSD was fundamental to a great number of these communal projects, shared houses, and squats. In part, this is because, as the historian Sarah Shortall has observed, the "pre-discursive" experience of psychedelics could serve to forge communal identities (although they generally did so by defining the community by comparing it to another).[49] LSD was crucial, for example, to the lifestyle at the Eel Pie Commune, based in the abandoned Eel Pie Hotel on an island in the River Thames in west London. By the 1970s, this was the UK's largest "hippie commune," with over forty young residents staying there in 1970. One former communard, Chris Faiers, has written about how psychedelics were used there to help communards bond and adapt to the communal lifestyle.[50] LSD was also, as was the case in many other communes, behind its eventual downfall, its excessive use being exploited by guru figures. While these experiments were not consistently successful, they could be very real manifestations of alternative lifestyles and were a response to calls for anarchists to "actually live out the alternative lives and lifestyles they're always rhetoricising about," to recruit people not by saying, "Vote for us and you will be living in a worker's paradise," but by saying, "Come down the road and see the way we live."[51] This was the same theory underpinning many of the "free festivals" of the 1970s and 1980s, which through their emphasis on "free" implemented a subversion of capitalist systems, often with psychedelic assistance.

Dwyer, through his organization of both communes and free festivals, as well as through his engagement with far-left circles, was an important conduit for these ideas to spread to diverse parts of Britain's radical community. In January 1972, however, he announced in *Freedom* and other alternative publications that he had been arrested with around 1,400 tabs of LSD.[52] He used his columns in part to advertise a letter that by that point had gathered fifty signatures of support to be sent to the underground press. Dwyer had decided to fight the case on the basis of no guilty intent and argued that his selling of LSD was a matter of conscience in which he believed that "acid is a holy sacrament which greatly assists the individual in cleaning himself of selfishness and the various million inhibitions bestowed upon us by an authoritarian, moralistic society." Dwyer announced that he was building evidence to prove that he was in no way motivated by personal profit, but rather lived "as an equal in a commune where the ambition was the growth of communes." What he needed, though, was "as many people as possible to testify in court the beneficial effects of acid in their own private lives." While in prison, he would also work on a novel, *Return of the Pagans*, that would explore the theme of "repossession by ordinary people of a cooperative, guilt-free and loving existence—a repossession from those forces which have alienated mankind from what I believe to be its birth-right."[53]

Simultaneously, Dwyer summarized a talk that he had recently given at Mansfield College, Oxford, entitled "People: Squares or Circles," part of a series on "Freedom and Control." He had been invited because of his "advocacy of psychedelic drugs in personality development and the conflict between such a position and the laws of the land." While Dwyer acknowledged that there would still be many anarchists who disagreed with his claims about LSD and other psychedelics, he called for more debate on the subject within anarchist networks. From his perspective, the aim was "personality development" in order to conceive of and arrive at new senses of self and to break out of conditioned patterns of thought and ways of behaving in the world—to help individuals "realise their full potential and in understanding their nature." Again, Dwyer appreciated that there were alternative routes to the same set of truths. However, he argued that "in a world where almost everyone is subjected to authoritarian and moralistic indoctrination from the very cradle we should at least carefully investigate ways of breaking away from such patterns of conditioning" and this deconditioning would be made much harder and longer without the catalyzing effects of the psychedelic experience.[54]

This was an overt political challenge; Dwyer recognized a move away from "confidence in authority," which was part of a broader postwar trend away from deference in the UK, and a declining willingness to "fight government's war" or "accept that the role for him or her is obedience."[55] What he identified as the "old society" appeared to him addled with sexual guilt and low self-worth. The "trend to communes," he argued, was a facet of the burgeoning new society where the prime motivation would be love. On the basis of personal experience and observation, Dwyer was "fully convinced" that LSD was "something to be approached with reverence and care. . . . Acid is a love machine in that it turns one on to life and everything positive in it." So for Dwyer, the words most crucial to understand when undergoing a psychedelic experience with LSD were "use only with love." Throughout most of his activist life, Dwyer demonstrated a profound belief in the politically radical potential of psychedelics and was committed to what he regarded as their subversive possibilities.

However, after 1972, Dwyer's main phase of contributions and *Anarchy*'s Acid Issue, the subject seldom came up again in anarchist magazines for the remainder of the 1970s, a reflection of how shallowly Dwyer had actually managed to penetrate the broader anarchist left with his brand of psychedelic philosophy in the early 1970s. In August 1972, the anarchist Terry Phillips pointed out in *Freedom* that Dwyer was facing possible imprisonment for possessing LSD and that "whilst many of us do not share his views on the desirability of drug use we defend his right to live as he chooses without being persecuted by the State."[56] At the end of 1972, *Freedom*'s editors announced an upcoming redesign and change of printers, but they assured readers that they were certainly not "going psychedelic."[57]

After his arrest, Dwyer addressed a British jury in 1973. He spoke passionately about his questioning in his early life of the "justice of a society based on Christian principles" and his discovery of LSD through which he "began to learn that tenderness and kindness to others was the prerequisite to any useful social action."[58] His conception of LSD as a "love machine" might be viewed as little more than a kind of basic utopian naivete, but he was convinced that the society in which he lived was characterized by warring factions and a moralism that inhibited an appreciation of the "splendour and beauty" of oneself and others, and LSD could be one potential "antidote" to the "cruelty and insensitivity" that pervaded modern society's pursuit of growth and profit. "I believe," Dwyer told the jury, "LSD is the most revolutionary weapon in the world. A weapon of peace and love. Millions of people all over the world are not merely realising the potential of LSD but are using it to assist themselves in founding a new civilization, a civilization which will eliminate the fearful loneliness of the bedsitting room and the emotional gas chamber nature of the family."[59] He envisioned a network of free, cooperative communes that would offer an alternative to the nuclear family. Therefore, while naivete is indeed one way to approach these ideas, a staunch conviction that psychedelics could be powerful tools for social change, and a desire to at least *try* to imagine other possibilities of arranging society is another, perhaps more interesting, interpretation.

At the 1974 Windsor Free Festival, which he had helped organize, Dwyer was arrested and charged with assault, criminal damage, and breach of the peace.[60] Several hundred police officers had moved to clear the gathering, which did not have permission from the crown estate that owned the land to hold the festival. Dwyer received a high court order banning him from organizing similar events at Windsor in the future.[61] He nevertheless attempted to stage the festival the next year and was again sent to prison.[62] He attempted yet another Windsor festival in 1978 and even managed to evade a police arrest warrant for two weeks by disguising himself as a priest. In the end, he spent a month in jail, apologized to a judge for his actions, and told the press that he would return to Windsor to look for a home the next year.[63] In fact, Dwyer moved back to southern Ireland, where he remained for the rest of his life. In the early 1980s, he was involved in a campaign to legalize cannabis—becoming known locally as the "High Priest of Pot"— and even stood unsuccessfully as a candidate in local elections, forming his own "Justice Party."[64] In the early 1990s, Dwyer was involved in a cycling accident from which he never fully recovered, and he died in 2001.[65]

The kind of ideas that Dwyer advocated did not disappear altogether from anarchist print networks. In November 1975, for instance, a contributor to Freedom, Dave Cuncliffe, offered a defense of countercultural values, arguing that ten years earlier, working-class youth had been largely excluded from the counterculture, but that now "alternative ideas have intruded into working-class consciousness," predicting future "anarchic change" in towns would come from "lumpen youth," including "the dropout, communard, acidhead, poet, freak."[66] The real revolution, thought Cuncliffe, would center on the "urban counter-culture newly removed to rural homestead and farm," a move that had been necessitated in large part by "ecological vandalism and scientific bankruptcy."

CONCLUSION

As the journalist and underground researcher David Nickles has observed, the 1960s are often portrayed as the period where psychedelics "got out of hand," their "escape from the lab" being retrospectively assessed as the death knell for their promising potential in medical, therapeutic, and psychiatric contexts.[67] Yet this narrative risks an overlooking of those advocates of the psychedelic experience who continued to recognize the healing potential of these drugs in a much broader sense than individual medicine (e.g., in the transformation of a society perceived to be sick, or the restoration of a degraded natural environment).[68] The "hippie" notion that the liberation of consciousness from capitalism was both desirable and necessary, channeled by activists like Dwyer into the radical left and anarchist movements, is again being taken seriously, and this chapter has examined how psychedelics and anarchism have previously intertwined. These precedents are important, and a focus on them might go some way toward counteracting the distortion of the radical history of psychedelic drugs via a disproportionate focus on the "stoned indolent hippies" of the counterculture and instances of countercultural replication of capitalist logic and structures (which were necessary for its survival).[69]

Key actors in the 1960s, 1970s, and beyond sought to employ psychedelics in their theoretical and practical efforts to form alternative societies to the one that they perceived to be characterized by the specter of nuclear war, bourgeois Christian values, the ascendency of capital, and a ceaseless fixation on economic growth; they represented and championed optimism for the *possibility* of radical change.[70]

NOTES

I would like to thank Andy Roberts for his thoughts, and Chris Elcock and Adrian Bingham for their insightful and extremely helpful comments on previous versions of this chapter.

1.	Dave Lee, "Life at No. 4 Havelock Square," Our Broomhall, March 9, 2021, https://www
.ourbroomhall.org.uk/content/latest-contributions/life-4-havelock-square-memories
-anarchist-commune.

2. Lee, "Life at No. 4."

3. Lee, "Life at No. 4."

4. There is little space here to explore the terms "counterculture" and "hippie" and their defects. For this, see Peter Braunstein and Michael Doyle, eds., *Imagine Nation: The American Counterculture of the 1960s & '70s* (London: Routledge, 2002), 7–10.

5. This point is made effectively in David Farber, "Intoxicated State/Illegal Nation," in *Imagine Nation*, ed. Peter Braunstein and Michael Doyle, 15–37 (London: Routledge, 2001), 15–37. For an example of arch-cynicism, see Gerald DeGroot, *The Sixties Unplugged* (London: Pan, 2013). For a more ambivalent approach, see Thomas Frank, *The Conquest of Cool* (Chicago: University of Chicago Press, 1997).

6. See Mark Fisher, *K-punk: The Collected and Unpublished Writings of Mark Fisher (2004–2016)*, ed. Darren Ambrose (London: Repeater, 2018); Mark Fisher, *Capitalist Realism: Is There No Alternative?* (Ropley: O Books, 2009).

7. Emma Stamm, "Turn On, Tune In, Rise Up," *Commune*, September 7, 2019, https:// communemag.com/turn-on-tune-in-rise-up/. On the psychedelic right, see Brian Pace, "Lucy in the Sky with Nazis: Psychedelics and the Right Wing," *Psymposia*, February 3, 2021, https://psymposia.com/magazine/lucy-in-the-sky-with-nazis-psychedelics-and-the -right-wing.

8. See, for instance, Jeremy Gilbert, "Why the Time Has Come for 'Acid Corbynism,'" *New Statesman*, October 24, 2017, https://www.newstatesman.com/politics/uk-politics/2017/10 /why-time-has-come-acid-corbynism.

9. On the psychedelic right, see Brian Pace, "Lucy in the Sky with Nazis: Psychedelics and the Right Wing," *Psymposia*, February 3, 2021, https://psymposia.com/magazine/lucy-in-the -sky-with-nazis-psychedelics-and-the-right-wing.

10. Marcus Collins and Willie Thompson, "The Revolutionary Left," in *The Permissive Society and Its Enemies*, ed. Marcus Collins (London: Rivers Oram, 2007), 155–169.

11. Tony Boraman, *Rabble Rousers and Merry Pranksters: A History of Anarchism in Aotearoa/New Zealand from the Mid-1950s to the Early 1980s* (Christchurch, New Zealand: Katipo Books and Irrecuperable Books, 2008), 18–19.

12. Boraman, *Rabble Rousers*, 23.

13. *Anarchy* 1:3 (Series 2, April 1971), 9–10.

14. Boraman, *Rabble Rousers*, 23.

15. Boraman, *Rabble Rousers*, 19.

16. Bill Dwyer, *Anarchy Now!* (Sydney: Federation of Australian Anarchists, 1968), 2.

17. Boraman, *Rabble Rousers*, 19–20.

18. For more information on free festivals, see Andy Roberts, *Albion Dreaming: A Popular History of LSD in Britain* (London: Marshall Cavendish, 2008), 184–209.

19. For postwar British anarchism, see David Goodway, *Anarchist Seeds beneath the Snow: Left-Libertarian Thought and British Writers from William Morris to Colin Ward* (Liverpool, UK: Liverpool University Press, 2006); Carissa Honeywell, *A British Anarchist Tradition: Herbert Read, Alex Comfort and Colin Ward* (New York: Continuum, 2011).

20. Ido Hartogsohn, *American Trip: Set, Setting, and the Psychedelic Experience in the Twentieth Century* (Cambridge, MA: MIT Press, 2020), 246–250.

21. *Anarchy* 68, 6:10 (October 10, 1966), 319.

22. In the US context, this was being mirrored by the Diggers in the Bay area.

23. Farber, "Intoxicated State," 15.

24. *Anarchy* 68, 6:10 (October 10, 1966), 319–320.

25. Alwyn W. Turner, *Crisis? What Crisis? Britain in the 1970s* (London: Aurum Press, 2008).

26. *Freedom* 31:37 (November 28, 1970), 4; *Anarchy* 1:3 (Series 2, April 1971), inside front cover.

27. *Anarchy* 1:3 (Series 2, April 1971), inside front cover.

28. Incidentally, in November 1970, Dr. Ivor Browne, then a professor of psychiatry at Dublin University and the chief advisor to the city's psychiatric services, told a public meeting that he had consumed LSD himself three times and it had a "profound" influence on his life, saying: "[F]or instance, I do not think I could ever be seriously interested in making money again." The next day, the chairman of the Dublin Mental Health Board called for his immediate dismissal. *Anarchy* 1:3 (Series 2, April 1971), inside front cover.

29. Original poster on newsprint, published by the East London Anarchist Group and printed by Richard Pugh.

30. *Freedom* 32:17 (May 29, 1971), 7.

31. *Freedom* 32:17 (May 29, 1971), 7.

32. *Anarchy* 1:3 (Series 2, April 1971).

33. *Oz* 27 (London: Oz Publications Ink. Ltd., April 1970).

34. *Anarchy* 1:3, 5–12.

35. *Anarchy* 1:3, 5–12.

36. *Anarchy* 1:3, 3.

37. *Anarchy* 1:3, 13–20.

38. *Anarchy* 1:3, 3.

39. The commune later split due to infighting. See "Anarchist Squatters Split 1970," RTÉ Archives, https://www.rte.ie/archives/2015/0505/698792-the-island-commune, accessed September 15, 2021.

40. See David Farber, "Building the Counterculture, Creating Right Livelihoods: The Counterculture at Work," *The Sixties* 6, no. 1 (2013): 1–24; David Farber, "Self-Invention in the

Realm of Production: Craft, Beauty, and Community in the American Counterculture, 1964–1978," *Pacific Historical Review* 85:3 (2016), 408–442.

41. Lee, "Life at No. 4"; Murray Bookchin, *Post-Scarcity Anarchism* (San Francisco: Ramparts, 1971).

42. *Anarchy* 78, 7:8 (August 1967), 225–260.

43. Sheila Rowbotham, *Promise of a Dream: A Memoir of the Sixties* (London: Allen Lane, 2000), 124–25.

44. *Oz* 6 (London: Oz Publications Ink., August 1967), 23.

45. Hartogsohn, *American Trip*, 183; Herbert Marcuse, *An Essay on Liberation* (London: Allen Lane, 1960).

46. Much of this philosophy of "play" was consolidated in Richard Neville, *Play Power* (London: Paladin, 1970).

47. On this theme, see David Buckingham, "Children of the Revolution? The Counter-culture, the Idea of Childhood and the Case of Schoolkids Oz," *Strenæ* 13 (2018), http://journals.openedition.org/strenae/1808, accessed February 15, 2021.

48. *The Listener* (August 20, 1970), 245.

49. Sarah Shortall, "Psychedelic Drugs and the Problem of Experience," *Past & Present* 222, Supplement 9 (2014), 187–206.

50. Chris Faiers, *Eel Pie Dharma* (2009), http://www.eelpie.org/epd.htm, accessed March 3, 2021.

51. *Freedom* 31:34 (October 31, 1970), 3.

52. *Freedom* 33:3 (January 15, 1972), 4.

53. *Freedom* 33:3 (January 15, 1972), 4.

54. *Freedom* 33:3 (January 15, 1972), 4.

55. *Freedom* 33:3 (January 15, 1972), 4.

56. *Freedom* 33:33 (August 12, 1972), 1.

57. *Freedom* 33:52 (December 23, 1972), 1.

58. "Bill Dwyer's Defence Notes," Anarchism in Australia, http://takver.com/history/aia/aia00034.htmb, February 2, 1998.

59. Ibid.

60. "Psilocybin Festival," UK Rock Festivals, http://www.ukrockfestivals.com/Psilocybin-Festival.html, accessed March 22, 2021; *Belfast Telegraph* (August 29, 1974), 5.

61. *Daily Mirror* (August 29, 1974), 11.

62. *Newcastle Journal* (May 30, 1975), 5.

63. *Reading Evening Post* (September 29, 1978), 3.

64. *Belfast Telegraph* (August 15, 1980), 5.

65. For a full obituary and collected memories of Dwyer, see "Bill 'Ubi' Dwyer," UK Rock Festivals, http://www.ukrockfestivals.com/UBI-DWYER.html, accessed April 10, 2021.

66. *Freedom* 36:46–47 (November 22, 1975), 3.

67. David Nickles, "The Dire Need for Systemic Critique within Psychedelic Communities," *Chacruna* (September 17, 2018), https://chacruna.net/dire-need-systemic-critique-within -psychedelics-communities, accessed February 7, 2021. Nickles's work has significantly shaped my thinking around the intersection between psychedelics and radical politics. There are many examples of this line of thinking. See, for instance, Ronald Sandison, "LSD Therapy: A Retrospective," in *Psychedelia Britannica: Hallucinogenic Drugs in Britain*, ed. Antonio Melechi (London: Turnaround, 1997), 74.

68. These points are powerfully argued in Nickles, "The Dire Need for Systemic Critique within Psychedelic Communities." For an exploration of the way psychedelic activists set out to transform society in a very practical way that benefited the community, see Morgan Shipley, "This Season's People: Stephen Gaskin, Psychedelic Religion, and a Community of Social Justice," *Journal for the Study of Radicalism* 9:2 (2015), 41–92.

69. For a more detailed critique, see Farber, "Self-Invention."

70. Similar sentiments are expressed in Beatriz C. Labate and Clancy Cavnar, *Psychedelic Justice* (Santa Fe, NM: Synergetic Press, 2021).

BIBLIOGRAPHY

Primary Sources

"Anarchist Squatters Split 1970." RTÉ Archives. Accessed on September 15, 2021. https://www .rte.ie/archives/2015/0505/698792-the-island-commune.

Anarchy 1:3 (Series 2, April 1971), inside front cover.

Anarchy 1:3 (Series 2, April 1971), inside front cover.

Anarchy 78, 7:8 (August 1967), 225–260.

Belfast Telegraph (August 15, 1980), 5.

Belfast Telegraph (August 29, 1974), 5.

"Bill 'Ubi' Dwyer'." UK Rock Festivals. Accessed on April 10, 2021. http://www.ukrockfestivals .com/UBI-DWYER.html.

"Bill Dwyer's Defence Notes." Anarchism in Australia, http://takver.com/history/aia/aia00034 .htm.

Daily Mirror (August 29, 1974), 11.

Faiers, Chris. "Eel Pie Dharma (2009)." Accessed on March 3 2021. http://www.eelpie.org/epd .htm

Freedom 31:34 (October 31, 1970), 3.

Freedom 31:37 (November 28, 1970),

Freedom 32:17 (May 29, 1971), 7.

Freedom 33:3 (January 15, 1972), 4.

Freedom 33:33 (August 12, 1972), 1.

Freedom 33:52 (December 23, 1972), 1.

Freedom 36:46–47 (November 22, 1975), 3.

Newcastle Journal (May 30, 1975), 5.

Oz 27 (London: Oz Publications Ink. Ltd., April 1970).

Oz 6 (London: Oz Publications Ink. Ltd., August 1967), 23.

"Psilocybin Festival." UK Rock Festivals. Accessed on March 22 2021. http://www.ukrockfestivals.com/Psilocybin-Festival.html

Reading Evening Post (September 29, 1978), 3.

The Listener (August 20, 1970), 245.

Secondary Sources

Bookchin, Murray. *Post-scarcity Anarchism*. San Francisco, CA: Ramparts Press, 1971.

Boraman, Tony. *Rabble Rousers and Merry Pranksters: A History of Anarchism in Aotearoa/New Zealand from the Mid-1950s to the Early 1980s*. Christchurch, New Zealand: Katipo Books and Irrecuperable Books, 2008.

Braunstein, Peter, and Michael Doyle, eds. *Imagine Nation: The American Counterculture of the 1960s and '70s*. London: Routledge, 2001.

Buckingham, David. "Children of the Revolution? The Counter-culture, the Idea of Childhood and the Case of Schoolkids Oz." *Strenæ. Recherches sur les livres et objets culturels de l'enfance* 13 (2018). Accessed on February 15, 2021. http://journals.openedition.org/strenae/1808.

Collins, Marcus, and Willie Thompson. "The Revolutionary Left and the Permissive Society." In *The Permissive Society and Its Enemies: Sixties British Culture*, edited by Marcus Collins, 158–169. London: Rivers Oram, 2007.

"Dear Psychedelic Researchers." *Psymposia*, updated April 4, 2020. Accessed March 9, 2021. https://www.psymposia.com/magazine/dear-psychedelic-researchers.

DeGroot, Gerard J. *The Sixties Unplugged: A Kaleidoscopic History of a Disorderly Decade*. Cambridge, MA: Harvard University Press, 2009.

Dwyer, Bill. *Anarchy Now!* Sydney: Federation of Australian Anarchists, 1968.

Farber, David. "Building the Counterculture, Creating Right Livelihoods: The Counterculture at Work." *The Sixties* 6, no.1 (2013): 1–24.

Farber, David. "Intoxicated State/Illegal Nation: Drugs in the Sixties Counterculture of the 1960s and 70s." In *Imagine Nation: The American Counterculture of the 1960s and '70s*, edited by Peter Braunstein and Michael Doyle, 15–37. London: Routledge, 2001.

Farber, David. "Self-invention in the Realm of Production: Craft, Beauty, and Community in the American Counterculture, 1964–1978." *Pacific Historical Review* 85, no. 3 (2016): 408–442.

Fisher, Mark. *Capitalist Realism: Is There No Alternative?* Ropley: O Books, 2009.

Fisher, Mark. *K-Punk: the collected and unpublished writings of Mark Fisher (2004–2016)*. London: Repeater, 2018.

Gilbert, Jeremy. "Why the Time Has Come for 'Acid Corbynism.'" *New Statesman*, October 24, 2017. Accessed on March 9, 2021. https://www.newstatesman.com/politics/uk-politics/2017/10/why-time-has-come-acid-corbynism.

Goodway, David. *Anarchist Seeds beneath the Snow: Left-Libertarian Thought and British Writers from William Morris to Colin Ward*. Liverpool, UK: Liverpool University Press, 2006.

Honeywell, Carissa. *A British Anarchist Tradition: Herbert Read, Alex Comfort and Colin Ward*. New York: Continuum, 2011.

Labate, Beatriz C., and Clancy Cavnar, *Psychedelic Justice*. Santa Fe, NM: Synergetic Press, 2021.

Lee, Dave. "Life at No 4 Havelock Square." Our Broomhall. Accessed March 9, 2021. https://www.ourbroomhall.org.uk/content/latest-contributions/life-4-havelock-square-memories-anarchist-commune.

Marcuse, Herbert. *An Essay on Liberation*. Boston: Beacon Press, 1971.

Neville, Richard. *Play Power: Exploring the International Underground*. London: Paladin, 1970.

Nickles, David. "The Dire Need for Systemic Critique within Psychedelic Communities." *Chacruna*, September 17, 2018. Accessed on February 7, 2021. https://chacruna.net/dire-need-systemic-critique-within-psychedelics-communities.

Roberts, Andy. *Albion Dreaming: A Popular History of LSD in Britain*. London: Marshall Cavendish, 2008.

Rowbotham, Sheila. *Promise of a Dream: A Memoir of the Sixties*. London: Allen Lane, 2000.

Sandison, Ronald. "LSD Therapy: A Retrospective." In *Psychedelia Britannica: Hallucinogenic Drugs in Britain*, edited by Antonio Melechi, 74. London: Turnaround, 1997.

Shortall, Sarah. "Psychedelic Drugs and the Problem of Experience." *Past & Present* 222, Supplement 9 (2014): 187–206.

Stamm, Emma. "Turn On, Tune In, Rise Up." *Commune*, September 7, 2019. Accessed on March 9, 2021. https://communemag.com/turn-on-tune-in-rise-up/.

Turner, Alwyn W. *Crisis? What Crisis? Britain in the 1970s*. London: Aurum Press, 2008.

III PSYCHEDELICS AS CULTURAL PHENOMENA

The final part of this volume urges readers to consider some of the ways that psychedelics have been used to produce generative experiences—those that inspire creative projects, innovative ways of thinking, designing, or being, and that provide provocative moments and insights that disrupt ordinary thinking. At times flirting with the history of psychiatry, reminiscent of discussions related to the perennial debate about the relationship between madness and genius, or madness and creativity, the chapters here provide examples of psychedelics and psychedelic experiences that inspired changes in the way we think, play, and create.

While these authors do not shy away from themes explored in the first two parts, on experience and networks of knowledge, they concentrate on exploring how psychedelics were inserted and reinserted into cultural artifacts: music, art, literature, fashion, politics, activism, and even business. Blending medical and cultural history, these chapters offer an optimistic framing of the legacy of psychedelics as both inspirational and aspirational, as they represent morsels of innovation and creativity better conducive to human flourishing than mere treatments for unwanted pathological conditions. The contexts are not all utopian fantasies; psychedelics still (and perhaps inevitably) conjure concerns about medical and legal risks. However, the authors here suggest that people continued to seek out psychedelic opportunities in diverse settings despite the articulated concerns and prohibitions. Indeed, as discussed in part I, psychedelics continue to have a double-edged cultural effect of conferring layers of cultural capital, a coolness factor that gives an artist her edge; and as ever, they can also introduce extrapsychological dangers as legal restrictions put bounties on those associated with psychedelic activities, especially those assumed to be stimulating countercultural or radical political perspectives.

The chapters in this part perhaps urge us to think the most expansively about psychedelics. While these psychoactive substances are implicated in a history of pharmaceuticals, they are also a deep part of our most recent cultural histories. Psychedelics as recreational drugs at times invite laughter, luxuriation, and levity (even dancing), and the authors here remind us of this playful side of these substances without detaching them entirely from the medicolegal and political contexts that mediated these experiences.

Readers are reminded that psychedelics are part of these profoundly subjective traditions of mind alteration, not exclusively for producing meaningful change through reorienting our relationship with spirituality, philosophy, heteronormativity, or explorations of sanity, but also a benign and universal search for fun. Without trivializing a desire for mind alteration as simplistic escape, these authors provide examples of intellectual, artistic, and activist pursuits that see psychedelics blend with other searching human qualities, whether through travel, personal transformation, or technological innovation. These more productive pursuits combat an image of recreational drug use that contributes to the adage of an aloof "dropping out" of society. Moving beyond those well-worn tropes, the authors reveal that there is a competing global history of engagement and enhancement with psychedelics that may just suggest that these individualized experiences have something to tell us about modern history and our place in it.

14 "VIDEO IS AS POWERFUL AS LSD": ELECTRONICS AND PSYCHEDELICS AS TECHNOLOGIES OF CONSCIOUSNESS

Peter Sachs Collopy

In the middle of the twentieth century, the invention and availability of new psychedelic drugs, and the growing cultural discourse around them, coincided with those of television, videotape, and computing. The technologies of psychedelics and electronics grew up together, and those using or thinking about one often implicated the other. When Sony and other Japanese manufacturers developed new portable videotape recorders in the late 1960s, for example, new communities of artists and tinkerers emerged around them, first in the US and Canada and then in Europe, Asia, North Africa, and Latin America. For the first time, declared these enthusiasts, many people could make their own television, breaking the broadcast oligopoly.

In describing the psychological and sociological implications of this new technology, many compared it to psychedelic drugs. "To write about . . . tape is explaining a trip to someone who's never dropped acid," wrote spiritual seeker Marco Vassi in the first issue of the hip, US-based video magazine *Radical Software*.[1] In the next issue, when philosopher and sociologist Victor Gioscia searched for methods of adapting to social change by helping people "accelerate the formation of generalization," he asked, "Does acid do it? Will videotape?"[2] Pages later, pioneering video artist Nam June Paik wondered, "Can we transplant this strange 'ontology' of drug experience to [a] 'safer' and more 'authentic' art medium?"[3] "Video is as powerful as LSD," answered a cartoon in the next issue by poet Edwin Varney.[4]

Materially, the two technologies were very different—one by now a blot of liquid on a paper tab, the other a complex optical and electronic

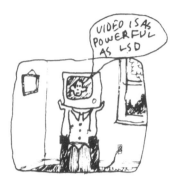

Figure 14.1
Edwin Varney, "Video Is as Powerful as LSD," 1971.

system—but, as Paik wrote, experimental videographers perceived a common underlying ontology. How did videotape and psychedelic drugs both come to be, to borrow a category of analysis from historian Fred Turner, "technologies of consciousness"?[5] In this chapter, I follow the common threads that bind the two technologies together. First, popular writers, including Aldous Huxley, Pierre Teilhard de Chardin, and Marshall McLuhan, depicted both psychedelics and electronic media as means to achieve the evolution of collective consciousness, and they found audiences among users of each. Meanwhile, in the 1950s, engineer Myron Stolaroff brought tape recording and psychedelic research together institutionally in a series of experiments on enhancing creativity, which he began at the magnetic tape firm Ampex. In the 1960s, the two technologies came together again in a variety of countercultural settings, including in the design of video synthesizers intended to be both aesthetically and functionally psychedelic.

MIND

Many users of both portable video and psychedelic drugs interpreted them in an intellectual framework of evolutionary panpsychism, in which they appeared as tools for connecting humanity into a single mind and directing human evolution toward collective consciousness. This worldview had a fundamentally transnational intellectual history. In his 1907 *Creative Evolution*,

French philosopher Henri Bergson argued that life, pushed by an inherent vitality, was evolving into a unity. The book had tremendous international influence, including among the next generations of writers about media and psychedelics. In his 1954 *Doors of Perception*, for example, English novelist and California resident Aldous Huxley speculated—citing Bergson—that "Mind at Large" was a shared phenomenon, but humans had evolved a limited, personal experience of it to focus on survival. Mescaline, added Huxley, might temporarily open the "reducing valve" and let universal consciousness flood in.[6]

Experimental videographers encountered similar ideas in the popular writings of French Jesuit paleontologist Pierre Teilhard de Chardin and Canadian media theorist Marshall McLuhan, each of whom also drew on Bergson. A devout but heterodox Catholic, Teilhard wrote his most influential work, *The Phenomenon of Man*, in religious exile in China, where he conducted paleontological fieldwork. In the book, published soon after he died in 1955, Teilhard argued that the development of human consciousness represented "a new era of evolution, the era of noogenesis," in which life could reflect on its own existence; that mind could be regarded as a layer of the Earth, the "noosphere"; and that, "thanks to the prodigious biological event represented by the discovery of electro-magnetic waves," humanity is rapidly evolving into "a harmonized collectivity of consciousness." Teilhard spent the last three years of his life in the US, where his work became increasingly influential after his death.[7]

In his 1964 *Understanding Media*, McLuhan cited this passage from Teilhard and further emphasized the role of electronic communications. "Our specialist and fragmented civilization of center-margin structure," he wrote, "is suddenly experiencing an instantaneous reassembling of all its mechanized bits into an organic whole. This is the new world of the global village." McLuhan thus formulated a new version of Bergson's organic community and Teilhard's noosphere, which substituted the sociological for the occult or biological. Computer-mediated communication, wrote McLuhan, might allow us "to by-pass languages in favor of a general cosmic consciousness which might be very like the collective unconscious dreamt of by Bergson."[8]

Upon reading *Understanding Media* "as a student during the seventies," writes Lance Strate, "it seemed only natural to ask if McLuhan himself was *on drugs*. McLuhan was an icon of the sixties, after all, a time when *electric* and *psychedelic* were used almost interchangeably."[9] McLuhan was indeed connected to psychedelic networks: In 1966, he met Timothy Leary for lunch at New York's Plaza Hotel and advised him on marketing the psychedelic experience, perhaps even coining Leary's phrase "turn on, tune in, drop out."[10] At Leary's Millbrook estate, artist Rudi Stern recalled, "I'd come down and Marshall McLuhan would be sitting at the table. We'd have some eggs together."[11] Leary told a journalist that he never introduced McLuhan to LSD, though, because McLuhan was already high on his own verbal expression; "he talks," said Leary, "in circles, and spirals, and flower forms and mandala forms."[12] Although McLuhan was curious about psychedelic experiences, his interest seems to have been detached and metaphorical rather than experiential.

McLuhan saw drugs and media—particularly television—as profoundly similar phenomena. "Look at the metaphor for getting high: turning on," he told *Playboy* in 1969. "One turns on his consciousness through drugs just as he opens up all his senses to a total depth involvement by turning on the TV dial." McLuhan also argued that being surrounded by electronic media motivated drug use, not necessarily as an escape from an overstimulating environment, but as an extension of the same experience. "Drug taking is stimulated by today's pervasive environment of instant information," he continued, "with its feedback mechanism of the inner trip. The inner trip is not the sole prerogative of the LSD traveler; it's the universal experience of TV watchers."[13]

For McLuhan, electronics and drugs were also similar because each interacted so directly with the brain. When Leary's archivist, Michael Horowitz, asked McLuhan to contribute to a Festschrift—never completed—in 1974, McLuhan wrote an abstract of an essay. "Electric technology, by virtue of its immediate relation to our nervous system," he suggested, "is itself a sort of inner trip, with drugs playing the role of sub-plot or alternate mode."[14] Electronic media were "extensions of man," externalizations of the human mind, but they were even more akin to ourselves than other media because they were made of electricity—literally the same stuff as our consciousness.

"The impulse to use hallucinogens is a kind of empathy with the electric environment," McLuhan wrote elsewhere, "but it is also a way of repudiating the old mechanical world." This sympathy between the electric and the psychedelic—both forms of postmechanical, organic, "tribal" engagement—led McLuhan to see links between social worlds that otherwise seemed at odds. "The computer," he wrote, "is the LSD of the business world, transforming its outlooks and objectives."[15] Similarly, but perhaps more profoundly, McLuhan's anthropologist collaborator Edmund Carpenter wrote that "TV is the psychic leap of our time. It's a trip far more potent than LSD. It turns thoughts inward, revealing new, unsuspected realities."[16]

Los Angeles art critic Gene Youngblood drew a similar connection in his 1970 book *Expanded Cinema*—the title of which, he wrote, "actually mean[s] expanded consciousness." Like McLuhan, Youngblood coined his own terminology for a gloss on Teilhard: "The videosphere," he wrote, "is the noosphere transformed into a perceivable state." Artists were using film and video to produce new ecological awareness of both a unified humanity and the natural world. Psychedelic drugs, with their origins in nature, were also contributing to this reconfiguration of awareness. "Because of mankind's inevitable symbiosis with the mind-manifesting hallucinogens of the ecology on the one hand," explained Youngblood, "and his organic partnership with machines on the other, an increasing number of the inhabitants of this planet live virtually in another world."[17]

New York philosopher and sociologist Victor Gioscia, whom I quoted earlier, argued more specifically that psychedelic drugs were tools for coping with new experiences of time brought about by the electronic age. In around 1965, he began two separate research programs, one on therapeutic uses of videotape and another on cultures of LSD use.[18] (Psychiatrist Harry Wilmer also combined these two agendas in his work at the Langley Porter Neuropsychiatric Institute in San Francisco.)[19] Two years later, as part of the Jewish Family Services' Village Project, "a sort of anti-clinic in the East Village," he "tried to use video playback to help people on dope see how they related to each other while badly stoned" and interviewed patients about the role of drugs in the counterculture. "Rap session participants at the Village Project were uniformly agreed," he found, "that 'dope' is central but not causal." The "drop-out phenomenon," they suggested, was instead primarily a product of "automation" and "cybernation," forms of electrification that made work obsolete (at least for some) and "created an era of global communication." Citing McLuhan, Gioscia argued that this new "electric environment" demanded cultural accommodation, and that "retribalization," communes, and the counterculture more generally were such human responses.[20]

"We now invent culture faster than we can transmit it," wrote Gioscia. "The psychedelic generation . . . have been forced to endure more rapid shifts in the rates of their experience than any before them."[21] LSD's capacity to alter one's experience of time, then, was central to its increasing popularity. "The world," Gioscia argued, "had better invent a way of comprehending itself that changes as fast as experience does. And that, I would argue, is exactly what psychedelics are—a psychochemical technology" that made it possible "to pay full emotional attention to events which in 'real' clock time would have sped by too rapidly for your empathy to catch hold."[22] Elsewhere, Gioscia wrote—again citing McLuhan—that "heads are trying to do psychologically what computers have done sociologically, that is, exponentially expand the ability to process vast quantities of experience very rapidly."[23] Both were technological means of adapting to accelerating social change.

Under the influence of writers like Huxley, Teilhard, and McLuhan, in the middle of the twentieth century many Americans believed that they had found tools that could deliver not only altered states of consciousness and greater insight into the self, but the ability to dissolve it, connect with others, and participate in a greater unity. For experimental videographers, video seemed not only a new medium, but one that would bring about a new kind of awareness, a new way of being human. "Our bodies cannot keep up with what evolution via our minds would have us do," wrote videographer Michael Shamberg. "So we are evolving through our technology."[24] Bergson's disciples became intellectual touchstones for the counterculture of the 1960s and 1970s, in part because they described a world in which the hippies' fascination with technologies of consciousness constituted a contribution to creative evolution.

CREATIVITY

Videotape and psychedelics also shared a history materially. The development of audiotape and recording followed the geography of the American military occupations that followed World War II. At the end of the war, US Army Signal Corpsman John Mullin shipped two German Magnetophon audiotape recorders—the first to record with high fidelity, and thus sound live—back to the US. When he demonstrated them in San Francisco in 1946, among those in the audience were engineers from the Ampex Corporation, based in what would become Silicon Valley, who had been building motors for the Navy but were looking for new markets. At Ampex, two engineers, Myron Stolaroff and Harold Lindsay, began designing their own high-fidelity tape recorder. The technology reshaped radio, enabling episodes to be prerecorded and reducing the necessity for live broadcast.[25]

Ampex then applied tape recording to other media. Stolaroff began developing "instrumentation recorders" for experimental plane and missile testing, and in 1951, he was among those to develop a videotape recorder, which similarly reshaped television in 1956, when Ampex released it as the VR-1000. However, that recorder weighed 1,465 pounds and cost $45,000 in 1956. The American companies Ampex and RCA introduced gradually smaller models and added color, electronic editing, and other technical improvements. But it was Japanese engineers at Sony who first encountered tape recorders during the US occupation who were most successful at miniaturizing them, eventually producing a 66-pound videotape recorder, the TCV-2010, in 1965, and an 11-pound battery-powered recorder, the VideoRover DV-2400, in 1967.[26]

Meanwhile, in the 1950s Stolaroff began participating in the Sequoia Seminar, a religious movement founded by Stanford University electrical engineer and lawyer Harry Rathbun and his wife Emilia, which incorporated the study of the Christian gospels, Jungian psychology, and the esotericism of British mystic Gerald Heard. "Harry convinced me of the enormity of human potential," wrote Stolaroff, "of the necessity to wake up and take charge of our evolution."[27]

It was from Heard, who had moved to Los Angeles in 1937 with his friend Aldous Huxley, that Rathbun borrowed his evolutionary rhetoric. The "limen," or boundary of individual consciousness, Heard believed, could be intentionally traversed using prayer and meditation, facilitating "the complete evolution of consciousness through unity." Heard drew not only on the Christianity in which he was raised, but on multiple religious traditions to explore this possibility. In Los Angeles, he and Huxley joined the Vedanta Society, a Hindu organization founded at the turn of the century by Swami Vivekananda, who had traveled from India to attend the World's Parliament of Religions in Chicago in 1893. In 1942, Heard founded Trabuco College, a monastery in the Santa Ana Mountains, to practice what he described as "a new syncretism of Vedanta, Buddhism, and some elements of Christianity"; it formed a kernel of California's emerging human potential movement until it dissolved in 1947.[28]

After meeting Heard in 1955, Stolaroff came to respect him as a mystic and was surprised to hear him speak about LSD. "I could not understand," Stolaroff later wrote, "why a person of his gifts who could freely explore the cosmos with his mind would want to take a drug."[29] Heard's answer, in the inaugural issue of *The Psychedelic Review* in 1963, was that LSD could facilitate "a free flow of comprehension beyond the everyday threshold of experience [through] a confronting of one's self, a standing outside one's self, a dissolution of the ego-based apprehensions that cloud the sky of the mind."[30]

Stolaroff was convinced, and at Heard's recommendation he met Al Hubbard, an eccentric promoter of psychedelics who collaborated with Huxley and pioneering psychiatrists Humphry Osmond and John Smythies, and tried methamphetamine and LSD. "I was familiar with the frontiers of many technological fields of knowledge," wrote Stolaroff, "for we were designing special magnetic recording equipment to aid research in most of those fields. . . . Yet after my first LSD experience, I stated with confidence about LSD: 'This is the greatest discovery that man has ever made.'" For Stolaroff, the experience included "profound revelations that God is absolutely real, and that there is only One Person, of which we are all a part."[31]

Inspired, Stolaroff formed a group of engineers and their wives who met every Monday to discuss philosophy and experiment with LSD. Under its influence, he later wrote, "fresh ideas and perspectives flow unhindered, presenting many new possibilities, often of great value. I felt that such heightened perceptions could be valuable in improving business operations." Stolaroff proposed to Ampex's management committee that they incorporate LSD into the company's operations, but he "immediately encountered enormous resistance" based on the concern that the drug would damage the employees' valuable minds. Stolaroff and Hubbard carried out their experiment with Ampex engineers anyway, taking eight to a cabin in the Sierra Nevada Mountains and giving them LSD. "All were impressed," wrote Stolaroff, "with the enormous openings of the mind, the ability to experience new levels of thought and comprehension, the gain in self-knowledge, and in some cases, the ability to solve technical problems. But much to my amazement, the results were totally ignored by management."[32]

In 1961, then, Stolaroff resigned from his job to found the International Foundation for Advanced Study (IFAS) in Menlo Park, a nonprofit that he funded by selling his Ampex stock. The IFAS conducted research in two areas. The first was essentially therapeutic, focused on treating mental illness and personal growth. In a process closely modeled on Hubbard's, over the course of a day a patient was given large doses of both LSD and mescaline, as well as methamphetamine. The result, wrote Stolaroff, electrical engineer Willis Harman, and physician J. N. Sherwood in an article on the efficacy of their treatment, was that a patient "sees that his own self is by no means so separate from other selves and the universe about him as he might have thought," leading them to value themself more and "accept the previously known self as an imperfect reflection." In an appendix, the researchers described this experience more speculatively, quoting Bergson and writing that patients perceived "that behind the apparent multiplicity of things . . . all beings are seen to be united."[33]

The IFAS also researched the effects of psychedelics on the creativity of engineers and other technical workers, including pioneering computing researcher Douglas Engelbart.[34] In a 1966 article, Harman, Stolaroff, and three other researchers placed this research in the context of humanistic psychologist Carl Rogers's theories of creativity. According to Rogers, creativity required low defensiveness, flexibility, personal rather than standardized judgment, and playfulness. Stolaroff and his colleagues found that, given an appropriate set and setting, mescaline use strengthened these traits both during sessions and in the weeks that followed them. Subjects reported in particular a lack of anxiety about their work and an ability to rapidly conceive new designs. Many also experienced their work more visually than usual. "I began to see an image of the circuit," reported one subject. "The gates themselves were little silver cones linked together by lines. I watched this circuit flipping through its paces. . . . The psychedelic state is, for me at least, an immensely powerful one for obtaining insight and understanding through visual symbolism." Projects designed during this research ranged from buildings for commercial and private clients to "a linear electron accelerator beam-steering device" and improvements to magnetic tape recorders.[35]

The IFAS was short-lived. In 1966, as public and press concern about the dangers of LSD developed, the US Food and Drug Administration instructed the group to cease their research. The association between LSD and technical creativity lived on through the continuing influence of IFAS researchers and their associates. In 2010, after forty-four years in other fields, psychologist James Fadiman returned to psychedelic research with a study on LSD microdosing, which, partly due to his advocacy, became a popular method for enhancing productivity in Silicon Valley. Beyond the group, Leary and IFAS research subject and *Whole Earth Catalog* editor Stewart Brand each followed McLuhan in associating LSD with computing. "The PC is the new LSD," wrote Leary in his 1994 book *Chaos and Cyberculture*. "Turn on, boot up, jack in."[36]

ART

The association of psychedelic drugs and electronics also influenced the art and performance of the 1960s. In New York, the USCO art troupe used strobe lights, slide projectors, and audiotape along with cannabis, peyote, and LSD to produce experiences of collectivity. In 1966, Brand, Ken Kesey, and the Merry Pranksters brought USCO's techniques to San Francisco for the Trips Festival, which, writes Turner, "represented a coming together of the Beatnik-derived San Francisco psychedelic scene and the multimedia technophilia of art troupes such as USCO." In an environment of LSD, dance, music, and projectors, attendees could watch themselves live on closed-circuit television.[37]

Psychedelic drugs and the discourse surrounding them went on to influence video most strongly in the artistic field of video synthesis, where they had both intellectual and aesthetic effects. While many saw video as a tool for documenting and networking the world, others were more interested in the artificial electronic space inside their monitors. Some of these artists and engineers built video synthesizers—machines that electronically manipulated either a video signal or a cathode ray tube to produce abstract or distorted images. I've previously explored in an article how they modeled these synthesizers on audio synthesizers, conceptualized them as analog computers, and interfaced them with digital minicomputers.[38] Here, I build on that analysis to focus specifically on the psychedelic dimension of video synthesis.

In the late 1960s, self-taught New York television technician Eric Siegel, like many videographers, experimented with visual feedback, pointing a camera at its own monitor to produce kaleidoscopic visual effects. He also built electronic devices to manipulate video signals, inverting light and dark and adding color to monochrome video. Siegel referred to his art as "psychedelevision," and his ambitions were indeed fundamentally psychedelic: he sought, he later told an interviewer, to "actually take a dream you had and make it visible to other people" or induce experiences like those he had while using cannabis and LSD. Even more ambitiously, Siegel told Gene Youngblood, "I see television as a psychic healing medium creating mass cosmic consciousness."[39]

In his 1968 video *Einstine*, Siegel distorted the scientist's face with feedback and pulsating color, reproducing one of his dreams to "transport the mind of the viewer into Einstein's multi-dimensional world." When *Einstine* appeared in one of the first video art exhibitions, *TV as a Creative Medium*, presented at New York's Howard Wise Gallery, it inspired other artists with its new psychedelic video aesthetic. "Something extraordinary happened

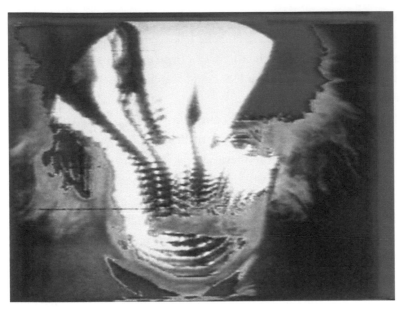

Figure 14.2
Still frame from Eric Siegel, *Einstine,* 1968, video, 5:22, *Surveying the First Decade: Video Art and Alternative Media in the U.S. 1968–1980,* vol. 2 (Chicago: Video Data Bank, 1995), DVD. An excerpt may be viewed at http://vdb.org/titles/einstine.

when we saw that flaming face of Einstein at the end of the corridor," wrote artist Woody Vasulka, "something finally free of film."[40]

In important ways, Siegel's media matched his message. If psychedelic drugs can increase color saturation and intensity beyond that perceived by the sober mind, Siegel's "psychedelevision" did the same for television. While cameras and broadcast television used only a portion of the range of color that television sets and video monitors were capable of displaying, Siegel's devices gave artists full access. In 1970, Siegel moved to Sweden and built the Electronic Video Synthesizer, which incorporated the same control over color but was also one of the first devices to integrate a variety of abstract video effects, including the ability to generate geometric shapes, without using a camera at all. "The images were not only 'free of film,'" writes Carolyn Kane, "but also free of optical media and therefore 'natural' vision altogether. Herein lies [a] rationale to understand how electronic color in video synthesis became magical and otherworldly: it literally was."[41]

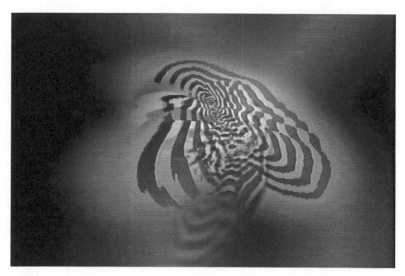

Figure 14.3
Still frame from Kris Paulsen, "In the Beginning, There Was the Electron," *X-TRA* 15, no. 2 (2013): http://x-traonline.org/article/in-the-beginning-there-was-the-electron/.Two performancesof *Illuminated Music*may be viewed at http://ubu.com/film/beckilluminated.html.

Nonetheless, Siegel's inventions did not meet his psychedelic ambitions, and he moved on to other video projects. "The motivation behind the creation of the video synthesizer," Siegel later explained, "was to create mandalas to alter states of consciousness, and I couldn't do that quite yet."[42]

Electrical engineer Stephen Beck was similarly inspired by the possibility of sharing his personal visions of light and color. "For as long as I can remember," he told a curator, "whenever I close my eyes, I see colors, shapes, forms, and swirling movements of textures, which I later learned are called *phosphenes*."[43] In the 1960s, he found that these experiences had a new cultural resonance. "There was a lot of experimentation with consciousness-altering substances such as cannabis, LSD-25, mescalin and shamanic rituals," he recalled. "We'd get together to chant and induce visions and hallucinations." In 1970, Beck became an artist-in-residence at the San Francisco public television station KQED's National Center for Experiments in Television, where he built his own synthesizers and performed with them on live broadcasts.[44]

Among those inspired by Siegel's work was Nam June Paik, perhaps the most prominent and successful early video artist.[45] Paik came to video synthesis in the midst of an itinerant international and multimedia artistic career, and much of his work reflected on the globalizing, multicultural, and media-saturated world that shaped him. Born in Seoul in 1932, Paik lived in Hong Kong and Tokyo as a young man and studied music history and composition. He spent much of his twenties in Germany, studying with composers including Karlheinz Stockhausen and John Cage, and he participated in the Fluxus avant-garde artistic movement. In the 1960s, Paik began modifying television sets with magnets, sometimes in collaboration with Japanese television engineer Shuya Abe. In 1964, he moved to New York. The next year, Paik purchased a Sony TCV-2010 video recorder and became one of the first artists to shoot their own video.[46]

When Paik articulated his own vision of video synthesis in 1970, he also responded directly to psychedelic experiences. "The 'attraction' of drug experience to young people," he wrote, "lies in the peculiar 'ontology' of this unfortunate medium. Generally speaking *art* consists of three different parties: . . . creator, . . . audience, . . . critics. . . . But in the drug experience, all three parties are united into one. . . . Drug is a short cut effort to recover the sense of participation."[47] For Paik, then, the video synthesizer was a psychedelic technology not due to its aesthetics or its capacity for inducing individual or collective altered states of consciousness in the viewer, but rather its capacity for facilitating a holistic creative experience for an artist, which it shared with psychedelic drugs.

Nonetheless, Paik's video synthesis aesthetics also borrowed from Siegel's psychedelic visions. Starting in 1969, Paik and Abe built the Paik-Abe Video Synthesizer, which combined signals from several monochrome cameras into a single color image, adding intense colorization reminiscent of Siegel's imagery. It also incorporated something called the "Wobbulator," a video monitor with additional electromagnets that could distort its image. The system was intentionally unpredictable and difficult to control—a "sloppy machine, like me," said Paik—in order to encourage Paik's vision of participation. When Paik debuted the system in the Boston television broadcast *Video Commune*, accompanying the catalog of the Beatles, he invited passers-by to enter the television studio and operate the synthesizer.[48]

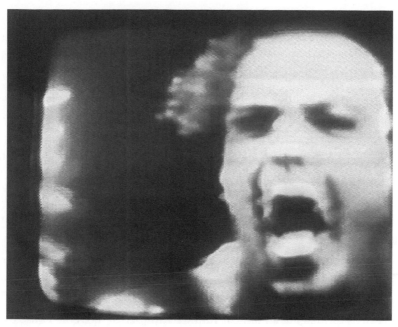

Figure 14.4

Still frame from John G. Hanhardt, *The Worlds of Nam June Paik* (New York: Guggenheim Museum, 2000), 191. An excerpt may be viewed at http://medienkunstnetz.de/works/video-commune/.

TECHNOLOGIES OF CONSCIOUSNESS

In a variety of ways, both for theorists like McLuhan and for artists like Paik, video technology and psychedelic drugs became analogous technologies. What tied together these two objects was that their users understood both as technologies of consciousness. These were not merely technologies that reshaped the thoughts and experiences of those that used them—as any technology does—but technologies that users themselves understood as doing so. "Technology typically is an outering of the inner being that feeds back into the self as it alters the environment," writes Strate, "but that feedback is a secondary, indirect effect, whereas in the case of drugs it is the primary effect; typically, we employ media without any awareness of the effects that they have on ourselves, whereas drugs are used with the conscious purpose of effecting a change on body, and maybe mind."[49] Video too was often used with the conscious purpose of effecting a change on mind.

In addition, the analogy between these technologies is useful for historians of each. The historiography of psychedelics has paid particular attention, most recently and extensively in Ido Hartogsohn's *American Trip*, to the dependence of drugs' psychological effects on set and setting.[50] Video and other media technologies have had similarly varied psychological effects depending on context; elsewhere, for example, I explore how artists and critics drew on the discourse of psychoanalysis to critique video for fostering narcissism, while psychotherapists, and later feminist scholars, drew on the same discourse to argue that video cured it.[51]

These material technologies did not have monolithic effects because they were entangled in complex networks in which the technologies themselves, techniques of their use, and ideas of their users shaped each other and collectively contributed to the experience of using them. "A collaborative model affords several advantages for studying drugs," writes David Lenson. "If consciousness is a *relationship* of subject and object, then it is possible to imagine an almost infinite number of 'possible consciousnesses.'"[52] The same is true of all technologies, but especially technologies of consciousness. It is on interactions within a system of people, ideas, emotions, practices, and things that we must focus in order to understand these technologies. And conversely, the history of consciousness—even the history of ideas about consciousness—is also the history of techniques for manipulating it.

NOTES

1. Marco Vassi, "Zen Tubes," *Radical Software* 1, no. 1 (1970): 18.

2. Vic Gioscia, "Frequency and Form," *Radical Software* 1, no. 2 (1970): 7.

3. Nam June Paik, "Video Synthesizer Plus," *Radical Software* 1, no. 2 (1970): 25.

4. Edwin Varney, "Video Is as Powerful as LSD," *Radical Software* 1, no. 3 (1971): 6.

5. Fred Turner, *From Counterculture to Cyberculture: Stewart Brand, the Whole Earth Network, and the Rise of Digital Utopianism* (Chicago: University of Chicago Press, 2006), 234, 258; Fred Turner, "The Pygmy Gamelan as Technology of Consciousness," in *Paul DeMarinis: Buried in Noise*, ed. Ingrid Beirer, Sabine Himmelsbach, and Carsten Seiffarth (Heidelberg, Germany: Kehrer Verlag, 2010), 23–27; Peter Sachs Collopy, "The Revolution Will Be Videotaped: Making a Technology of Consciousness in the Long 1960s" (PhD diss., University of Pennsylvania, 2015), 41–47.

6. Collopy, "The Revolution Will Be Videotaped," 3–13; Aldous Huxley, *The Doors of Perception* (New York: Harper, 1954), 17–21. On evolutionary psychedelic rhetoric beyond Huxley, see Chris Elcock, "From Acid Revolution to Entheogenic Evolution: Psychedelic Philosophy in the Sixties and Beyond," *Journal of American Culture* 36, no. 4 (2013): 301–303.

7. Susan Kassman Sack, *America's Teilhard: Christ and Hope in the 1960s* (Washington, DC: Catholic University of America Press, 2019), 5–17; Pierre Teilhard de Chardin, *The Phenomenon of Man*, trans. Bernard Wall (1959; New York: Harper Torchbooks, 1965), 4, 182, 240, 251.

8. Marshall McLuhan, *Understanding Media: The Extensions of Man* (1964; Cambridge, MA: MIT Press, 1994), 80, 93, 247.

9. Lance Strate, "Drugs: The Intensions of Humanity," in *Drugs & Media: New Perspectives on Communication, Consumption, and Consciousness*, ed. Robert C. MacDougall (New York: Continuum, 2012), 19. Emphasis in original.

10. Timothy Leary, *Flashbacks: An Autobiography, a Personal and Cultural History of an Era* (Los Angeles: Jeremy P. Tarcher, 1990), 251–253; Stephen Siff, *Acid Hype: American News Media and the Psychedelic Experience* (Urbana: University of Illinois Press, 2015), 148.

11. Rudi Stern, interview by David Gigliotti, December 1999, Early Video Project, May 24, 2001, http://davidsonsfiles.org/rudisterninterview.html.

12. Philip Marchand, *Marshall McLuhan: The Medium and the Messenger* (1989; Cambridge, MA: MIT Press, 1998), 218.

13. Marshall McLuhan, interview, *Playboy*, March 1969, 66.

14. Lisa Rein and Michael Horowitz, "Timothy Leary and Marshall McLuhan, Turned On and Tuned In," *Boing Boing*, June 3, 2014, http://boingboing.net/2014/06/03/timothy-leary-and-marshall-mcl.html.

15. Marshall McLuhan and Quentin Fiore, *War and Peace in the Global Village* (New York: Bantam Books, 1968), 77, 83.

16. Edmund Carpenter, *Oh, What a Blow That Phantom Gave Me!* (New York: Holt, Rinehart and Winston, 1973), 65.

17. Gene Youngblood, *Expanded Cinema* (New York: Dutton, 1970), 41, 47, 78.

18. Gioscia, "Frequency and Form," 7; Victor Gioscia, "LSD Subcultures: Acidoxy Versus Orthodoxy," *American Journal of Orthopsychiatry* 39, no. 3 (1969): 428–436.

19. Carmine Grimaldi, "Televising Psyche: Therapy, Play, and the Seduction of Video," *Representations* 139 (2017): 95–117.

20. Vic Gioscia, "Notes on Videotherapy," *Radical Software* 2, no. 4 (1973): 2; Victor Gioscia, "Groovin' on Time: Fragments of a Sociology of the Psychedelic Experience," in *Psychedelic Drugs: Proceedings of a Hahnemann Medical College and Hospital Symposium Sponsored by*

the Department of Psychiatry, ed. Richard E. Hicks and Paul Jay Rink (New York: Grune & Stratton, 1969), 170–172.

21. Victor Gioscia, "Psychedelic Myths, Metaphors, and Fantasies," in *Origin and Mechanisms of Hallucinations: Proceedings of the 14th Annual Meeting of the Eastern Psychiatric Research Association held in New York City, November 14–15, 1969* (New York: Plenum, 1970), 444–445.

22. Gioscia, "Groovin' on Time," 174–175.

23. Gioscia, "Psychedelic Myths, Metaphors, and Fantasies," 440.

24. Michael Shamberg and Raindance Corporation, *Guerrilla Television* (New York: Holt, Rinehart and Winston, 1971), section I, p. 5.

25. Collopy, "The Revolution Will Be Videotaped," 53–63.

26. Collopy, "The Revolution Will Be Videotaped," 63–64, 74–91.

27. Myron J. Stolaroff, *Thanatos to Eros: Thirty-Five Years of Psychedelic Exploration* (Berlin: Verlag für Wissenschaft und Bildung, 1994), 18–20; Steven M. Gelber and Martin L. Cook, *Saving the Earth: The History of a Middle-Class Millenarian Movement* (Berkeley: University of California Press, 1990), 36–37, 46, 65–68.

28. Alison Falby, *Between the Pigeonholes: Gerald Heard, 1889–1971* (Newcastle upon Tyne, UK: Cambridge Scholars, 2008), 17, 66–69, 88, 103–106; Timothy Miller, "Notes on the Prehistory of the Human Potential Movement: The Vedanta Society and Gerald Heard's Trabuco College," in *On the Edge of the Future: Esalen and the Evolution of American Culture*, ed. Jeffrey J. Kripal and Glenn W. Shuck (Bloomington: Indiana University Press, 2005), 82–92.

29. Myron Stolaroff, "How Much Can People Change?" in *Higher Wisdom: Eminent Elders Explore the Continuing Impact of Psychedelics*, ed. Roger Walsh and Charles S. Grob (Albany: State University of New York Press, 2005), 55; Stolaroff, *Thanatos to Eros*, 21.

30. Gerald Heard, "'Can This Drug Enlarge Man's Mind?'" *Psychedelic Review* 1, no. 1 (1963): 10.

31. Stolaroff, *Thanatos to Eros*, 18, 22, 24; Erika Dyck, *Psychedelic Psychiatry: LSD from Clinic to Campus* (Baltimore: Johns Hopkins University Press, 2008), 97.

32. Stolaroff, *Thanatos to Eros*, 24–25.

33. J. N. Sherwood, M. J. Stolaroff, and W. W. Harman, "The Psychedelic Experience: A New Concept in Psychotherapy," *Journal of Neuropsychiatry* 4 (1962): 69, 71, 73, 77–78. For accounts of the foundation focusing on Harman, see Bretton Fosbrook, "How Scenarios Become Corporate Strategies: Alternative Futures and Uncertainty in Strategic Management" (PhD diss., York University, 2017), 99–104; Malina Aronov, "(Micro-) 'Psychedelic' Experiences: From the 1960s Creativity at the Workplace to the 21st Century Neuro-Newspeak," *Ethnologie française* 49, no. 4 (2019): 702–705.

34. Ido Hartogsohn, *American Trip: Set, Setting, and the Psychedelic Experience in the Twentieth Century* (Cambridge, MA: MIT Press, 2020), 153.

35. Willis W. Harman et al., "Psychedelic Agents in Creative Problem-Solving: A Pilot Study," *Psychological Reports* 19 (1966): 211–212, 219–226.

36. Hartogsohn, *American Trip*, 153, 158, 257–58; Tim Doody, "The Heretic," *Morning News*, July 26, 2012, http://www.themorningnews.org/article/the-heretic; Aronov, "(Micro-) 'Psychedelic' Experiences," 701.

37. Turner, *From Counterculture to Cyberculture*, 49, 65–66.

38. Peter Sachs Collopy, "Video Synthesizers: From Analog Computing to Digital Art," *IEEE Annals of the History of Computing* 36, no. 4 (2014): 74–86.

39. Collopy, "Video Synthesizers," 75.

40. Collopy, "Video Synthesizers," 75; Marita Sturken, "TV as a Creative Medium: Howard Wise and Video Art," *Afterimage*, May 1984, 7.

41. Collopy, "Video Synthesizers," 75; Eric Siegel, interview by Woody Vasulka, January 21, 1992, Vasulka Archive, last modified June 2, 2008, http://vasulka.org/archive/RightsIntrvwInstitMediaPolicies/IntrvwInstitKaldron/74/Siegel.pdf, 8; Carolyn Kane, *Chromatic Algorithms: Synthetic Color, Computer Art, and Aesthetics after Code* (Chicago: University of Chicago Press, 2014), 73–75.

42. Collopy, "Video Synthesizers," 75.

43. Stephen Beck, interview by Glenn Phillips, March 23, 2007, in *California Video: Artists and Histories*, ed. Glenn Phillips (Los Angeles: Getty Research Institute, 2008), 42. Emphasis in original.

44. Collopy, "Video Synthesizers," 77.

45. Collopy, "Video Synthesizers," 75.

46. Eva Keller, "Biographical Notes," in *Nam June Paik: Video Time—Video Space*, ed. Toni Stooss and Thomas Kellein (New York: Harry N. Abrams, 1993), 133; Collopy, "The Revolution Will Be Videotaped," 86.

47. Paik, "Video Synthesizer Plus," 25. Paik also wrote in "Video Synthesizer Plus" that in drug use, "there is no room for comparison or grading, such as 'first class drug taker' or 'second rate pot smoker.'" He did not succeed in making the video synthesizer an instrument without skill or judgment—and even before his manifesto, scholars recognized that drug use too involves learned skill. Howard S. Becker, "Becoming a Marihuana User," *American Journal of Sociology* 59, no. 3 (1953): 235–242.

48. Collopy, "Video Synthesizers," 76; Edith Decker-Phillips, *Paik Video*, trans. Karin Koppensteiner, Marie-Genviève Iselin, and George Quasha (Barrytown, NY: Barrytown, 1998), 154.

49. Strate, "Drugs," 28.

50. Hartogsohn, *American Trip*, esp. ch. 8.

51. Peter Sachs Collopy, "Video and the Self: Closed Circuit | Feedback | Narcissism," in *Video Theories: A Transdisciplinary Reader*, ed. Dieter Daniels and Jan Thoben (London: Bloomsbury, 2022), 108–118.

52. David Lenson, *On Drugs* (Minneapolis: University of Minnesota Press, 1995), 56. Emphasis in original.

BIBLIOGRAPHY

Primary Sources

Beck, Stephen. "Interview by Glenn Phillips, March 23, 2007." In *California Video: Artists and Histories*, edited by Glenn Phillips, 42–45. Los Angeles: Getty Research Institute, 2008.

Becker, Howard S. "Becoming a Marihuana User." *American Journal of Sociology* 59, no. 3 (1953): 235–242.

Carpenter, Edmund. *Oh, What a Blow That Phantom Gave Me!* New York: Holt, Rinehart and Winston, 1973.

Gioscia, Victor. "Frequency and Form." *Radical Software* 1, no. 2 (1970): 7.

Gioscia, Victor. "Groovin' on Time: Fragments of a Sociology of the Psychedelic Experience." In *Psychedelic Drugs: Proceedings of a Hahnemann Medical College and Hospital Symposium Sponsored by the Department of Psychiatry*, edited by Richard E. Hicks and Paul Jay Rink, 167–176. New York: Grune & Stratton, 1969.

Gioscia, Victor. "LSD Subcultures: Acidoxy versus Orthodoxy." *American Journal of Orthopsychiatry* 39, no. 3 (1969): 428–436.

Gioscia, Victor. "Notes on Videotherapy." *Radical Software* 2, no. 4 (1973): 1–4.

Gioscia, Victor. "Psychedelic Myths, Metaphors, and Fantasies." In *Origin and Mechanisms of Hallucinations: Proceedings of the 14th Annual Meeting of the Eastern Psychiatric Research Association held in New York City, November 14–15, 1969*, 435–447. New York: Plenum, 1970.

Harman, Willis W., Robert H. McKim, Robert E. Mogar, James Fadiman, and Myron J. Stolaroff. "Psychedelic Agents in Creative Problem-Solving: A Pilot Study." *Psychological Reports* 19 (1966): 211–227.

Heard, Gerald. "'Can This Drug Enlarge Man's Mind?'" *Psychedelic Review* 1, no. 1 (1963): 7–17.

Leary, Timothy. *Flashbacks: An Autobiography, a Personal and Cultural History of an Era*. Los Angeles: Jeremy P. Tarcher, 1990.

McLuhan, Marshall. Interview, *Playboy*, March 1969, 53–74, 158.

McLuhan, Marshall. *Understanding Media: The Extensions of Man*. 1964. Cambridge, MA: MIT Press, 1994.

McLuhan, Marshall, and Quentin Fiore. *War and Peace in the Global Village*. New York: Bantam Books, 1968.

Paik, Nam June. "Video Synthesizer Plus." *Radical Software* 1, no. 2 (1970): 25.

Shamberg, Michael, and Raindance Corporation. *Guerrilla Television*. New York: Holt, Rinehart and Winston, 1971.

Sherwood, J. N., M. J. Stolaroff, and W. W. Harman. "The Psychedelic Experience: A New Concept in Psychotherapy." *Journal of Neuropsychiatry* 4 (1962): 69–80.

Siegel, Eric. *Einstine*. 1968. In *Surveying the First Decade: Video Art and Alternative Media in the U.S. 1968–1980*. Vol. 2. Chicago: Video Data Bank, 1995. DVD Video, 5:22.

Siegel, Eric. "Interview by Woody Vasulka. January 21, 1992." Vasulka Archive. Last modified June 2, 2008. http://vasulka.org/archive/RightsIntrvwInstitMediaPolicies/IntrvwInstitKaldron /74/Siegel.pdf.

Stern, Rudi. "Interview by David Gigliotti. December 1999." Early Video Project. May 24, 2001. http://davidsonsfiles.org/rudisterninterview.html.

Stolaroff, Myron. "How Much Can People Change?" In *Higher Wisdom: Eminent Elders Explore the Continuing Impact of Psychedelics*, edited by Roger Walsh and Charles S. Grob, 55–67. Albany: State University of New York Press, 2005.

Stolaroff, Myron J. *Thanatos to Eros: Thirty-Five Years of Psychedelic Exploration*. Berlin: Verlag für Wissenschaft und Bildung, 1994.

Teilhard de Chardin, Pierre. *The Phenomenon of Man*. Translated by Bernard Wall, 1959. New York: Harper Torchbooks, 1965.

Varney, Edwin. "Video Is as Powerful as LSD." *Radical Software* 1, no. 3 (1971): 6.

Vassi, Marco. "Zen Tubes." *Radical Software* 1, no. 1 (1970): 18.

Youngblood, Gene. *Expanded Cinema*. New York: Dutton, 1970.

Secondary Sources

Aronov, Milana. "(Micro-) 'Psychedelic' Experiences: From the 1960s Creativity at the Workplace to the 21st Century Neuro-Newspeak." *Ethnologie française* 49, no. 4 (2019): 701–718.

Collopy, Peter Sachs. "The Revolution Will Be Videotaped: Making a Technology of Consciousness in the Long 1960s." PhD diss., University of Pennsylvania, 2015.

Collopy, Peter Sachs. "Video and the Self: Closed Circuit | Feedback | Narcissism." In *Video Theories: A Transdisciplinary Reader*, edited by Dieter Daniels and Jan Thoben, 108–118. London: Bloomsbury, 2022.

Collopy, Peter Sachs. "Video Synthesizers: From Analog Computing to Digital Art." *IEEE Annals of the History of Computing* 36, no. 4 (2014): 74–86.

Decker-Phillips, Edith. *Paik Video*. Translated by Karin Koppensteiner, Marie-Genviève Iselin, and George Quasha. Barrytown, NY: Barrytown, 1998. https://www.worldcat.org/title/37725629

Doody, Tim. "The Heretic." *Morning News*, July 26, 2012. http://www.themorningnews.org /article/the-heretic.

Dyck, Erika. *Psychedelic Psychiatry: LSD from Clinic to Campus*. Baltimore: Johns Hopkins University Press, 2008.

Elcock, Chris. "From Acid Revolution to Entheogenic Evolution: Psychedelic Philosophy in the Sixties and Beyond." *Journal of American Culture* 36, no. 4 (2013): 296–311.

Falby, Alison. *Between the Pigeonholes: Gerald Heard, 1889–1971*. Newcastle upon Tyne, UK: Cambridge Scholars, 2008.

Fosbrook, Bretton. "How Scenarios Become Corporate Strategies: Alternative Futures and Uncertainty in Strategic Management." PhD diss., York University, 2017.

Gelber, Steven M., and Martin L. Cook. *Saving the Earth: The History of a Middle-Class Millenarian Movement*. Berkeley: University of California Press, 1990.

Grimaldi, Carmine "Televising Psyche: Therapy, Play, and the Seduction of Video." *Representations* 139 (2017): 95–117.

Hanhardt, John G. *The Worlds of Nam June Paik*. New York: Guggenheim Museum, 2000.

Hartogsohn, Ido. *American Trip: Set, Setting, and the Psychedelic Experience in the Twentieth Century*. Cambridge, MA: MIT Press, 2020.

Kane, Carolyn. *Chromatic Algorithms: Synthetic Color, Computer Art, and Aesthetics after Code*. Chicago: University of Chicago Press, 2014.

Keller, Eva. "Biographical Notes." In *Nam June Paik: Video Time—Video Space*, edited by Toni Stooss and Thomas Kellein, 133–137. New York: Harry N. Abrams, 1993.

Lenson, David. *On Drugs*. Minneapolis: University of Minnesota Press, 1995.

Marchand, Philip. *Marshall McLuhan: The Medium and the Messenger*. 1989. Cambridge, MA: MIT Press, 1998.

Miller, Timothy. "Notes on the Prehistory of the Human Potential Movement: The Vedanta Society and Gerald Heard's Trabuco College." In *On the Edge of the Future: Esalen and the Evolution of American Culture*, edited by Jeffrey J. Kripal and Glenn W. Shuck, 80–98. Bloomington: Indiana University Press, 2005.

Paulsen, Kris. "In the Beginning, There Was the Electron." *X-TRA* 15, no. 2 (2013). http://x-traonline.org/article/in-the-beginning-there-was-the-electron/.

Rein, Lisa, and Michael Horowitz. "Timothy Leary and Marshall McLuhan, Turned On and Tuned In." Boing Boing. June 3, 2014. http://boingboing.net/2014/06/03/timothy-leary-and-marshall-mcl.html.

Sack, Susan Kassman. *America's Teilhard: Christ and Hope in the 1960s*. Washington, DC: Catholic University of America Press, 2019.

Siff, Stephen. *Acid Hype: American News Media and the Psychedelic Experience*. Urbana: University of Illinois Press, 2015.

Strate, Lance. "Drugs: The Intensions of Humanity." In *Drugs & Media: New Perspectives on Communication, Consumption, and Consciousness*, edited by Robert C. MacDougall, 19–34. New York: Continuum, 2012.

Sturken, Marita. "TV as a Creative Medium: Howard Wise and Video Art." *Afterimage*, May 1984, 5–9.

Turner, Fred. *From Counterculture to Cyberculture: Stewart Brand, the Whole Earth Network, and the Rise of Digital Utopianism*. Chicago: University of Chicago Press, 2006.

Turner, Fred. "The Pygmy Gamelan as Technology of Consciousness." In *Paul DeMarinis: Buried in Noise*, edited by Ingrid Beirer, Sabine Himmelsbach, and Carsten Seiffarth, 23–31. Heidelberg: Kehrer Verlag, 2010.

15 FROM PSYCHIATRIC CLINICS TO MAGICAL CENTER: LSD IN THE NETHERLANDS

Stephen Snelders

Onno Nol truly believed in "the message": the use of LSD was the panacea to solve the world's problems. If only the Soviet leader Nikita Khrushchev and the American president Lyndon Johnson would have a psychedelic experience, they would never start a nuclear war.[1] In 1964, Nol, an idealistic student of first medicine and later physics, started to recruit investors from the Amsterdam beatnik and drug scene to build his own underground laboratory.[2] A first test run produced a tube containing a liquid with only 50–80 dosage units. Three months later, Nol's lab produced a bottle containing 40,000 dosage units of LSD. (He did not make it solid enough to crystallize it.) The liquid LSD was dripped on sugar cubes with a pipette. These LSD cubes, priced between 5 and 10 Dutch guilders (around 15–30 USD today), were made available in bars and other locations in Amsterdam where the alternative youth and drug scene gathered. Nol's LSD was possibly also a major source of supply for the underground UK market. His lab had to discontinue operations, however, because Nol turned into a major consumer of his own product, taking a staggeringly high dose of 900 μg each day for a period of eight months. By the next year, he had become completely paranoid and went to Germany to recuperate.[3]

Nol's activities stood at a watershed in the diffusion of LSD in the Netherlands. The drug had arrived in Dutch psychiatric clinics in the 1950s. It crossed boundaries between medical and public domains through psychiatric treatments and psychological experiments involving intellectuals and artists. Taken up by a bohemian beatnik drug scene in the larger cities, especially Amsterdam, Rotterdam, and The Hague, LSD was reconfigured from a drug that caused or mimicked psychosis into a mind-liberating drug that would revolutionize the world. At the same time, its use came to be perceived as a major threat to society, creating a cultural legacy that lives on today. While similar developments took place in other Western countries, Dutch psychedelic history had its own characteristics.[4] In psychiatry, LSD therapy was used for the management of the traumas of World War II; in Dutch society, overlapping groups of activists and psychedelics users were involved in a playful transformation of society into a "Magical Center"; and in economics, the Netherlands became a key player in the illegal production and distribution of LSD worldwide.

THE RISE OF LSD IN PSYCHIATRY

LSD found its first Dutch users in psychiatric clinics in the 1950s. Until LSD was regulated under the Dutch drug law (the *Opiumwet*) in 1966, the drug was therapeutically used in eight clinics and at least three private practices in the Netherlands.[5] This was made possible by the existence of a medical setting in which contemporary managerial concepts such as team-work, evidence-based medicine, and quality indicators were unknown. In the 1950s, psychiatrists ruled their departments as feudal lords and developed the accompanying personality styles. Early LSD therapy in psychiatry was framed by these dominant structures. To many patients, pioneering LSD psychiatrists such as Kees van Rhijn (b. 1918), Willy Arendsen Hein (1912–1995), and Jan Bastiaans (1917–1997) were authoritarian father figures to whom they turned for help. It is characteristic that psychiatric publications of the time fail to mention the importance of the nurses (male and female) who nursed patients through their rebirths, nurturing more positive experiences and minimizing the risks of bad trips.[6]

Van Rhijn was the first Dutch psychiatrist to experiment with LSD on a systematic basis, in the Brinkgreven psychiatric clinic, outside the city of Deventer. In 1952, a salesperson from the Sandoz pharmaceutical company visited Van Rhijn, bringing some samples of LSD. The next year, the psychiatrist started to give LSD therapy to chronic alcoholics admitted to his clinic.

Neither the clinic's managing director, nor the staff, nor the patients exerted much influence on Van Rhijn's treatments.[7] This situation of virtually free experimentation with LSD was made possible by the comparatively low social status of the patients, as was the case with the work of Van Rhijn's fellow researcher, Arendsen Hein.[8] Arendsen Hein began giving LSD therapy in 1959 as chief psychiatrist at the Salvation Army clinic Groot Batelaar in Lunteren. This clinic admitted so-called criminal psychopaths sentenced by the judicial courts to psychiatric treatment. Only after perceiving success with this class of patients did Arendsen Hein give LSD therapy to other patients in his own private clinic, Veluweland in Ederveen. Most of these latter patients were classified as "neurotics" and came from wealthier social backgrounds. They were registered as "guests," not as "patients," indicating their higher social status.[9]

Apart from the availability of both the drug and patients, there were substantive reasons for psychiatrists such as Van Rhijn, Arendsen Hein, and later Bastiaans (who began LSD and psilocybin therapy in 1961 at the University of Amsterdam, and who continued this therapy from 1963, as a psychiatry professor at the University of Leiden, in the Jelgersma clinic in Oegstgeest) to experiment with LSD. A key factor contributing to the diffusion of LSD in psychiatry was that its use stood in continuity with earlier developments in therapy and research and was not seen as something completely new. LSD seemed to provide answers and strategies that could be adopted within existing psychiatric frameworks. Since psychiatry was at this time dominated by psychoanalytic schools of thought, LSD was incorporated within their frameworks, providing a tool to break through the mental barriers that patients erected against their own treatment.

Van Rhijn formulated the following indications for LSD therapy: to loosen a stagnated situation in treatment; to strive for quick results in emergency cases; and to give love and security to acceptance-frustrated neurotics.[10] This way of working became known as "psycholytic" therapy, differentiated from "psychedelic" therapy. Psycholytic therapy involved administering low dosages of LSD to gain access to the patient's unconscious, whereas psychedelic therapy required high dosages to elicit a peak healing experience. However, in practice, Dutch psycholytic therapists did not hesitate to administer high doses to make their patients talkative and cooperative if they considered it useful.[11]

ARENDSEN HEIN

Arendsen Hein, who was heavily influenced by the psychoanalytic ideas of Alfred Adler (1870–1937), treated his "psychopathic" patients with a combination of individual and group therapy and resocialization. However, he encountered a number of so-called refractory patients, who failed to respond to all therapeutic efforts. To break down their barriers of resistance, Arendsen Hein experimented with chemical means. The 1950s were, after all, the decade of the psychopharmaceutical revolution in psychiatry.[12] Carbon dioxide inhalation, narcoanalysis with sodium pentothal, and administration of methamphetamine were all tried by Arendsen Hein, but with limited success. Inspired by publications by psycholytic therapists such as the German Hanscarl Leuner and the Brit Ronald Sandison, Arendsen Hein began administering LSD in 1959.[13] He claimed considerable results: a majority of his "tough guys" showed a notable reduction of resistance, intensive abreaction of repressed emotional material, allegoric and symbolic presentation of conflicts, lucid insights into hitherto misunderstood attitudes, reorganization of values, marked improvement in behaviors, and intensification of human contact.[14]

In Arendsen Hein's work, the distinction between psycholytic and psychedelic therapy disappeared. In the LSD experiences of both his patients and himself (he regularly took LSD to "cleanse his mind"), Arendsen Hein started to recognize the "peak-experience" transcending normal ego-boundaries: an experience of the "cosmic consciousness." In his words: "It is as if lightning strikes and the inner panorama is suddenly bright illuminated."[15] This peak experience transformed the experiencer and gave him a positive self-image. Arendsen Hein wrote: "Have not most of us been living in a state of complete unawareness of our roots in the transcendental, until we saw this clearly under the influence of LSD?"[16] The concept was again not new in Dutch psychiatry. Both Arendsen Hein and Van Rhijn had studied with H. C. Rümke, the influential professor of psychiatry at Utrecht

University, who taught that an intensive feeling of happiness could bring one to the brink of dissolution in the whole of being.[17]

BASTIAANS

The therapeutic use of LSD also provided an answer to the problems that Jan Bastiaans was having in his attempts to treat a special kind of patient: survivors of the German and Japanese concentration camps and prisons of World War II. After attempting to treat them after the war, Bastiaans discovered that many of these victims suffered from alexithymia, an inability to talk about their feelings. Traumatizing experiences, such as torture by SS hangmen, were suppressed in their memories. Moreover, many patients did not have faith in their therapists, who had not themselves been in the camps and prisons and therefore could not understand how it had really been.

Bastiaans, working from a theoretical framework that combined psychoanalysis and psychosomatic medicine, at first tried to open up his patients by using narcoanalysis in combination with psychoanalysis and psychodrama. However, he felt that he did not achieve sufficient results with his most rigid patients. Moreover, the patients did not always remember what they had said during narcosis. In 1961, therefore, Bastiaans began incorporating psychedelic drugs into his treatments: mainly LSD, but also psilocybin. When he deemed it necessary, he used psychodrama techniques in the drug sessions as well. Nazi paraphernalia, images of German war leaders, and recordings of Adolf Hitler's speeches were used to make patients consciously relive their experiences in the prisons and camps. Bastiaans treated around 300 patients in total with psychedelics, mainly with success (so he claimed) until his retirement in 1988.[18]

DOUBTING THE MEDICAL BENEFITS OF LSD

The LSD molecule could diffuse itself in psychiatric settings because it offered solutions to the therapeutic problems of psychiatrists. But as in other countries, the diffusion of LSD within psychiatric settings that started promisingly in the 1950s and early 1960s soon encountered limitations. In the

Netherlands, the first problems arose around Arendsen Hein, whose personality style led to conflicts. In a public scandal involving a personal dispute between a doctor at his Groot Batelaar clinic and this doctor's wife, Arendsen Hein tried to force the doctor into psychiatric treatment. The latter divulged to the press that Arendsen Hein drove his patients insane with secret LSD experiments. This negative media attention compromised his position in the clinic. Arendsen Hein had to leave Groot Batelaar in 1960, but he continued LSD therapy in his private clinic.[19]

In his 1960 textbook on psychiatry, Rümke stressed the dangers of using LSD and mentioned two examples of treatment that led to negative effects—one patient fell into a months-long severe depression, and another committed suicide. Rümke's personal Calvinist convictions, moreover, made him opposed to actively seeking ecstasy.[20] As the 1960s wore on, news of a psychedelic movement originating in the US that threatened the fabric of society served to increase Rümke's fears of LSD. Just before his death in 1967, in a new edition of his textbook, he even gave as an example of the negative effect of LSD on people's mental health the fact that two of his own patients experienced "paranoid delusions" about the drug, even though they had never used it. Rümke thought that these delusions were caused by the public advocacy of LSD by the movement by Timothy Leary and Richard Alpert.[21] (As will be seen next, Leary had indeed reached out to the Netherlands, but Rümke could not have known this.) However, within psychiatry, there was no consensus about either the benefits or the disadvantages of LSD therapy in psychiatry, as witnessed by a discussion in the influential *Nederlands Tijdschrift voor Geneeskunde* (Dutch journal of medicine) in 1968.[22]

As it happened, the medical benefits of LSD were also doubted in public media. In a recent analysis of a digitized database of Dutch newspapers, David Claessen (2020) showed that after the media coverage of Arendsen Hein's work in Groot Batelaar, LSD was regularly mentioned in the newspapers, but not always in a positive sense. LSD therapy was even described in one newspaper as "creepy."[23] Nonmedical use of LSD became a feature of media coverage from 1962 onward. In 1965, newspapers suggested a relationship between drug addiction and the death of a drug addict (but not because of LSD) on the one hand, and the diffusion of LSD use on the other. Such negative publicity led a right-wing party to pose questions in parliament in February 1966 about the necessity of ending trade in LSD, and it contributed to the prohibition of the drug in the same month, as discussed next.[24]

THE DECLINE AND FALL OF LSD IN PSYCHIATRY

Medical use of LSD in the Netherlands declined after 1966. Only two psychiatrists (Arendsen Hein and Bastiaans) applied for and received permits to continue LSD therapy when doing so became obligatory in 1966. Arendsen Hein now kept out of the public eye, even though one of his patients published a book in 1968 discussing her LSD treatment in his clinic and the peak experience that helped her overcome her neurotic inability to cope with life.[25] Bastiaans went on to gain a high public profile in the 1970s. On the one hand, he was seen as a hero and a last resort for healing by members of the former Dutch Resistance, who viewed him as the psychiatrist who gave hope to the victims of the war. On the other hand, his work became even more controversial when a weekly magazine in 1976 revealed that the heroic memories elicited in his LSD sessions by one of Bastiaans's patients and published in a book had been fantasized.[26] Bastiaans's emotional involvement with his patients also made him suspect for many colleagues who worked more from a position of professional detachment.

Moreover, in the 1980s, Bastiaans's personality style alienated him from a more informal and democratic new generation of psychiatrists; his students and successors were not interested in continuing his method. In 1985, the government asked its Council of Health for advice on the continuation of LSD therapy after his retirement. All the consulted experts considered the use of psychedelics unnecessary. The positive effects of LSD therapy were attributed to Bastiaans's professional competence, not to his method. One expert even made clear that "the continuation of apparently legitimate therapeutic uses of LSD detracts from the work of people trying to contain the enormous drug problem"; he also resented the "metaphysical speculations" found in Bastiaans's work, for which he saw no use in medicine.[27] Ultimately, LSD therapy was discontinued when Bastiaans left his clinic in

1988. Disillusioned, he wrote: "It does appear as if medieval fears for insanity or for the confrontation with psychotics are evoked again, leaving one with the impression that society has a need for eliminating as swiftly as possible that which seems to pose a threat to its own existence."[28]

To a postwar generation of psychiatrists, LSD had seemed to answer the problems of their therapeutic practice. But to their post-1960s successors, the drug had become irrelevant and dangerous.

LSD'S SPILLOVER INTO SOCIETY

While Bastiaans's work developed independently from any psychedelic revolution in Dutch society more broadly, the public image of this revolution had negative effects on the continuation of his work. Ironically, at the same time, it was psychiatry that introduced people outside the medical domain to the possibilities and benefits of LSD. In the Netherlands, a key catalyst in this process was the experiments of the psychiatrist Frank van Ree, who was interested in the relationship between the nature and extent of the LSD experience and the personality structure of the experiencer. He designed an experiment testing the effects of the drug on voluntary, healthy subjects.

Volunteers for these experiments, conducted in an Amsterdam hospital in 1958–1959, were recruited from the city's literary and artistic circles.[29] They included two men who in the following years would play prominent roles in the Dutch psychedelic movement: the writer and poet Simon Vinkenoog and a medical student named Bart Huges. Both participated in the so-called *pleiner* scene that had evolved in Amsterdam in the 1950s, with similar scenes in other Dutch cities such as Rotterdam and The Hague. The nucleus of this scene was a group of artists, writers, university and high school students, and dropouts who gathered in the bars around Amsterdam's Leidseplein square (hence the name *pleiner*) in the center of town. These people constituted a self-conscious bohemia in the classical sense of the word. They shared attitudes such as "seize the day" hedonism and contempt for "straight" and respectable citizens.

The mainstream media reported negatively on the *pleiners*, but to Vinkenoog, these "Barbarians of the Leidseplein" were a healthy antidote to the bourgeois world: "The encyclopedia describes Barbarians as having no part in civilization . . . with their own precepts, without revolution, and as normal as can be in a neurotic world."[30] Out of this scene, the psychedelic movement in the Netherlands grew. An essential factor in this development was the *pleiners'* penchant for drug use and their imperative to get high by any possible means, foremost by using cannabis, but also by taking other drugs such as ether, amphetamines, and opium. Since cannabis use had been prohibited in 1953 and had become the object of police persecution, this contributed to the *pleiners'* sense of alienation from Dutch society. Police raids on their houses and apartments were a familiar occurrence. Prison sentences of three to twelve months were imposed for possession of marijuana. Vinkenoog himself spent six weeks in prison for illegal possession in 1965 (but he smuggled LSD into his cell and took eight trips behind bars during these weeks).[31]

LSD spilled out of the medical domain into society first through the *pleiners.* The experiments of Van Ree were the original catalyst, but it took a few years before a regular supply became available. In 1962, LSD became available on an "extralegal" market: its use was not yet illegal, but the drug was not purchasable in a legal way (e.g., in a pharmacy).[32] The only source for LSD until the activities of Onno Nol and his friends emerged was the Switzerland-based Sandoz, which provided the drug for scientific and medical purposes to doctors and scientists. As has often been the case with medicinal drug supplies, some of the Sandoz LSD turned up in a nonmedical market, but it took LSD's production in underground laboratories for Dutch consumers to have a regular supply and establish the psychedelic revolution on a firm basis.[33]

INTERPRETING THE PSYCHEDELIC EXPERIENCE

LSD was not just one drug of many in the *pleiners'* cupboard. To Vinkenoog and Huges, and many after (and before) them, LSD gave new and overwhelming experiences, not only placing users apart from the bourgeois world but offering them a tool to transcend and transform the world. They were not interested in the interpretations of their LSD experiences offered by the doctors who gave them the drug. To van Ree in 1959, the LSD experience was a form of psychosis, and one of the tasks of the psychiatrists was to categorize the specific form the user experienced.[34] Typical LSD experiences, in which the boundaries between the "I" of the user and the "One" of the universe blurred, van Ree classified as "degenerative" forms of psychosis. Later he revised these conclusions: in 1971, he referred to these experiences as "cosmic-transcendental," in the terminology of the American theologian and psychedelic researcher Walter Pahnke. In his famous Good Friday experiment in 1962, Pahnke had attempted to elicit religious and mystical experiences in an experimental group that was administered psilocybin.[35] But in 1959, van Ree was scathing about these kinds of experiences, dismissing one such report by a test subject as an "exalted kind of Christmas mood."[36]

Vinkenoog experienced a rebirth when participating in the experiment: "I looked for the switch to eternity. You become aware of things you don't know, as your lungs labor your entire life without you knowing that you're breathing. With great effort I was (re)born."[37] But he felt he could share this experience with very few people.[38] For Huges, his two experiences in the experiment seemed to elude all meaning, and he perceived the attendant scientists as devils, monkeys, and liars, growing bored with them.[39]

Over time, both men developed their own influential interpretations of the psychedelic experience. For Vinkenoog, the key was his interactions with the American physician Steve Groff (not to be confused with the well-known LSD psychiatrist Stanislav Grof), who in 1962 or 1963 came to Amsterdam for medical training before returning to the US in 1967. Groff was a member of the emerging international psychedelic network that formed around Timothy Leary, to whom Groff introduced Vinkenoog. Of considerable influence on Vinkenoog was the *Psychedelic Review*, the journal of the Leary group, the first issue of which was published in 1963. After a visit to the Leary commune in Millbrook in upstate New York in 1965, Groff returned as one of two "apostles" sent out with the last stock of Sandoz LSD to turn on the world. (The other was Michael Hollingshead, who went to London.) Groff and Vinkenoog collaborated on a Dutch translation of the Leary-Metzner manual *The Psychedelic Experience*, published in 1969.[40]

REALITY AS A GAME

Of particular importance to Vinkenoog was Leary's "game theory" of reality, operationalized in what the American psychologist had named an "applied mysticism." The idea of the game-character of reality linked the psychedelic movement closely to more politically oriented activists in Amsterdam, who derided the bourgeois world as well, such as the anarchist Provo group. A major source of inspiration on these activists was the work of the Dutch historian Johan Huizinga. In *Homo ludens*, published in 1938, Huizinga had analyzed the importance of games to the development of culture. To him, behavior (e.g., of medieval knights) was, even when this was not consciously perceived as such by the participants, a kind of game with its own rules.[41]

The 1960s counterculture became imbued with this idea of life as a game. The influence of Huizinga, for example, is explicitly acknowledged in *Play Power*, published by the Australian journalist Richard Neville in 1970. Neville was the editor of the influential London underground magazine *Oz* and a central figure in the international counterculture. His book offers an overview of countercultural attitudes and seeks the unifying element in all the currents within the "politics of the game." The key element is a sense of freedom that fosters creativity: high-level performance is achieved in art and science environments wherein people play, not in work, which involves an element of coercion or obligation.[42]

Psychedelic game theory went still a step further than the political activism of Provo and Neville. For Leary and kindred spirits such as Vinkenoog, not only culture but the whole of the reality we experience was a game. They developed distinctly religious and mystical views in which psychedelics were the means of making us aware of the game character of reality, in which a pantheistic divinity plays hide and seek with itself.[43]

TURNING AMSTERDAM INTO A MAGICAL CENTER

The idea of game reality, whether in a sociocultural or metaphysical sense, inspired Dutch *pleiners* between 1962 and 1966 to undertake public activities aimed at transforming Amsterdam into a Magical Center: a city full of play, leisure, creativity, and magic events rather than boring workdays. Leading roles were played by Huges and his friend Robert-Jasper Grootveld, a window cleaner who did not like LSD but was a compulsive cannabis smoker. They staged public happenings to create ambiences where people could go collectively out of their mind and unleash their creative power. They also designed the symbol of the Magical Center: an apple with a dot on it. Reality is, after all, an apple ready for you to bite into.

Grootveld heralded the coming of a man called "Klaas," who would satisfy everyone's needs even while nobody knew who he was. From their shared house, Huges and Grootveld also designed a game in which the police could participate: the Marihu game. Marihu was everything that looked like marijuana but was not. Packages of Marihu circulated, and one could win a considerable number of points in this game by provoking police raids and arrests on the ground of possession of marihu. In 1964, Grootveld started to hold antitobacco smoking events on the Spui in the center of the city, a square containing a statue paid for by the tobacco industry.

The next summer, members of the anarchist group Provo began to participate in these happenings. *Provo* stood for "provocation," and just like Grootveld, these group members wished to provoke the police and other authorities in violent and disproportionate reactions to unmask their authoritarian character. This led to a hot summer of happenings and riots. Amazingly, the magic worked. Not only did youngsters start to question authority, but Klaas even materialized in the person of Prince Claus von Amsberg, the new fiancé of Crown Princess Beatrix and, during World War II, an officer in the German Wehrmacht.

The peak of Provo's provocative revolt occurred in the first three months of 1966 in a campaign against the marriage of Beatrix and Claus. The ceremony was to be held in Amsterdam. The city's population had been liberated from the Wehrmacht only twenty years before and held a deep-seated resentment to anything representing Germany. Provo argued that the ceremony was a symbol of the authoritarian character of Dutch society that lurked behind its supposedly democratic façade.

In the atmosphere of provocation and repression that ruled the capital, Provo's confrontation reached its pinnacle in the streets on March 10, 1966, and continued in the aftermath. In February, Provo had proclaimed the day of the marriage a "Day of Anarchy" and jokingly threatened to dope the horses of the mounted police with LSD. The national authorities did not take this provocation as a joke. It became the occasion to prohibit the production, distribution, and use of LSD and eighteen other psychedelic drugs, including mescaline and psilocybin. Even before the law came into effect, Peter ten Hoopen, the leading Amsterdam LSD dealer and friend of Huges and the Provo group, was arrested.[44]

Ironically, Provo was itself divided on the issue of LSD. Referencing the famous words of Karl Marx, the editors of issue no. 7 of *Provo* magazine, published in 1966, wrote that "unfortunately," drugs such as marijuana and LSD were the "opium for the provotariat" and they were "nervous" about these drugs. But the same issue also published a defense of LSD by Vinkenoog, while *Lynx,* the magazine of the Hague Provo group, cited in September 1966 the already (in)famous Leary slogan "Turn on, tune in, drop out," first uttered at the Human Be-In that had occurred in January that year in San Francisco.[45] This lack of consensus within Provo reflected the general debate on politics and drugs in the 1960s counterculture: did drugs lead away from revolutionary struggle, or was self-liberation through drug use imperative for a successful transformation of society?

HUGES AND THE THIRD EYE

In the meantime, Huges developed his own remarkable, and to some extent influential, interpretation of the psychedelic experience. In 1962, he authored the scroll *Homo Sapiens Correctus,* in which he developed his theory that the use of LSD leads to a temporary increase of blood volume in the brain. There was, according to him, a method for permanently inducing this increase: trepanation (drilling a hole in the skull), which he associated with opening up a "third eye." This practice would permanently produce a third of the effect of an LSD trip, he claimed. A society that was trepanned would therefore be a utopian society.[46]

In January 1965, Huges bored a third eye in his skull using a dental drill. (However, according to one doctor, X-rays showed that the self-trepanation had not succeeded.) Ten days after his trepanation, at a happening called "Stoned in the Streets," Huges unwrapped a 32-m bandage from his head, on which were written the words "HA HA HA HA"—while a beautifully painted girl (and later clothing designer for The Beatles) did a striptease. But for most of his friends in the drug scene, Huges took his theories too seriously, a position contrary to the idea of reality as a game. Nevertheless, he found followers, especially in England, where he spent some time.[47] This event links the 1960s psychedelic movement to today's psychedelic renaissance: one of his followers was the noted trepanation enthusiast Amanda Feilding, whose Beckley Foundation is a major financer of today's scientific research into psychedelics.[48]

CONCLUSION: THE LEGACY OF 1960s LSD USE

Dutch psychiatrists developed their methods of doing LSD therapy in an attempt to liberate neurotic and traumatized patients. Taken up by a drug-using, bohemian, beatnik crowd, LSD was reconfigured into a mind-liberating drug that would change society. This transformation was influenced by the rise of an underground production and distribution of the drug, as well as by the influence of the psychedelic thought and actions of Timothy Leary.

In 1966, LSD made a fresh career start as an illegal drug. As in most Western countries, the use of LSD grew exponentially from the Summer of Love of 1967 onward, notwithstanding its prohibition. Surveys of the early 1970s suggest that the number of LSD users had risen into the thousands by then.[49] After the arrival of the heroin epidemic in 1971, the drug fell out of fashion but never completely disappeared from the illegal drug circuits. In 1985, the International Narcotics Control Board suggested that Dutch underground laboratories were the biggest suppliers of LSD in Europe.[50] While the drug kept a low profile, the legacy of Onno Nol lived on.

LSD use in the Netherlands had its own characteristics. LSD therapy in psychiatry was closely connected to the culture of Dutch psychiatry of the time, and to the traumas and heritage of the German occupation in World War II. Dutch artists and political activists pioneered new, nonviolent, provoking tactics based on game theory to expose the authoritarianism in Dutch society and to turn the city of Amsterdam into a magical center. The LSD experience both strengthened the idea of reality as a game and fitted into these disaffected young people's antiauthoritarian tactics.

The LSD molecule successfully spread through Dutch culture by eliciting hopes and insights in different settings and among users with different mindsets. Because of its plasticity, not any single group of users was able to monopolize the drug that continued and still continues to flow into and out of medical and public domains. However, its diffusion also elicited opposition among state authorities and medical professions. LSD became inseparably linked to 1960s revolt and excess, a drug leading to madness such as that experienced by Nol. This produced a legacy that many of its advocates are still struggling to undo today.

NOTES

1.   A similar sentiment was expressed by Aldous Huxley in 1962. See Nicholas Murray, *Aldous Huxley: A Biography* (New York: St. Martin's Press, 2002), 447. (Thanks to Chris Elcock for the reference.)

2.   Underground laboratories were by this time starting to produce LSD in several Western countries. In 1963, for instance, a "green" and only 60 percent pure form of LSD appeared on the US market. See Stephen Snelders, *Drug Smuggler Nation: Narcotics and the Netherlands, 1920–1995* (Manchester, UK: Manchester University Press, 2021), 221.

3.   On Nol and underground LSD, see Herman Cohen, *Drugs, druggebruikers, en drug-scene* (Alphen aan den Rijn, Netherlands: Samsom, 1975), 63; D. van Weerlee, ed., *Allemaal rebellen: Amsterdam 1955–1965* (Amsterdam: Tabula, 1984), 74–79; S. A. M. Snelders, LSD en de psychiatrie (PhD thesis, VU-University Amsterdam, 1999), 149; A. Roberts, *Albion Dreaming: A Popular History of LSD in Britain* (Singapore: Marshall Cavendish, 2012), 126.

4.   For similar developments in other Western countries such as the US, see Martin A. Lee and Bruce Shlain, *Acid Dreams: The Complete Social History of LSD* (New York: Grove Press, 1985); Jay Stevens, *Storming Heaven: LSD and the American Dream* (New York: Grove Press, 1998); and for the UK, Roberts, *Albion Dreaming*.

5.   On LSD and psychiatry in the Netherlands, see Stephen Snelders, *LSD-therapie in Nederland. De experimenteel-psychiatrische benadering van J. Bastiaans, G. W. Arendsen Hein en C.H. van Rhijn* (Amsterdam: Candide, 2000); Stephen Snelders, "The Use of Psychedelics in Dutch Psychiatry 1950–1970: The Problem of Continuity and Discontinuity," *Curare* 18 (1995): 415–425; Stephen Snelders, "The LSD Therapy Career of Jan Bastiaans, M.D.," in *Welten des Bewusstseins*, vol. 10, *Pränatale Psychologie und Psycholytische Therapie*, ed. Michael Schlichting (Berlin: VWB, 2000), 135–141; Stephen Snelders and Charles Kaplan, "LSD Therapy

in Dutch Psychiatry: Changing Sociopolitical Settings and Cultural Sets," *Medical History* 46 (2002): 221–240.

6.   For instance, see Stephen Snelders, "Kin Spruijt: A Psychedelic Nurse in a Psychiatric Clinic," https://chacruna.net/a-psychedelic-nurse-in-a-dutch-psychiatric-clinic/.

7.   On Van Rhijn, see Snelders, *LSD-therapie*, 103–127.

8.   Compare chapter 3 in this volume.

9.   On Arendsen Hein, see Snelders, *LSD-therapie*, 128–160.

10. C. H. Van Rhijn, "Variables in Psycholytic Treatment," in *The Use of LSD in Psychotherapy and Alcoholism*, ed. H. A. Abramson (Indianapolis: Bobs-Merrill, 1967): 208–222.

11. Cf. Snelders, *LSD-therapie*.

12. For a critical history of this revolution, see David Healy, *The Creation of Psychopharmacology* (Cambridge, MA: Harvard University Press, 2002).

13. On Sandison, see chapter 5 in this volume.

14. G. W. Arendsen Hein, "LSD in the Treatment of Criminal Psychopaths," in *Hallucinogenic Drugs and Their Psychotherapeutic Uses*, ed. R. Crocket, R. A. Sandison, and A. Walk (London: H. K. Lewis, 1963): 101–106; G. W. Arendsen Hein. "Treatment of the Neurotic Patient, Resistant to the Usual Techniques of Psychotherapy, with Special Reference to LSD," *Topical Problems of Psychotherapy* 4 (1963), 50–57; Stephen Snelders, "Het gebruik van psychedelische middelen in Nederland in de jaren zestig. Een hoofdstuk uit de sociale geschiedenis van drug-gebruik," *Tijdschrift voor Sociale Geschiedenis* 21(1995):1, 37–60.

15. G. W. Arendsen Hein, "LSD als hulpmiddel bij de behandeling van psychisch gestoorden," *Nederlands Tijdschrift voor Criminologie* 7 (1965): 61–77; 72 (my translation).

16. G. W. Arendsen Hein, "Dimensions in Psychotherapy," in *Use of LSD*, 572.

17. C. H. van Rhijn, personal communication to the author.

18. Snelders, *LSD-therapie*, 161–210.

19. Snelders, *LSD-therapie*, 147–149; David A. A. Claessen, "LSD: Van wondermiddel tot gevaarlijke drug. Nederlandse kranten over LSD 1951–1966" (BA thesis, Leiden University, 2020), 11. Many thanks to David Claessen for sharing his research.

20. H. C. Rümke, *Psychiatrie*, vol. 2 (Amsterdam: Scheltema & Holkema, 1960), 222; H. C. Rümke, *Psychiatrie*, vol. 3 (Amsterdam: Scheltema & Holkema, 1967), 318–323.

21. Rümke, *Psychiatrie*, vol. 3, 321–323.

22. Snelders, *LSD-therapie*, 249–270; Snelders and Kaplan, "LSD Therapy," 235–256.

23. Claessen, "LSD," 17.

24. Claessen, "LSD," 28. Compare the media coverage of LSD in the US, as described in Stephen Siff, *Acid Hype: American News Media and the Psychedelic Experience* (Champaign: University of Illinois Press, 2015).

25. Tina Fransen, *De nacht heeft armen* (Hilversum, Netherlands: Paul Brand, 1968).

26. Wim Wennekes, Jan Bastiaans and Willem van Salland, *Allemaal rottigheid, allemaal ellende. Het KZ-syndroom van Willem van Salland* (Amsterdam: wetenschappelijke Uitgeverij, 1975); Snelders, *LSD-therapie*, 191–198; Bram Enning, *De oorlog van Bastiaans: De LSD-behandeling van het kampsyndroom* (Amsterdam: Augustus, 2009); Bastiaans: Leo van Bergen, *Bevrijd. Het concentratiekampsyndroom en de LSD behandeling van Jan Bastiaans* (Nijmegen, Netherlands: QV Uitgeverij, 2022).

27. Malcolm Lader, in "Advies inzake de toepassing van hallucinogenen behandeling van slachtoffers van oorlog en geweld," *Gezondheidsraad* 1985/33.

28. J. Bastiaans, "Mental Liberation Facilitated by the Use of Hallucinogenic Drugs," unpublished paper, 16.

29. On Van Ree and his experiments, see Snelders, *LSD-therapie*, 218–236.

30. Simon Vinkenoog, "Barbaren van het Leidseplein," in *Twen* 1 (1960), 43.

31. On the *pleiner* scene in general, see Van Weerlee, ed., *Allemaal rebellen*; Hans, het leven voor de dood. Een film van Louis van Gasteren (Amsterdam, 1985); Eric Duivenvoorden, *Magiër van een nieuwe tijd. Het leven van Robert Jasper Grootveld* (Amsterdam: De Arbeiderspers, 2009); Eric Duivenvoorden, *Rebelse jeugd. Hoe nozems en provo's Nederland veranderden* (Amsterdam: Nieuw Amsterdam, 2005). On the *pleiners* and drugs, see Cohen, *Drugs*, 53ff. On Dutch cannabis policies, Marcel de Kort, *Tussen patiënt en delinquent. Geschiedenis van het Nederlandse drugsbeleid* (Hilversum, Netherlands: Verloren, 1995). On Vinkenoog's LSD experiences in prison, see Simon Vinkenoog, *Tegen de wet. Zes weken Huis van Bewaring, maart, april 1965* (Maasbree, Netherlands: Corrie Zelen, 1980).

32. On the concept of extralegality, see Alan Smart and Filippo M. Zerilli, "Extralegality," in *A Companion to Urban Anthropology*, ed. Donald M. Nonini (John Wiley and Sons, 2014), 222–238.

33. Stephen Snelders, "Het gebruik van psychedelische middelen in Nederland in de jaren zestig. Een hoofdstuk uit de sociale geschiedenis van druggebruik," *Tijdschrift voor Sociale Geschiedenis*, 21 (1995): 37–60; 46–48. For a contemporary account of a LSD dealer, see Peter ten Hoopen, *King Acid: Hoe Amsterdam begon te trippen* (Amsterdam: Contact, 1999).

34. F. van Ree, *LSD-25. Een experimenteel psychopathologisch onderzoek* (Deventer, Netherlands: Kluwer, 1966).

35. R. Doblin, "Pahnke's 'Good Friday Experiment': A Long-Term Follow-up and Methodological Critique," *Journal of Transpersonal Psychology*, 23 (1991): 1–28.

36. Van Ree, *LSD-25*, 59–60. For the evolution of Van Ree's thoughts about these kind of experiences, see Snelders, *LSD-therapie*, 229–235.

37. Bibeb, interview with Vinkenoog in *Vrij Nederland*, July 18, 1964.

38. Simon Vinkenoog, letter to the author, December 11, 1991.

39. Bart Huges, *The Book with the Hole: Autobiography* (Amsterdam: Foundation for Independent Thinking, 1972).

40. Letters, Vinkenoog to Groff, August 18, 1963 and September 18, 1963; Leary to Vinkenoog, September 18, 1963; Groff to Vinkenoog, December 1964 (these letters or copies of them were shown by Vinkenoog to the author); Groff to the author, January 19, 1997; also see Timothy Leary, Ralph Metzner, and Richard Alpert, *De psychedelische ervaring. Een handboek gebaseerd op "Het Tibetaanse Dodenboek"* (Amsterdam: De Bezige Bij, 1969). On Hollingshead, see Michael Hollingshead, *The Man Who Turned on the World* (London: Abelard-Schuman, 1973); Andy Roberts, *Divine Rascal: On the Trail of LSD's Cosmic Courier, Michael Hollingshead* (London: Strange Attractor Press, 2019).

41. Johan Huizinga, *Homo ludens* (Haarlem, Netherlands: Tjeenk Willink & Zoon, 1938).

42. Richard Neville, *Play Power: Exploring the International Underground* (New York: Random House, 1970).

43. Simon Vinkenoog, *Weergaloos. Ontdekkingsreizen naar de waarheid* (Matchless: Voyages of discovery into truth) (Hilversum, Netherlands: Paul Brand, 1968), 235. See also Simon Vinkenoog, *Vogelvrij. Bouwstenen 1963–1967* (Amsterdam: De Bezige Bij, 1967); Simon Vinkenoog, "A Rap on the High Road to Happiness," in *Counterculture: The Creation of an Alternative Society,* ed. Joseph Berke (London: Peter Owen Limited, 1969), 144–68; Simon Vinkenoog, *Timothy Leary magiër. Het ABZ van de psychedelische avant-garde* (Den Haag: Sijthof, 1972).

44. A good English-language introduction to Provo is still Rudolf de Jong, "Provos and Kabouters," in *Anarchism Today,* ed. D. E. Apter and J. Joll (London: Macmillan, 1971), 164–180. For a contemporary account, see Dick P. J. van Reeuwijk, *Damsterdamse extremisten* (Amsterdam: De Bezige Bij, 1965). More detailed histories of the happenings and events leading to the prohibition of 1966 include Coen Tasman, *Louter Kabouter. Kroniek van een beweging* (Amsterdam: Babylon-De Geus, 1996); Duivenvoorden, *Magiër,* Duivenvoorden, *Rebelse jeugd.* On the prohibition of LSD, see De Kort, *Tussen patiënt en delinquent,* 172–173. On media and LSD, see Claessen, "LSD," 22–30. On the arrest of Peter ten Hoopen, see Ten Hoopen, *King Acid.*

45. *Provo* 7 (1966); *Lynx,* September 1966.

46. Hugo Bart Huges, "Homo sapiens correctus," in *Suikergoed & marsepein* (mimeograph, Amsterdam 1968).

47. Hugo Bart Huges, *Suikergoed & marsepein* (Amsterdam: Barbara Huges, 1968); Huges, *Book with the Hole.* On the trepanation, see Van Reeuwijk, *Damsterdamse extremisten,* 33–34.

48. Feilding was one of the English translators of Huges's autobiography, *The Book with the Hole.*

49. For a discussion of the evidence, see Snelders, "Gebruik van psychedelische middelen," 54–55; Stephen Snelders, "Het gebruik van psychedelische middelen in Nederland in de jaren zestig. Een hoofdstuk uit de sociale geschiedenis van druggebruik," *Tijdschrift voor Sociale Geschiedenis,* 21(1995): 1, 37–60.

50. Snelders, *Drug Smuggler Nation,* 225.

BIBLIOGRAPHY

Primary Sources

Bibeb. Interview with Simon Vinkenoog in Vrij Nederland, July 18, 1964.

Letters. Simon Vinkenoog to Steve Groff. August 18, 1963 and September 18, 1963.

Letters. Timothy Leary to Simon Vinkenoog. September 18, 1963.

Letters. Steve Groff to Simon Vinkenoog. December 1964.

Letters. Steve Groff to the author. January 19, 1997.

Simon Vinkenoog, letter to the author, December 11, 1991.

Secondary Sources

Hein. G. W. Arendsen.

Bastiaans, J. "Mental Liberation Facilitated by the Use of Hallucinogenic Drugs." Unpublished typewritten article from Bastiaans's personal archive.

Claessen, David A. A. "LSD: Van wondermiddel tot gevaarlijke drug. Nederlandse kranten over LSD 1951–1966." BA thesis, Leiden University, 2020.

Cohen, Herman. *Drugs, druggebruikers, en drug-scene.* Alphen aan den Rijn, Netherlands: Samsom, 1975.

De Jong, Rudolf. "Provos and Kabouters." In *Anarchism Today*, edited by D. E. Apter and J. Joll, 164–80. London: Macmillan, 1971.

De Kort, Marcel. *Tussen patiënt en delinquent. Geschiedenis van het Nederlandse drugsbeleid.* Hilversum, Netherlands: Verloren, 1995.

Doblin, R. "Pahnke's 'Good Friday Experiment': A Long-Term Follow-up and Methodological Critique." *Journal of Transpersonal Psychology* 23 (1991): 1–28.

Duivenvoorden, Eric. *Magiër van een nieuwe tijd. Het leven van Robert Jasper Grootveld.* Amsterdam: De Arbeiderspers, 2009.

Duivenvoorden, Eric. *Rebelse jeugd. Hoe nozems en provo's Nederland veranderden.* Amsterdam: Nieuw Amsterdam, 2005.

Enning, Bram, *De oorlog van Bastiaans: De LSD-behandeling van het kampsyndroom.* Amsterdam: Augustus, 2009.

Fransen, Tina. *De nacht heeft armen.* Hilversum, Netherlands: Paul Brand, 1968.

Healy, David. *The Creation of Psychopharmacology.* Cambridge, MA: Harvard University Press, 2002.

Hein, G. W. Arendsen. "LSD in the Treatment of Criminal Psychopathy." In *Hallucinogenic Drugs and Their Psychotherapeutic Uses*, edited by R. Crocket, R. A. Sandison, and A. Walk, 101–6. London: H. K. Lewis, 1963.

Hein, G. W. Arendsen. "LSD als hulpmiddel bij de behandeling van psychisch gestoorden." *Nederlands Tijdschrift voor Criminologie* 7 (1965): 61–77.

Hein, G. W. Arendsen. "Treatment of the Neurotic Patient, Resistant to the Usual Techniques of Psychotherapy, with Special Reference to LSD." *Topical Problems of Psychotherapy* 4 (1963): 50–57.

Hein, G. W. Arendsen. "Dimensions in Psychotherapy," In *The Use of LSD in Psychotherapy and Alcoholism*, edited by H. A. Abramson, 569–576. (Indianapolis: Bobs-Merrill, 1967).

Hollingshead, Michael. *The Man Who Turned on the World*. London: Abelard-Schuman, 1973.

Hoopen, Peter ten. *King Acid: Hoe Amsterdam begon te trippen*. Amsterdam: Contact, 1999.

Huges, Bart. *The Book with the Hole: Autobiography*. Amsterdam: Foundation for Independent Thinking, 1972.

Huges, Hugo Bart. *Suikergoed & marsepein*. Amsterdam: Barbara Huges, 1968.

Huizinga, Johan. *Homo ludens*. Haarlem, Netherlands: Tjeenk Willink & Zoon, 1938.

Lader, Malcolm. "Advies inzake de toepassing van hallucinogenen behandeling van slachtoffers van oorlog en geweld." *Gezondheidsraad* 33 (1985).

Leary, Timothy, Ralph Metzner, and Richard Alpert. *De psychedelische ervaring. Een handbook gebaseerd op "Het Tibetaanse Dodenboek."* Amsterdam: De Bezige Bij, 1969.

Lee, Martin A., and Bruce Shlain. *Acid Dreams: The Complete Social History of LSD*. New York: Grove Press, 1985.

Murray, Nicholas. *Aldous Huxley: A Biography*. New York: St. Martin's Press, 2002.

Neville, Richard. *Play Power: Exploring the International Underground*. New York: Random House, 1970.

Roberts, Andy. *Albion Dreaming: A Popular History of LSD in Britain*. Singapore: Marshall Cavendish, 2012.

Roberts, Andy. *Divine Rascal: On the Trail of LSD's Cosmic Courier, Michael Hollingshead*. London: Strange Attractor Press, 2019.

Rümke, H. C. *Psychiatrie*, vol. 2. Amsterdam: Scheltema & Holkema, 1960.

Rümke, H. C. *Psychiatrie*, vol. 3. Amsterdam: Scheltema & Holkema, 1967.

Siff, Stephen. *Acid Hype: American News Media and the Psychedelic Experience*. Champaign: University of Illinois Press, 2015.

Smart, Alan, and Filippo M. Zerilli. "Extralegality." In *A Companion to Urban Anthropology*, edited by Donald M. Nonini 222–38. John Wiley and Sons, 2014.

Snelders, Stephen. *Drug Smuggler Nation: Narcotics and the Netherlands, 1920–1995*. Manchester, UK: Manchester University Press, 2021.

Snelders, Stephen. "Het gebruik van psychedelische middelen in Nederland in de jaren zestig. Een hoofdstuk uit de sociale geschiedenis van druggebruik." *Tijdschrift voor Sociale Geschiedenis* 21 (1995): 37–60.

Snelders, Stephen. "Kin Spruijt: A Psychedelic Nurse in a Psychiatric Clinic." Women in the History of Psychedelic Plants. https://chacruna.net/a-psychedelic-nurse-in-a-dutch-psychiatric-clinic/

Snelders, S. A. M. *LSD en de psychiatrie*. PhD thesis, VU-University Amsterdam, 1999.

Snelders, Stephen. *LSD-therapie in Nederland. De experimenteel-psychiatrische benadering van J. Bastiaans, G.W. Arendsen Hein en C.H. van Rhijn*. Amsterdam: Candide, 2000.

Snelders, Stephen. "The LSD Therapy Career of Jan Bastiaans, M.D." In *Welten des Bewusstseins, Pränatale Psychologie und Psycholytische Therapie,* vol. 10, edited by Michael Schlichting, 135–41. Berlin: VWB, 2000.

Snelders, Stephen. "The Use of Psychedelics in Dutch Psychiatry 1950–1970: The Problem of Continuity and Discontinuity." *Curare* 18, no. 2 (1995): 415–425.

Snelders, Stephen, and Charles Kaplan. "LSD Therapy in Dutch Psychiatry: Changing Sociopolitical Settings and Cultural Sets." *Medical History* 46 (2002): 221–240.

Snelders, Stephen. "Het gebruik van psychedelische middelen in Nederland in de jaren zestig. Een hoofdstuk uit de sociale geschiedenis van druggebruik." *Tijdschrift voor Sociale Geschiedenis* 21(1995): 1, 37–60.

Stevens, Jay. *Storming Heaven: LSD and the American Dream*. New York: Grove Press, 1998.

Tasman, Coen. *Louter Kabouter. Kroniek van een beweging*. Amsterdam: Babylon-De Geus, 1996.

Van Bergen Leo. *Bevrijd. Het concentratiekampsyndroom en de LSD behandeling van Jan Bastiaans*. Nijmegen: QV Uitgeverij, 2022.

Van Ree, F. *LSD-25. Een experimenteel psychopathologisch onderzoek*. Deventer, Netherlands: Kluwer, 1966.

Van Reeuwijk, Dick P. J. *Damsterdamse extremisten*. Amsterdam: De Bezige Bij, 1965.

Van Rhijn, C. H. "Variables in Psycholytic Treatment." In *The Use of LSD in Psychotherapy and Alcoholism*, edited by H. A. Abramson 208–222. Indianapolis: Bobs-Merrill, 1967.

Van Weerlee, D. ed. *Allemaal rebellen: Amsterdam 1955–1965*. Amsterdam: Tabula, 1984.

Van Weerlee, D. ed. *Allemaal rebellen; Hans, het leven voor de dood. Een film van Louis van Gasteren*. Amsterdam, 1985.Vinkenoog, Simon. "Barbaren van het Leidseplein." *Twen* 1 (1960).

Vinkenoog, Simon. "A Rap on the High Road to Happiness." In *Counterculture: The Creation of an Alternative Society*, edited by Joseph Berke, 144–168. London: Peter Owen, 1969.

Vinkenoog, Simon. *Tegen de wet. Zes weken Huis van Bewaring, maart, april 1965*. Maasbree, Netherlands: Corrie Zelen, 1980.

Vinkenoog, Simon. *Timothy Leary magiër. Het ABZ van de psychedelische avant-garde*. Den Haag, Netherlands: Sijthof, 1972.

Vinkenoog, Simon. *Vogelvrij. Bouwstenen 1963–1967*. Amsterdam: De Bezige Bij, 1967.

Vinkenoog, Simon. *Weergaloos. Ontdekkingsreizen naar de waarheid* (Matchless: Voyages of discovery into truth). Hilversum, Netherlands: Paul Brand, 1968.

16 AMONG DOCTORS, ARTISTS, AND POLICE: THE HISTORY OF LSD IN BRAZIL

Henrique Carneiro and Júlio Delmanto

The history of LSD in Brazil, as in many countries, begins with its use in medicine and psychiatry and extends to the spheres of arts and culture, including 1960s counterculture, before finding itself embroiled in political and judicial domains through its regulation, prohibition, and persecution, aggravated, in the Brazilian case, by the peculiar conditions of a long military dictatorship (1964–1985).

LSD's history in Brazil during this time can be divided into two distinct phases: 1954–1964, characterized by its legal, medical (psychiatric), and then psychoanalytic use during a democratic regime, and the period from after 1964's military coup until 1985, when it became prohibited, giving rise to a clandestine supply network associated with countercultural movements. During this second phase, 1968 was a major turning point when, on December 9, the "coup within the coup", when military government by means of the AI-5 (Institutional Act 5), effectively closed the congress and strengthened the dictatorship that had started four years earlier. Under the military regime, the government fundamentally changed the drug laws by introducing equal criminal sanctions for users and traffickers, an unprecedented policy in Brazil that occurred, not by coincidence, during the era of the regime's greatest repressive violence.

INITIAL MEDICAL STUDIES

LSD initially arrived in Brazil at the end of the 1950s in psychiatrists' medical offices, which received it from the Swiss pharmaceutical company

Sandoz as free samples for experimental treatment of mental illnesses such as psychoses. In return, the pharmaceutical company only asked for data about any experiments using it in order to consolidate a model of medical application that would guarantee large-scale production and trade. Sandoz's international approach to LSD research necessarily makes the early history of LSD transnational in character.

The first scientific article published in Brazil on LSD's medicinal use appeared in 1954, in the *Jornal Brasileiro de Psiquiatria*, and was written by the psychiatrist Eustachio Portella Nunes Filho (1929–2020). Nunes Filho was born in the northwestern state of Piauí and had graduated with a medical degree from the Federal University of Rio de Janeiro one year before publishing his article. His article reports the effects in eight patients, which included diagnoses of hebephrenic schizophrenia, catatonic schizophrenia, manic-depressive psychosis, and alcoholism in the stage of delirium tremens. The reappearance of schizophrenia symptoms during their sessions in almost all but one of the patients caused Nunes Filho to conclude that LSD was "schizogenic."

In addition to these psychiatric patients, many other doctors engaged in self-experimentation or experimented with their colleagues, practices that were also typical in the US, Europe, and other South American countries such as Argentina and Chile. These researchers were enthusiastic about the potential applications of hallucination-causing drugs in their investigations of mental processes, consciousness, and creativity, not only in people with psychiatric disorders but in psychotherapy in general.

In this way, doctors, artists, and writers were part of the first wave of Brazilian LSD experimentation in the early 1960s, and their stories constitute a considerable amount of the primary sources available for investigating the drug's arrival in the country. This nonclinical experimentation allowed LSD to escape from the clinics, since some of the patients who experienced the drug later maintained their consumption, but no longer on a therapeutic basis. Some of these initial LSD-experimenting doctors included among their guinea pigs prominent Brazilian artists, such as the writers Paulo Mendes Campos and Clarice Lispector.

One of the most outstanding LSD practitioners was Murilo Pereira Gomes, who had dosed Campos and Lispector. We have few records of his work, but from a 2020 article by Elvia Bezerra,[1] we know that Gomes got his medical degree in 1954 in Recife, in the northeastern state of Pernambuco. He moved to Rio de Janeiro in 1957, where he worked as a psychiatrist until his early death in the mid-1960s. Gomes was part of a generation of pioneering psychiatrists in Brazil who studied and disseminated LSD for therapeutic purposes. His work gained media attention, and an article describing a meeting of psychiatrists in the 1960s records that he first used LSD himself in 1961, the year that he started using it with his patients.[2] He died in 1966, while undergoing cardiac surgery.

Along with Nunes Filho and Gomes, other Brazilian psychiatrists also worked with LSD. In 1961, Paulo Luiz Viana Guedes, the psychiatrist, musician, and founder of the Psychoanalytic Society of Porto Alegre, published an article in the journal *Arquivos de Neuro-Psiquiatria* reporting on LSD experiences with five patients. Summarizing his work, he described observing "the appearance, in an intensely dramatic way, of conflicting childhood situations and fantasies."[3]

In 1964, the year of the military coup, Clovis Martins (1920–2011) presented a thesis to ascend as a full professor in psychiatry at University of São Paulo Medical School, entitled "Psicose lisérgica: Psicopatologia da percepção do espaço, da percepção do tempo e da despersonalização" (*Lysergic Psychosis: Psychopathology of the Perception of Space, the Perception of Time and Depersonalization*). Martins describes research conducted in Brazil between 1958 and 1963 at an important public hospital in São Paulo. Another doctor, Jamil Almansur Haddad, translated the Argentinian researcher Alberto Fontana's studies on psychedelics and participated in a debate about psychedelics in the late1960s. Haddad wrote articles for the popular Brazilian periodical *O Pasquim* about LSD and other substances, and he even expressed public opposition to the highly popular military regime. Resistance to the military dictatorship resulted in severe consequences. For example, another doctor, Benedicto Arthur Sampaio, was arrested for his political combativeness in resisting the dictatorship. However, psychedelics had not yet permeated the political counterculture, and it was at his hospital in Santo André on São Paulo's outskirts, that his own pioneering psychiatric clinical experiments with LSD were carried out.

Martins criticized the psychotomimetic theory of psychedelics, which states that substances like LSD create a supposedly chemically induced psychosis (also reflected in Nunes Filho's term "schizogenic").

These early publications describe small sets of studies that aligned Brazilian psychedelic research with similar research emerging from abroad and attracted psychiatrists, psychoanalysts, and other thinkers curious about the relationship between altered states of consciousness and healing. However, beginning in 1964, Brazil's promising LSD research was cut short by the repressive military regime.

LSD AND PSYCHOANALYSIS AMONG WRITERS AND ARTISTS

In the Brazilian context, the most influential framework for therapeutic research with LSD was the psychoanalytic approach, especially among artists and intellectuals. In August 1962, in Rio de Janeiro, Gomes conducted an LSD experiment with the writer Paulo Mendes Campos, who later joined Gomes as important voices in the public debate on the medical use of psychedelics. Newspaper records indicate that these two men collaborated in lectures and debates on the topic.

Between November and December 1962, the magazine *Manchete* published a series of articles by Campos where he presented his ideas about an "intimate similarity" between LSD and schizophrenia. Psychoanalytic concepts are evident as he defined both as sources of "forgotten childhood experiences" and "old primitive images of the collective unconscious," such as the "archetype of the serpent." In his second piece, he summarized a report by the Argentinian doctors Alberto E. Fontana, Luísa de Alvarez Toledo, and Francisco Pérez Morales, who since 1956 had been experimenting with LSD on several patients in Buenos Aires. Their work, Campos wrote, resulted in "prenatal regression, in which he [the patient] has oceanic experiences of identity with the analyst (with the mother), with the cosmos, feeling at the height of omnipotence, outside of time and space."[4] For Fontana's group, however, the primary use of LSD for therapeutic purposes occurred mainly with facilitating the "transfer" between patient and analyst: the substance allowed for the breaking down of barriers and a deep investigation of traumas, which facilitated positive therapeutic outcomes. In 1969, Jamil Almansur Haddad translated the Fontana's Argentinian edition to portuguese.[5] Similarly, Cesário Morey Hossri, another physician working in São Paulo in the 1960s, employed LSD as an adjunct to the psychoanalytic technique of "intrauterine regression." In 1968, he published *Treinamento Autógeno e LSD* (Autogenic training and LSD), in which he promoted using LSD alongside hypnosis and intrauterine regression, the latter a technique developed in 1932 by the controversial German psychiatrist J. H. Schultz, a member of the Nazi Göring Institute. The book also includes a discussion of extrasensory perception and LSD and resulted from classes by the author in the Medical Associations of Santos and Santo André and in the Psychology Society of São Paulo.[6] In addition to Campos, a respected writer and poet prominent in Brazilian cultural public debates in the 1960s, Gomes treated several other artists, including the actors Fauzi Arap and Joana Fomm, the plastic artists Mário Gruber, Wesley Duke Lee, and Marcelo Grassman, and the writer Clarice Lispector, a major figure in the history of Brazilian literature.

Lispector tried LSD under Gomes's direction, in the company of Campos; she claimed that the LSD had no effects on her. This is remarkable, as she depicts a raw, narrative account of an altered state of consciousness in what many consider to be her greatest novel, *A Paixão Segundo G. H.* (The Passion According to G. H.), published in 1964. When staging excerpts from her novel in the theater for the first time, Lispector told the actor and director Fauzi Arap that she had felt absolutely nothing when she tried it, and she even offered to go buy sandwiches for the rest of the group. Arap wrote that "It took many years, and becoming his friend, for me to discover that the strong impression I had had that *The Passion According to G. H.* related a lysergic experience had not been gratuitous."[7]

Arap's 1998 autobiography *Mare Nostrum* focuses on his experiences with LSD, which started with Murilo Pereira Gomes in his psychiatric office in 1961 and continued underground in the 1970s. His book provides a compelling picture of the oppressive political climate of the time. Faced with the ruthless policies of a dictatorial regime, a younger part of the left turned to armed struggle, which developed into a cultural and social split between those pursuing active political resistance and those opting for a more personal break with society's dominant values.

In Arap's account, the LSD experience was associated with new intellectual influences emerging in the 1960s: spiritualism, Jungian psychology, astrology, Umbanda (an Afro-Brazilian religion), and mystical traditions, among them the Brazilian ayahuasca religions, especially the União do Vegetal. The psychiatrist Murilo Pereira Gomes also included elements of yoga and Zen Buddhism when referring to the psychedelic experience. This broad interpretative approach is characteristic of other adepts of LSD's medicinal use in Brazil in this early period. However, despite the variety of approaches and even political and philosophical positions in the medical community, there were other psychiatrists, such as Jamil Almansur Haddad and Cesário Morey Hossri, who were identified with extramedical, "alternative" practices, such as traditional healing techniques from China and India. Haddad employed hypnosis and Hossri included parapsychology in sessions. In this dependence on Eastern philosophies and alternative medical practices in psychedelic therapy, the Brazilian context shared much in common with the international phenomenon known as "counterculture."

BRAZILIAN COUNTERCULTURE

The historiography of postwar counterculture in Brazil situates this movement as part of the Global Sixties, but also draws attention to the national peculiarities of a peripheral country in the process of modernization under a dictatorship. These circumstances made the Brazilian counterculture more of a cultural phenomenon—affecting art, music, and popular forms of expression—than a political one.[8]

The military government promoted a modernization of national infrastructure that expanded the economy but rejected and repressed social and cultural characteristics inherent in the emancipatory values of modernity, such as the social movements of youth, women, artists, homosexuals, and black people. Thus, the link seen in other countries between modernization and modernism was severed, driving the Brazilian counterculture into a search for subjectivity, alternative communities, in some cases strongly individualist and libertarian, in defiance of the rationalization of daily life.

The Brazilian counterculture, therefore, distinguished itself from an American-style countercultural movement, which had a strong political component, due to the limitations created by a lack of democracy, and a left political movement that aligned itself with hostility toward drug experiences. Homosexuality was also a problematic issue among leftist movements, being part of the counterculture identity of a more open sexuality that not everyone on the left welcomed.[9] In addition, the urban middle and upper classes made up the bulk of countercultural activities, in a country that was until the late 1960s largely dominated by rural communities.[10]

In the cities, vanguard theatrical groups, especially the Teatro Oficina, led by José Celso Martinez Correa, included the use of LSD in their performances. In July 1971, its members were arrested for possession of marijuana in the city of Ouro Preto, along with the American stage duo Julian Beck and Judith Malina and several other members of the New York–based Living Theater.

Psychedelia also manifested in Brazilian cinema in the 1960s, in both explicit and subtle ways. Glauber Rocha, one of Brazil's most important directors in the 1960s and 1970s, evoked the trance of messianic traditions and the social *bandoleirismo* of the Brazilian northeast, in depictions of altered states of consciousness, but only personally came to experience LSD in 1971. Despite his antihippie rhetoric in interviews and public statements, Rocha's films spurred an ecstatic movement in Brazilian cinema, which was popular in Brazil's so-called marginal cinema, in which psychedelic aesthetics were used to depict themes of drug use, such as in the film *Meteorango Kid* (1969), directed by André Luiz de Oliveira.

LSD's significant influence in Brazilian cinema is also notable in Rocha's 1975 short film *Claro*, when while on location in Italy, Rocha and the actors took LSD together.[11] While he was personally open to psychedelic experimentation, his interests did not extend to the emancipatory politics seen in other countries. In an interview that same year, he accused the counterculture—"hippism, feminism, gay-powerism, psychoanalyticism, and ecology"—of aiming to "alienate popular consciousness from the main contradictions of society that are economic."[12]

A major figure in São Paulo's marginal cinema scene, José Mojica Marins, known as Zé do Caixão (Coffin Joe), directed the 1970 film *O Despertar da Besta* (The awakening of the beast), in which a psychiatrist appears to inject LSD into his patients to investigate their alleged "sexual perversions." While the psychiatrist manages to convince his patients that they're experiencing an LSD trip, the injection turns out to be a placebo. Famous for his low-budget horror films and his unusual persona, which included never cutting his nails, Zé do Caixão became a cult director in Brazilian cinema, producing countless films until his death in February 2020.

Perhaps even more significant than cinema to Brazil's early psychedelic history are music and poetry. Beginning in the early 1960s, a group of poets from São Paulo, as Roberto Piva and Claudio Willer, known as the "brand new generation," were responsible for some of the first translations of novels and poems by authors associated with the American Beat movement.[13] Like their cousins in the Northern Hemisphere, these poets made extensive use of drugs, including their practices as objects of some of their works.

However, despite being pioneers, these "brand new" poets came nowhere near the notoriety that writers like Allen Ginsberg, Jack Kerouac, and William Burroughs obtained in the US. By this criterion, it was not the writers and poets that would hold a decisive countercultural significance, but rather the Tropicalistas, a group of musicians and other artists who gravitated around the figures of the Bahians Caetano Veloso and Gilberto Gil, who lived in São Paulo and Rio de Janeiro before being exiled by the dictatorship.

In his 2009 book *Brutalidade Jardim* (Brutality garden), Cristopher Dunn defines tropicalism as "a cultural movement of short duration, but of great impact," which came to prominence in 1968. Dunn describes a movement that was primarily associated with popular music but reflected as a broad cultural phenomenon that found expressions in cinema, theater, visual arts, and literature.[14]

Tropicalism also had political objectives: to revolt against the military regime and its "conservative modernization," and to counteract the national populism dominant among the Brazilian left, which had even organized a march against the use of electric musical instruments. In December 1968, the country was experiencing a wave of renewed oppression by the military regime, with the promulgation of the notorious legislation AI-5, which resulted in systematic arrests, torture, and censorship.[15] Psychedelic drugs, especially LSD, contributed to creating countercultural scenes in several cities, many of which were targeted by political militancy and ultimately stifled by armed repression and censorship. However, there were still young people interested in other ways of living and doing politics who continued to experiment with psychedelic drugs. Notably, Rita Lee, an iconic Brazilian rock star associated with the tropicalism scene, later said in an interview that, "one can survive a dictatorship like the one in Brazil, only by taking a lot of LSD."[16]

The concept of a "social scene," referred to in anthropology as "ethnocenology," helps to capture a phenomenon that appeared in some Brazilian cities at this exact moment of political oppression. [17] In 1971, psychedelic scenes begin to appear as LSD reached the broader swaths of youth from the middle and upper classes. This moment coincided with the toughest period of the dictatorship, characterized by a particularly acute persecutory context for those experimenting with illicit drugs. The formation of psychedelic scenes in Brazil was associated with the global hippie culture adapted in different ways to the Brazilian reality.

Psychedelic drugs had varying impacts on Brazilian musicians. The prominent musician and political activist Gilberto Gil stated in an interview that marijuana "gave me a lot of fluency, the perception of intricacies, nuances and chromatic sounds. And I would say semiotic fluency too, in terms of words and such." Regarding LSD, he said that "the acid trip did not give me the same openness of perception as marijuana. Marijuana is very musical. The acid led to a world of fantasies, mental images, interventions in the sense of reality."[18]

In São Paulo, the musician Raul Seixas and his songwriting partner (and later a writer of international prominence), Paulo Coelho, became famous for promoting an "alternative society." Seixas, although he consumed alcohol and cocaine, said: "I never took LSD, and I would never take it. I'm scared to death. My business is black-and-white film. I don't like color film."[19] Paulo

Coelho, on the other hand, describes his first time trying LSD in 1971, in Spain, in his 2018 book *Hippie*. Both Seixas and Coelho were arrested and tortured during two weeks in 1974 by the political police.[20]

LSD AS A POLICING AND LEGAL MATTER

In 1965, in response to pressure mainly from the US government and the first steps in its disastrous "war on drugs," the Swiss pharmaceutical firm Sandoz stopped producing and legally distributing LSD. However, young people in the counterculture were already obtaining LSD from other sources. Scientific researchers seeking legitimate supplies were left with no alternatives. In 1968, the Brazilian government introduced even tighter controls through a more restrictive set of laws, not only against experiment and research, but by effectively banning public debate around these substances, whether in the press or in artworks.

This moment of prohibition had consolidated government and regulatory efforts that began in the mid-1960s that depicted LSD as an especially dangerous drug. The new laws introduced a provision that allowed the prosecution of individuals involved in LSD use, whether production, distribution, or consumption. The first person to be charged for possession and trafficking of LSD was the artist Antonio Peticov in January 1970. That year also marked a high point in modern Brazilian nationalism, when the Brazilian soccer team, led by the iconic Pelé, won the World Cup in Mexico for an unprecedented third time. This achievement happened during a moment of significant propaganda by the military government that extolled its authoritarian, nationalist, and conservative policies. While the country's economic indexes grew, supported by foreign loans, the average Brazilian's wages fell while the cost of living rose. Unbeknownst to most urban dwellers, large projects in rural areas, such as roads and hydroelectric plants, devastated the environment, reflecting policies that effectively aimed at Indigenous genocide. So while the national soccer team's accomplishment portrayed Brazil as a winning nation, the average rural Brazilian experienced much loss.

From that period on, the press began publishing sensational accounts of the dangers of LSD. In January 1970, the newspaper *O Estado de São Paulo* featured the headline: "LSD traz agente do FBI ao país" (LSD brings FBI agent to the country) reporting on an alleged investigation of a Miami–Rio de Janeiro LSD smuggling route. It was early days, and Brazil's primary technical expertise body, the Institute of Forensics, did not have the technical capacity to test the substance.[21]

The allure of psychedelic stories in Brazil is reflected in the 1972 publication of *LSD: Alucinógenos e a Lei* (LSD: Hallucinogens and law), written by Geraldo Gomes, the judge who presided over Peticov's LSD case. Gomes's book reviews the literature and theories that attempt to explain the peculiarities of this new drug, and it concludes by condemning the substance in all its uses, even arguing that LSD was capable of causing "addiction," although this was not reflected in the pertinent legislation. The laws introduced by the dictatorship in 1968 created the legal space for this type of selective interpretation, by grouping together substances that cause "physical or psychic dependence" as susceptible to prohibition. The selective invocation of this clause is clear, given the omission of alcohol, tobacco, and other common drugs sold in drugstores.

Judge Gomes based his decision in the Peticov case on a purely moral argument.[22] In his legal opinion, he describes some of the defendants as "misfits," "depressed," and "losers" due to their alleged drug use, and praises family values and female virginity. In addition, case records in this instance, as well as other sources, reveal evidence of physical and psychological torture of the defendants (and even some witnesses) during all the stages of legal proceedings. Judge Gomes's condemnatory sentence of Peticov of one year, eleven months, and twenty-four days in prison exemplifies how the Brazilian judiciary handled these cases; not only did Gomes ignore allegations of torture made by the defense lawyers, but he dismissed their relevance by reasoning that if torture had occurred, such abuse would not void the validity of the police evidence. That the ends would justify the means was an official government position.

Another victim of this LSD witch hunt was the journalist Lucy Dias. In her 2004 memoir, *Enquanto Corria a Barca* (While the Boat Was Running), Dias recounts being arrested for possession of LSD in São Paulo in March 1971 and her subsequent torture by police. The government's National Security Law gave police wide latitude to carry out such actions.

Just how wide a latitude is reflected in the case of the police officer Angelino Moliterno, who arrested Peticov and six other defendants. Born in 1924 and known by his nickname Russinho, he was an investigator with São Paulo's Civil Police force in the 1950s. In the 1960s, he joined both the narcotics unit and a special unit responsible for the violent repression of organizations and militants among the Brazilian left. He was a prominent figure within the so-called death squads, groups of corrupt police officers who executed people for money or revenge, and he later became involved in São Paulo's underground drug and illegal gambling scene.[23] In 1971, eight police officers involved in the execution of three people were fired. Among them was Moliterno, who, expelled from the police, spent approximately a year in prison before being acquitted by a jury, just like the others, in the late 1970s.[24]

It can be a challenge to determine exactly what happened during Brazil's military dictatorship, in force from 1964 until 1985. In 2011, President Dilma Roussef established a National Truth Commission to piece together the innumerable gaps in information and documentation during this period. Its final report, delivered in 2014, lists the names of those murdered and disappeared, and in some cases, it also names the perpetrators of these state-sanctioned crimes. Moliterno's name is there, having been identified by several informants as a torturer.

Brazil's war on drugs implicated police in mafia-related crimes and enforcing dictatorial security measures largely with impunity. Under these persecutory conditions, LSD was targeted and seized by the police, which along with other illicit drugs was associated with a supposed strategy of the international communist movement to corrupt youth.[25] This association is ironic, as almost all the genuine communists in the country were puritans against drug use of any kind. The military regime had disseminated the conspiracy theory of leftist drug dependence to cast them as antisocial activists working against the good of the country. A confidential document in 1973 produced by the National Information Service stated that "drug addiction" was "one of the most subtle and sinister weapons in the varied arsenal of the International Communist Movement . . . in its continuous and surreptitious striving for the dominion of the world and the slavery of mankind."[26]

The historian Antonio Brito has recently shown how "drug addiction as a communist strategy is out of step with memories and works that indicate that the communists and the left had a severe attitude towards the use of drugs, associating them with escape, alienation and desbunde [dropping out]."[27] Despite this significant aversion to illicit drug use, Brazil's counter-culture was nevertheless seen as "a ruse created by Soviet communism," and the "hippies would have been created by Moscow."[28]

Reports about drug use in the press were similarly sensationalized; Brito (2021) notes that "the authorities qualified the problem of toxics and narcotics in Brazil as of the same seriousness as the elimination of terrorism."[29] These reports were mirrored in official documents produced by high-level governing bodies, including the Aeronautics Information Center's 1972 text "Drug Addiction and National Security," written by the psychiatrist A. C. Pacheco e Silva.[30] Similarly, in 1981, the army published an internal document titled "Toxins and Corruption as an Instrument of Subversion," in which it characterizes the figure of an "ideological drug dealer."[31]

In a state of dictatorial exception, with the increasing policing of morals and everyday life, LSD no longer had space to be the experimental psychiatric drug it had been. Its use was brutally repressed and served as a pretext for a specter of moral panic: communists handing out drugs in order to politically subvert young people.

CONCLUSION

The psychiatrist Murilo Gomes, the judge Geraldo Gomes, and the police officer Angelino Moliterno represent significant characters involved in the arrival of LSD in Brazil, and yet their stories reveal very different aspects of this history. Beginning with its medical use in the 1950s, LSD and other psychedelics grew to have a relatively significant impact among artists and intellectuals before being violently maligned and repressed in the early 1970s. Brazil's psychedelic history is not just a site of the burgeoning war on drugs of this period; rather, it happened in the context of a military dictatorship that beginning in late 1968 wielded political violence to repress psychedelics and their users, whether real or alleged. Emblematic of this persecution were the changes to Brazil's drug laws that same year, which for the first time equated possession and trafficking with consumption.

As in many other countries, Brazilian doctors received LSD free of charge from Sandoz, which was looking for psychiatric research and possible future commercial application for the substance. This all changed following its categorization as an illegal drug and Brazil's ratification of an international treaty, the Convention on Psychotropic Substances, in 1971. But, unlike other countries, Brazilians experienced psychedelics in the atmosphere of a dictatorship in which policemen like Moliterno, a typical product of the Brazilian repression apparatus, with its origins and brutal practices rooted in colonialism and slavery, became agents of an arbitrary and violent drug enforcement policy.

It does not appear that the doctor Murilo Gomes, the judge Geraldo Gomes, and the police officer Moliterno knew each other, nor did they run in the same social circles, but their trajectories intersect in Brazil's LSD history, which is yet to be fully documented and has only recently begun to be studied. This history involved doctors, artists, judges, police, and smugglers. In doctors' offices, hospitals, and laboratories, LSD was a legal therapeutic remedy for a time. In prisons and in courts, on the other hand, LSD use could be fatal. In the press and the arts, association with LSD could result in the tragic consequences of repression and surveillance.

Although LSD's trajectory is marked by the international context, its particular arrival, diffusion, and repression in Brazil involved significant local characteristics. A most notable example was the military dictatorship, with its violent and corrupt practices that affected not only politics, but also police, justice, culture, and media across the country. Furthermore, there are significant differences between the Cold War and capitalist context of the US and the context of Brazil's authoritarian modernization, which aspired to rapidly develop national industry and boost Brazil's international standing. However, in this effort, the country became subordinate to foreign capital, and the cultural, educational, and material development of the poorest classes was neglected. When the military dictatorship finally gave way to civilian democracy in 1985, at the end of a long, negotiated transition, the country was more unequal and in debt than ever.

Another interesting difference between LSD in Brazil and in the US and Europe, regarding both its counterculture and medicinal uses, is the time delay between what happened outside and inside the country. While LSD in the US began in 1949 with the experiments of the psychiatrist Max Rinkel, in Brazil, similar studies first began appearing in the mid-1950s. Similarly, in relation to its countercultural use and its subsequent repression, we also see that although very similar in some aspects, psychedelics in Brazil are some years behind the US and Europe. While the US counterculture becomes visible between 1963 and 1965, with Timothy Leary and Richard Alpert's 1963 departure from Harvard, Brazil's tropicalism movement begins fostering hippie aesthetics only in 1968, and the first lawsuit for LSD trafficking takes place only in 1970. In a decade, from its use as a potential treatment in psychiatry and psychology, LSD became an influential drug in artistic and intellectual circles, and later, part of a more diffuse Brazilian popular counterculture.

It is difficult to quantify the scale of LSD use in Brazil. There is no data on the quantities of legal shipments of LSD by Sandoz to Brazil. Post-Sandoz, there are no estimates of the volume of LSD circulating in the country owing to its being supplied through clandestine domestic producers and international smugglers. The magnitude of clandestine manufacturing, for obvious reasons, also remains unknown. Police statistics of LSD-related apprehensions provide possibly valuable evidence, but a statistical analysis of LSD consumption statistics remains elusive. In the later era of raves and Internet culture, at the end of the twentieth century, its use had become widespread, alongside MDMA and other synthetic substances. The emergence of MDMA in Brazil is described by Ann and Alexander Shulgin in their book *TIHKAL* (1997), in a chapter called "The Brazil Caper," where they recount coming to Rio de Janeiro in the late 1980s, after the end of the dictatorship, to produce MDMA for a group of doctors and businessmen. Brazil's psychedelic counterculture also formed around psilocybin mushrooms and ayahuasca, which probably supplied a much larger volume of substances available for the formation of the psychedelic scene.

Brazilian ayahuasca religions have been an important contribution to the psychedelic revival of the twenty-first century, even though most practitioners in Brazil do not recognize themselves as users of "psychedelics." It was, however, the legalization of the religious use of ayahuasca in 1992 that helped reduce LSD's stigma as a cursed and dangerous drug. The similarity of the effects of DMT, ayahuasca's psychoactive ingredient, and LSD also helped to legitimize the beneficial potential of both drugs in religious or psychotherapeutic contexts remerging in scientific research.

As with other countries in this moment, Brazil is seeing increasing interest in psychedelic topics, most recently reflected in the journalist Marcelo Leite's 2021 publication *Psiconautas: Viagens com a ciência psicodélica brasileira* (Psychonauts: Trips in Brazilian Psychedelic Science), which compiles Brazilian research on drugs such as ayahuasca, MDMA, LSD, ibogaine, and psilocybin. Also recently, Brazil has seen its first double-blind LSD studies since the 1960s, with twenty-four healthy volunteers participating in trials at Unicamp (the University of Campinas). The results of this study were published in July 2021, and its authors concluded that "the LSD state resembles a psychotic experience and offers a tool for healing. The link between psychosis model and therapeutic model seems to lie in mystical experiences. The results point to the importance of meaning attribution for the LSD psychosis model and indicate that psychedelic-assisted therapy might benefit from therapeutic suggestions fostering mystical experiences."[32]

After decades of repression, Brazil is reassessing LSD and other psychedelics as potential psychotherapeutic remedies, and even as tools for cognitive freedom. In so doing, they are finally picking up a thread of curiosity and inquiry that had been broken under the country's dictatorial regime.

NOTES

This chapter summarizes research described in Julio Delmanto's 2018 doctoral thesis in history, supervised by Dr. Henrique S. Carneiro at the University of São Paulo, and published in 2020: Júlio Delmanto, *História Social do LSD no Brasil* (São Paulo: Elefante, 2020). https://teses.usp.br/teses/disponiveis/8/8138/tde-11122018-161707/pt-br.php.

1. Elvia Bezerra, "Cadernos do LSD: Paulo Mendes Campos," *Instituto Moreira Salles*, December 14, 2020. https://ims.com.br/por-dentro-acervos/caderno-do-lsd-paulo-mendes-campos-por-elvia-bezerra/.

2. Murilo Pereira Gomes, "Configurações de uma psicoterapia com o uso do LSD 25," *A Folha Médica* 46, no. 2 (February 1963).

3.   Delmanto, *História Social do LSD no Brasil*, 235.

4.   Paulo Mende Campos, Apud Elvia Bezerra, "Cadernos do LSD: Paulo Mendes Campos," *Instituto Moreira Salles*, December 14, 2020. https://ims.com.br/por-dentro-acervos/caderno -do-lsd-paulo-mendes-campos-por-elvia-bezerra/.

5.   Alberto Fontana et alli, Psicoterapia com LSD e outros alucinógenos, tradução Jamil Almansur Haddad, São Paulo, Editoria Mestre Jou, 1969.

6.   Cesário Morey Hossri, *Prática do Treinamento Autógeno & LSD*, São Paulo: Editora Mestre Jou, 1968.

7.   Fauzi Arap, Mare Nostrum, São Paulo: Editora Senac, 1998, p. 71, "Foram precisos muitos anos, e ter me tornado seu amigo, para descobrir que a forte impressão que eu tivera de que A paixão segundo G. H. relatava uma experiência lisérgica não havia sido nada gratuita."

8.   On the history of conterculture in Brazil, see Sheyla Castro Diniz; *Desbundados e marginais: MPB e contracultura nos Anos de Chumbo* (Campinas, Brazil: Unicamp, 2017); Cesar Augusto de Carvalho, *Viagem ao mundo alternativo: a contracultura nos 80* (São Paulo: Edunesp, 2008); Christopher Dunn, *Brutalidade Jardim* (São Paulo: Unesp, 2009); Marco Alexandre Capellari, *O discurso da contracultura no Brasil: o underground através de Luiz Carlos Maciel* (São Paulo: University of São Paulo, 2007); Cláudio Novaes Pinto Coelho, *A transformação social em questão: as práticas sociais alternativas durante o regime militar* (São Paulo: University of São Paulo, 1990); Carlos Alberto Messeder Pereira, *O que é contracultura?* (São Paulo: Brasiliense, 1984).

9.   About homosexuality and politics in Brazil, see James Naylor Green, *Beyond Carnival: Male Homosexuality in Twentieth-Century in Brazil* (Chicago: University of Chicago Press, 2001).

10. The evolution of drug policies in the broad political space of the Brazilian left since the 1960s was analyzed in Julio Delmanto, *Camaradas Caretas* (Straight comrades) (São Paulo: Alameda, 2015).

11. Ivonete Pinto, "Memórias de um Glauber muito louco," Cinema Escrito, November 2, 2020. https://www.cinemaescrito.com/2020/11/44a-mostra-de-sp-2020-glauber-claro/.

12. Glauber Rocha: "A partir de 1968 . . . o fenômeno da 'contra-cultura' tentacular . . . nas [nações] subdesenvolvidas, hipismo, feminismo, gaypowerismo, psicanalismo, ecologia . . . tem como objetivo alienar a consciência popular das contradições principais da sociedade que são econômicas." "Glauber em Paulo Francis," *Revista Status*, São Paulo, março de 1975, p. 17.

13. Delmanto, *História Social do LSD no Brasil* (São Paulo: Elefante, 2020).

14. Christopher Dunn, *Brutalidade Jardim*, São Paulo: Editora Unesp, 2009. "Tropicália, um movimento cultural de curta duração, mas de grande impacto, que se consolidou em 1968" p.17; "A Tropicália foi um movimento cultural articulado priordialmente na música popular, mas com significativas manifestações em outros campos artísticos", p.142.

15. The institutional acts were made to legally formalizedictatorial measures to increase repression, close the Congress and arrest members of the regime's opposition.

16. Luis Freitas Branco "Rita Lee: Para sobreviver a uma ditadura como a que houve no Brasil só tomando muito LSD," *Observador*, July 8, 2017. https://observador.pt/especiais/entrevista-autobiografia-rita-lee/.

17. Christine Greiner and Armindo Bião, *Etnocenologia: Textos Selecionados* (São Paulo: Annablume, 1999).

18. Sérgio Cohn (org.), *Gilberto Gil. Encontros* (Rio de Janeiro: Beco do Azougue, 2007, 278–279).

19. Apud Lucy Dias, *Anos 70. Enquanto corria a barca* (São Paulo: Editora Senac, 2004, p.156).

20. Coelho's 1988 novella *O Alquimista* (The alchemist) is the best-selling and most translated book by a Brazilian writer of all time.

21. Delmanto, *História Social do LSD no Brasil*, 289.

22. Delmanto, *História Social do LSD no Brasil*, 363.

23. Delmanto, *História Social do LSD no Brasil*, 302.

24. "Quem é quem no enfumaçado submundo do jogo." Antônio Carlos Fon. *Jornal da República*, São Paulo, edição 58, 1979.

25. Antonio Maurício Freitas Brito, "A droga da subversão: Anticomunismo e juventude no tempo da ditadura," *Revista Brasileira de História* 41, no. 86 (2021): 45. https://www.scielo.br/j/rbh/a/NQnHQgpdRHwmnfQymwbvh9z/#.

26. Brito, "A droga da subversão," 40." Uma das mais sutis e sinistras armas do variado arsenal do Movimento Comuista internacional (. . .) em sua busca contínua e subreptícia pela dominação do mundo e escravidão da humanidade (Ministério da Justiça, 1973)."

27. Brito, "A droga da subversão," 42. "A toxicomania como estratégia comunista está em descompasso commemórias e trabalhos que indicam que os comunistas e a esquerda tinham uma atitude severa e/ou depreciativam o uso de drogas, associando-as à fuga, à alienação e ao desbunde."

28. Leon Frederico Kaminski, "O movimento hippie nasceu em Moscou": imaginário anticomunista, contracultura e repressão no Brasil dos anos 1970 (Antíteses, v.9, n.18, 2017: 467); Brito, "A droga da subversão."

29. Brito, "A droga da subversão," 46.

30. Brito, "A droga da subversão," 49.

31. Brito, "A droga da subversão," 55.

32. Isabel Wießner, Marcelo Falchi, Fernanda Palhano-Fontes, Amanda Feilding, Sidarta Ribeiro, Sidarta, and Luiz Fernando Tófoli, "LSD, Madness and Healing: Mystical Experiences as Possible Link between Psychosis Model and Therapy Model," *Psychology Medicine* (July 2021): 1–15. https://doi.org/10.1017/S0033291721002531.

BIBLIOGRAPHY

Bezerra, Elvia. "Cadernos do LSD: Paulo Mendes Campos." Instituto Moreira Salles, December 14, 2020. https://ims.com.br/por-dentro-acervos/caderno-do-lsd-paulo-mendes-campos-por-elvia-bezerra/.

Branco, Luis Freitas. "Rita Lee: Para sobreviver a uma ditadura como a que houve no Brasil só tomando muito LSD." *Observador*, July 8, 2017. https://observador.pt/especiais/entrevista-autobiografia-rita-lee/.

Brito, Antonio Mauricio Freitas. "A droga da subversão: Anticomunismo e juventude no tempo da ditadura1." *Revista Brasileira de História* 41 (2021): 39–65.

Capellari, Marco Alexandre. *O discurso da contracultura no Brasil: o underground através de Luiz Carlos Maciel.* São Paulo: University of São Paulo, 2007.

Carlos, Fon Antônio. "Quem é quem no enfumaçado submundo do jogo." *Jornal da República* 58 (1979).

Coelho, Cláudio Novaes Pinto. *A transformação social em questão: as práticas sociais alternativas durante o regime militar.* São Paulo: University of São Paulo, 1990.

Cohn, Sérgio (org.) *Gilberto Gil: Encontros.* Rio de Janeiro: Beco do Azougue, 2007.

de Carvalho, Cesar Augusto. *Viagem ao mundo alternativo: a contracultura nos anos 80.* São Paulo: Edunesp, 2006.

Delmanto, Júlio. *Camaradas Caretas* (Straight comrades). São Paulo: Alameda, 2015.

Delmanto, Júlio. *História social do LSD no Brasil: os primeiros usos medicinais e o começo da repressão.* São Paulo: Editora Elefante, 2020. https://teses.usp.br/teses/disponiveis/8/8138/tde-11122018-161707/pt-br.php.

Dias, Apud Lucy. *Anos 70. Enquanto corria a barca.* São Paulo: Editora Senac, 2004.

Diniz, Sheyla Castro. *Desbundados e marginais: MPB e contracultura nos Anos de Chumbo.* Campinas, Brazil: Unicamp, 2017.

Dunn, Christopher. *Brutalidade Jardim.* São Paulo: Unesp, 2009.

Fontana, Alberto et alli. *Psicoterapia com LSD e outros alucinógenos.* tradução Jamil Almansur Haddad, São Paulo, Editoria Mestre Jou, 1969.

Gomes, Murilo Pereira. "Configurações de uma psicoterapia com o uso do LSD 25." *A Folha Médica* 46, no. 2 (February 1963).

Green, James N. *Beyond Carnival: Male Homosexuality in Twentieth-Century Brazil.* Chicago: University of Chicago Press, 1999.

Greiner, Christine, and Armindo Bião. *Etnocenologia: Textos Selecionados.* São Paulo: Annablume, 1999.

Hossri, Cesário Morey. *Prática do Treinamento Autógeno & LSD.* São Paulo: Editora Mestre Jou, 1968.

Kaminski, Leon Frederico. "O movimento hippie nasceu em Moscou: imaginário anticomunista, contracultura e repressão no Brasil dos anos 1970." *Antíteses* 9, no. 18 (2016): 467–493.

Pereira, Carlos Alberto Messeder. *O que é contracultura?* São Paulo: Brasiliense, 1984.

Pinto, Ivonete. "Memórias de um Glauber muito louco." Cinema Escrito, November 2, 2020. https://www.cinemaescrito.com/2020/11/44a-mostra-de-sp-2020-glauber-claro/.

Rocha, Glauber. "Glauber em Paulo Francis." São Paulo: *Revista Status* março de 1975, p.13–17.

Wießner, Isabel, Marcelo Falchi, Fernanda Palhano-Fontes, Amanda Feilding, Sidarta Ribeiro, Sidarta, and Luiz Fernando Tófoli. "LSD, Madness and Healing: Mystical Experiences as Possible Link between Psychosis Model and Therapy Model." *Psychology Medicine*, (July 2021): 1–15. https://doi.org/10.1017/S0033291721002531.

17 PSYCHEDELICS IN ISRAEL: A BRIEF HISTORY

Ido Hartogsohn and Itamar Zadoff

As of 2021, Israel is positioned at the forefront of a global revival of psychedelic research and culture. The small Middle Eastern country hosts clinical trials with psychedelics, generates multiple psychedelic start-ups, and hosts a pioneering psychedelic therapy training program. Popular interest in psychedelics is surging throughout the country as well, with multiple conferences, podcasts, magazines, and online communities dedicated to the subject. This vibrant scene reflects the radical transformations underwent by the formerly conservative and socialist country over the past half-century as it grew increasingly receptive to global influences.

This chapter examines the growth and evolution of psychedelic culture in Israel, showing how historical and sociocultural conditions molded the reception of psychedelics into Israeli society. It focuses on the period between 1960–2000, when psychedelics first appeared in Israel, concluding with the rapid evolution and growth of the psychedelic scene there since the turn of the millennium.

This research contributes to a nascent but growing body of literature that provides global perspectives on psychedelics by portraying how the political, ethnic, and sociocultural dynamics of Israeli society produced a distinct psychedelic culture mixing both global and local trends. It thereby provides a compelling example for the sociocultural embeddedness of psychedelics.

EARLY EXPERIMENTS WITH PSYCHEDELICS
IN 1960s ISRAEL

Israel's foundation in 1948 was the crowning achievement of the Zion-ist movement, a nationalist Jewish renewal campaign that emerged in nineteenth-century Europe, advocating for the "return" of the Jews to their biblical homeland. The intensity of antisemitism in the nineteenth and twentieth centuries, culminating in the Holocaust, catalyzed the success of Zionism, which promised an old-new homeland where the Jewish people would be free of persecution. Zionist settlement in Palestine, however, was riddled with violent confrontations with the native Palestinian population, which viewed the Zionist project as colonialist and racist.

At the center of the Zionist project stood an ambition to mold a new Jewish identity. Unlike the rootless diaspora Jews, the new Jews proudly worked the land and defended their new borders. Values of agrarianism, socialism, and military strength were central in the country's first decades of existence.[1] By the end of the twentieth century, however, the country had opened itself up to global currents promoting Western liberal values and a post-Zionist perspective.[2] This perspective, nevertheless, competed with other religious, nationalist, and ethnocentric forces within Israeli society. Like much else, this intricate interplay of both global and local forces has shaped the reception of psychedelics in Israeli society and culture.[3]

Psychedelics first appeared in modern Israel as psychiatric drugs. During the 1960s, two Israeli psychiatric institutions engaged in psychedelic research and therapy: the Geha Mental Health Center in Petah-Tikva just east of Tel Aviv, and the Talbieh Psychiatric Hospital in Jerusalem.

A 1960 paper by the psychiatrists Henricus Wijsenbeek and Ruth Lan-dau detailed an LSD trial conducted at the Geha Center,[4] briefly surveying the experimental use of LSD, which they described as a psychotomimetic or psychosis-inducing drug.[5] The investigators explored the drug's thera-peutic potential, offering it on multiple occasions to ten patients diagnosed with diverse medical conditions including schizophrenia, neurosis, depres-sion, anxiety, and hysteria. They concluded that LSD exacerbated psychotic symptoms in schizophrenics, but they were impressed with its effectiveness in treating neurosis.

The same year, David Karsilovsky published about LSD experimentation at Talbieh Psychiatric Hospital in *Medical Pages*, a bimonthly journal published by the Israeli Labor Union (Histradrut Haovdim Beretz-Israel).[6] Karsilovsky warned against simply equating the "LSD psychosis" with schizophrenia—a position that echoed prevalent discussions in psychotomimetic psychiatry in this period.[7] Karsilovsky's subjects included psychotic patients, epileptics, and healthy volunteers (who were medical students). The psychiatrist kept the setting as natural as possible, allowing the subjects to write, draw, lie down, or sit as they wished, and found the drug's effects to depend on the personality of the participants and their specific experimental situations.

The use of LSD for therapy at the Talbieh Psychiatric Hospital continued during the early to mid-1960s. The story of the Israeli poet Yona Wallach (1944–1985), who was hospitalized in Talbieh in 1965, illustrates the transition from psychiatric uses of psychedelics (which were soon discontinued) to their emergence outside the clinic. Much like elsewhere, psychedelics attracted cultural figures. Wallach's experience at Talbieh produced the first Israeli psychedelic cultural artifact.

An icon of twentieth-century Israeli poetry, Wallach is known as the enfant terrible of Israeli literature. In 1965, the young poet admitted herself into the Talbieh Psychiatric Hospital, reporting hallucinations and horrible, homicidal impulses. She was diagnosed as exceptionally creative but unruly and suffering from compulsive anxieties, hallucinations, and substance abuse disorder.[8]

Wallach later admitted that she had hospitalized herself out of curiosity for drugs: "I had a book about drugs, and I thought I'd take drugs there. . . . I had a doctor there that did me a favor and performed all sorts of drug experiments with me. Anything I wanted."[9] Marcel Asael, a psychiatrist at the hospital, eagerly helped and was fascinated by the young, unconventional, and exceedingly bright patient. Wallach's first experience with LSD, described in the journalist Igal Sarna's biography of her, began beatific and became horrific. The poet received 100 μg of LSD. Soon, she glanced out the window and was moved to tears by the beauty of it all. Later, however, she opened a tap and saw blood coming out, cascading over the sink and towels. Looking out the window again, she now saw a guillotine and became convinced that she was about to be decapitated for an unknown crime.[10] Wallach continued her experimentations with LSD and other drugs during her three-month stay at the hospital. She later described these LSD experiences as "wonderful";[11] however, her best-known poem on the subject, "If you go tripping on LSD," is overwhelmingly grim.

During the 1960s, the literary scene was liberating itself from the collectivist and nationalist discourse that dominated Israeli literature.[12] Writers embraced a growing willingness to explore subjective experience, which bred new pharmacoliterary encounters. The modernist David Avidan (1934–1995), considered one of the three big poets of Israel's state-founding generation, also experimented with LSD. In 1967, he went on an extended LSD trip (involving multiple ingestions amounting to about 400 μg), accompanied by a dictaphone that he used to document the events of his trip. These recordings were later transcribed in the book *Personal Report on an LSD Trip*, published in 1968.[13]

Avidan's account showed awareness of the American psychedelic scene by referencing Timothy Leary and the US counterculture, but it was critical of the unbridled hippie enthusiasm for the drug. One potential application that the author suggested was to use LSD for military purposes. LSD, he argued, could be given to generals to orchestrate their minds together and produce superior military performance; indeed, the book evinced a bellicose spirit. A recurring theme was Avidan's attempt to overcome the effects of LSD using the power of language. He portrays his mind as a battlefield between the disorienting, ominous forces of the feminine "drug array" and the discerning, control-oriented forces of the masculine "verbal array." Battling the psychedelic effects with all his manly and poetic might, Avidan resisted the LSD experience rather than surrender to it. His psycholiterary experiment, therefore, feels botched. As the literary critic Nadav Neuman recently has written: "If we were to examine the result based on the poet's ability to 'overpower' the drug and produce coherent poems carrying Avidanic poesy, the result is a resounding defeat for Avidan at the hands of the drug array. In fact, it is difficult to call the fragments in 'Personal report on an LSD Trip' poems. These are better characterized as schizophrenically

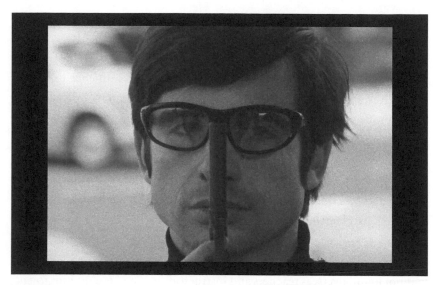

Figure 17.1
David Avidan, in a still from the movie *Everything Is Possible*, 1969.
The Lotam-Avidan family collection.

tinged murmurs and fragments of interesting ideas incessantly diverted by bizarre associations."[14] Misguided and flawed as it may be, the book nevertheless remains a landmark in the cultural reception of psychedelics in 1960s Israel.

BIRTH OF AN ISRAELI COUNTERCULTURE

In the summer of 1967, the psychedelic movement reached international cultural prominence. In Israel, the period coincided with a war that changed the history of Israel and the Middle East. On June 5, 1967, after months of escalating tensions, Israel embarked on an extraordinarily successful military campaign. In less than a week, it defeated and seized control over territories formerly belonging to Egypt, Syria, and Jordan, including the old city of Jerusalem, the Temple Mount, and other biblical holy sites. While Americans allegedly bathed in a "summer of love," for Israelis this period led to a swell of national pride and messianic dreams. The young country was suddenly a regional power enjoying international admiration.[15]

This military success expedited the percolation of international liberalizing influences, including that of the hippie movement. "After the Six-Day war, proud soldiers traveled to Europe like backpackers today travel to India and Thailand. It was a cultural shock that would influence us for our entire lives, releasing us from the Israeli khaki uniform to colors we didn't know, the psychedelia of King's Road and Cranberry Street," writes the Israeli author and songwriter Yehonatan Geffen (1947–).[16] Young international volunteers—many of them hippies—traveled to Israel from Europe and North America carrying countercultural ideas, pulling the young country out of its former isolation, and ushering in a torrent of Western, liberalizing, and often psychedelic elements. Drugs like hashish, formerly condemned, suddenly appealed to Israeli bohemia.[17] "It is doubtful whether the average Israeli would have been tempted to indulge in a psychedelic experience if he had not found overseas teachers and instructors who had taught him to take full advantage of [these drugs]," noted one observer.[18]

Two prominent bohemian groups were active in Tel Aviv during the late 1960s and early 1970s, whose psychedelic use presents interesting counterpoints. The Lul Group consisted of culturally prominent filmmakers, songwriters, and musicians (e.g., Arik Einstein, Uri Zohar, Shalom Hanoch, and Boaz Davidson) who produced an impressive flow of iconic films, television shows, and albums. Its members came predominantly from the cohorts of Israeli Defense Force (IDF) bands that dominated Israeli music until the 1970s, and they embodied the iconic figure of the *Sabra*, the new, locally bred Israeli: proud, self-confident, and cheeky.[19] The group was a culturally updated version of the Israeli institution of the *chevre*, a term that dates to preindependence Zionist pioneers and paramilitary groups like the Palmach and connotes intimate group camaraderie and cheerful fooling around.[20]

In the early 1970s, members of Lul presented classic Palmach-style *chevre* humor with a psychedelic tinge on Israeli TV programs that became instant classics. Inspired by Bob Dylan, the Beatles, and Pink Floyd, Lul members integrated psychedelic elements into Israeli music and culture, mixing them with distinct local flavors. The group occasionally promoted countercultural ideals but stopped short of withdrawing from state obligations. "We talked of love and peace, but we never stopped serving in our combat units," writes

Geffen. "We were a company with multiple personality. A soldier lying in an ambush on the Dead Sea or crawling towards an Egyptian sniper in the Suez Canal listening to 'Imagine' and 'Give peace a chance' on his radio earphones. [Israeli prime minister] Golda Meir and John Lennon raging in one head, but a few tokes [of hash] will sort that too."[21]

Importantly, the group's primary drug of choice was not psychedelics but hashish, as the title of Geffen's book *Chomer Tov* (Good Dope) indicates. Although many of Lul's members experimented with psychedelics, they did so only casually, haphazardly, without ascribing much importance to the experience. The Lul Group's interest in psychedelics was not spiritual, political, or even creative. Their trip adventures sound more like a *chevre*-style fooling around, hardly distinguishable from their tales of cocaine use. Hashish and psychedelics functioned mostly as an escape from the dreary, uninspiring, and sometimes oppressive reality of Zionist society.

A contrasting case is found in the Third Eye Group, active in Tel Aviv around the same time. If Lul were the proud embodiment of the locally grown *Sabra*, the Third Eye Group represented a mixture of newly arrived immigrants with an as-yet-unsettled relationship to Israeli society. The leader was the artist and filmmaker Jacques Katmor (1938–2001). Born into a wealthy Jewish family in Cairo, Katmor received a cosmopolitan education and was well read and acutely aware of the international world of art and culture.[22]

Katmor had his first taste of psychedelics at age nineteen, when he ingested mescaline after reading Henry Michaux's *Miserable Miracle* (1956).[23] He became interested in the writings of William S. Burroughs, Aleister Crowley, Aldous Huxley, and Timothy Leary. After emigrating to Israel in 1960 and serving in the Israeli army, Katmor moved to Tel Aviv and immersed himself in local bohemian circles. The handsome, charismatic, young man soon emerged as the leader of a dissident cultural group.

The Third Eye Group focused on self-liberation and -transformation through art. Its members spent days and nights debating philosophical issues, making art, and consuming vast amounts of drugs. Unlike the Lul Group, theirs was markedly international in both biographical origins and artistic influences. They also approached drugs differently: "[Katmor's] understanding of drugs as spiritual tools catalyzed perpetual exploration" writes his biographer, Ori Drumer.[24] "Drugs were central to the ideology," said Katmor's wife, Ann Tuchmeyer, "they were meant to open up the mind and help people become artists."[25]

In 1969, Katmor's film *A Woman's Case* was the first Israeli film to screen at the Venice Film Festival. Drawing from the avant-garde style of French New Wave directors like Jean-Luc Godard, the film features extensive nudity and the Israeli psychedelic band The Churchills (which gained international success under the name Jericho Jones). Katmor's short film *The Hole* (1973) was created under the influence of LSD. The film featured Katmor himself, digging a burial hole in a field, cut with blurred, broken images. It offered a "Jewish, hippie, psychedelic combination within a theological model."[26] While Drumer interprets the film as an excavation dismembering Jewish-Israeli identity, it could alternatively be understood as symbolizing psychedelic ego-death. Either way, the experience of digging his own grave while on acid appears to have shaken Katmor for months following the event.

Kamor and his group were challenging Zionist morals. They traveled to socialist kibbutzim, small, intentionally created communities with socialist-Zionist principles that emerged around the turn of the century, and challenged kibbutznik mentality using sensory bombardment, avant-garde theater, nudity, and psychedelic visuals. In one particularly notorious event in Tel Aviv's Artists House, the group combined deafening noise cascades, psychedelic lighting, and dildo-wearing female models as Katmor moved through the crowd riding a heavy motorcycle. These provocative exhibitions elicited public outrage. The Israeli press covered the events with a mixture of voyeurism and condemnation. The spartan Israeli society did not buy into the ideas of peace, love, sex, drugs, and rock 'n' roll. Interest in hallucinogens was frowned upon as symptomatic of an individualist inward turn that threatened to undermine Zionist ideals.

In 1972, following economic hardships, the group opened an alternative cultural center. The Third Eye shop in central Tel Aviv functioned as an embassy for the international countercultural movement. Its merchandise included rock albums, Indian incense, mystical titles, and books by countercultural favorites like Leary, Carlos Castaneda, Jerry Rubin, and Hermann

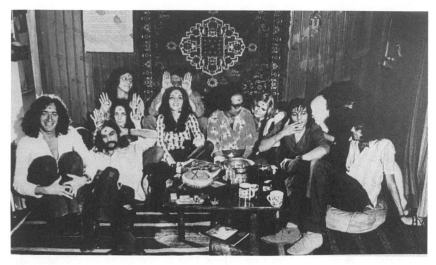

Figure 17.2
Members of the Third Eye Group in Jacque Mory-Katmor's home in Tel Aviv, 1972.
Unknown photographer.

Hesse.[27] Persistent police raids, burglaries, and a steady stream of unwanted, nonpaying visitors led to its closure.

The Lul Group and the Third Eye Group symbolized two divergent approaches to drugs and culture and were generally disdainful of one another. Lul members considered Third Eye members to be pretentious and weird; Third Eye members viewed Lul members as parochial ignoramuses. One group, based in local *Sabra* culture and lore, regarded psychedelic use as a mere pastime. The other, orienting itself toward international cultural movements, regarded these drugs as spiritual, creative, mind-expanding tools.[28]

PSYCHEDELICS AFTER THE YOM KIPPUR WAR

In 1973, Israeli's confidence suffered a fatal blow after a near-defeat in the Yom Kippur War. At a time when the American counterculture was facing a war on drugs, Israel's cultural highs and lows were again dictated by the results of military confrontation. The 1973 war shook the integrity of the Lul Group. Members of the Third Eye Group refused to join the military effort and later emigrated to San Francisco, to "the heart of the movement we tried so hard to import."[29] Katmor eventually moved to the Netherlands, ending his life embittered and dependent on narcotic drugs.

In 1977, Israel elected the nationalist Likud Party, replacing the socialist Mapai Party that had ruled the country in its first thirty years. Supported by non-European ethnic minorities, the new ruling party challenged Israel's power structures. For many in the old elite, the loss of political control and fears of cultural decline led away from political engagement and toward an esoteric search for spiritual redemption. The author Gabi Zohar (1992) speaks of a crisis of Zionism that emerged, identifying participants in new sects and religious movements as coming from the old elite: ". . . those young people whose world descended into the twilight of a profound crisis. Their identity twitching and bleeding. Their fate in the traditional leadership unsettled. They search meaning for their lives."[30]

Psychedelics converged with these new cultural trends. The poet and later cult leader Rina Shani (1937–1983) was a bright and charismatic poet in 1960s Tel Aviv bohemia. In 1973, she had a revelatory LSD experience that radically shifted her perspective of the world. "An explosion of consciousness . . . I feel and know everything," she wrote. "LSD enlightened me. That's how it happened to the Baal Shem Tov [the founder of Hasidism], to Shimon Bar Yochai [a second-century Jewish mystic]. I was out of the cave. I found my true self which is God."[31] Shani felt reincarnated. She renamed her newly transformed self Rain Shine. The beautiful, charismatic leader, whose teaching merged Buddhism, psychoanalysis, and hippie counterculture together with Jewish concepts and symbols, soon attracted a following. She believed in the transformative power of LSD and the liberal use of cannabis. Police identified the group as the first Israeli cult.[32]

The suicide of a group member, who was also a kibbutz member, led to growing public scrutiny and condemnation. Shani traveled to India, where she died alone at age forty-six. Like Katmor, Shani's encounter with the Zionist establishment was crushing. She had been a spiritual leader, but her writings disappeared from bookstores. "Zionist Bolshevism erased her," says Yaakov Rotblitt, her former lover.[33] Rotblitt, a member of the Lul Group, characterized Shani's engagement with LSD as another example of the versatility of psychedelics in Israeli bohemia. "If Uri Zohar and Lul did it for the laughs, Katmor used it as a tool for inner and artistic exploration, and Rina, she used it for her spiritual development, to talk with god."[34]

By the end of the 1970s, the cultural prominence of psychedelics in Israel waned. As 1960s flower power became passé, new cultural movements gained popularity in Israeli society, from disco to punk. These new movements had new, nonpsychedelic drug preferences.[35]

One noteworthy exception that brought psychedelics back into the limelight and linked revelatory hallucinations with modern Jewish trauma was the LSD treatment of the Polish-born author Yehiel De-Nur (known by his pen name, Ka-Tzetnik). An Auschwitz survivor, De-Nur was Israel's most respected Holocaust author, with multiple works exploring the horrors of the Nazi death camps.

In 1976, De-Nur traveled to Leiden, Netherlands, and went through a series of LSD treatments under the supervision of the Dutch psychiatrist Jan Bastiaans.[36] Bastiaans had treated traumatized Holocaust survivors since the 1960s; however, De-Nur was his most prominent patient. After the treatment, De-Nur declared himself cured from his persistent nightmares. Using LSD, he had been able to heal the traumatic wounds of the Holocaust. However, the event did not become publicly known until 1987, when he published a book detailing his LSD therapy. The October 6 issue of the controversial but influential weekly *HaOlam Haze* featured De-Nur on the cover with a headline reporting the miraculous healing of Holocaust trauma using LSD. A copy of De-Nur's book *Shivitti: A Vision* was included.[37] The book was also later included in collection of KaZetnik's Holocaust books produced by the Israeli Ministry of Education and aimed at teachers and students.

De-Nur's early writings refer to Auschwitz as "A different planet"—a parallel reality beyond the laws of this world. Following his LSD experiences, he reversed his perspective on Auschwitz. In a 1988 interview he famously stated: "Neither Satan nor God built Auschwitz, but I and you."[38] Holocaust memory in Israel historically veered between the universalist humanist perspective and the particularistic, nationalist perspective. Through LSD, De-Nur came to embrace a wholly universalist interpretation of Auschwitz.[39]

THE 1990s ISRAELI BACKPACKERS AND THE TRANCE SCENE

By the late 1980s, a new global psychedelic subculture was brewing. Psy-trance, a musical style that developed in the late 1980s and early 1990s on the Indian coasts of Goa, soon reached Israeli shores.

The background for this new emerging phenomenon was a growing movement fueled by Israeli backpackers who traveled to the Indian sub-continent seeking adventure and spiritual fulfillment. Israeli backpacking culture has been linked to Zionist traditions running all the way to 1940s Palmach,[40] and indeed, early travelers belonged to socially strong elements of Israeli society, including kibbutz members and veterans of elite IDF units. Many of these backpackers immersed themselves in the Goa trance scene, becoming successful DJs, producers, and record label owners. They carried the new culture back to their homeland during the 1990s and 2000s as backpacking spread across the strata of Israeli society.

Israeli backpackers' penchant for mind-altering drugs has often been tied to the oppressive experience of the two to three years of compulsory military service mandated for all Israeli citizens.[41] Having sacrificed several of the most crucial years of their young adulthood inside an authoritarian system, Israelis rushed to India and South and Central America to make up for lost time and medicate the trauma of their military service.[42] Their gung-ho approach to risk-taking and desire to use up a preciously short period of liberty from life's obligations led them on the path to devil-may-care drug adventures. A 2008 BBC program titled "Flipping Out: Israel's Drug Generation" investigated "why so many young Israelis use their National Service discharge bonus to go backpacking in India, with a high propor-tion experimenting with drugs."[43] Many sold drugs to finance their travels, earning reputations as resourceful, reliable drug dealers.[44] The backpacking anthropologist Tamir Leon writes that when asking Israelis in India how to recognize a drug dealer, he received the answer: "Approach an Israeli. Every Israeli is a dealer. (Meaning that in every Israeli social circle there is a person with access to commercial quantities of drugs.)"[45]

With the break of the first Intifada (1987–1993), Palestinian resistance to Israeli occupation of the West Bank and Gaza sent many young men to participate in patently unheroic missions of policing civilian populations. This led to an intensification of the internal discussions about the need for an Israeli-Palestinian peace treaty (leading to the Oslo peace process, starting in 1993). By that time, parts of Israeli society were entering a post-Zionist phase.[46] The Israeli sociologist Oz Almog speaks of a disengagement from the old Zionist model and an "implosion of Zionistic Charisma," leading to a greater willingness to engage with Zionism critically.[47] "It was under the pressure of these traumas [e.g., the Lebanon war, the Intifada, the Gulf War, and suicide bombings] that a sense of impotence began to take hold, a disbelief in the possibility of having an impact on political and societal realities," writes the scholar Assaf Sagiv (2000), who describes the rise of an Israeli Dionysian culture embracing mind-altering drugs. "These sentiments left deep scars, especially among veterans of combat units . . . one result was the steady withdrawal of young adults from engagement in national concerns and their retreat into the sphere of the exclusively private."[48]

Sagiv blamed the vulnerability of Israeli youth to the allure of drugs on the failure of Israeli society to "provide its young with a viable alternative ethos."[49] Like their bohemian predecessors in the 1970s, Israeli youth wished to disengage from the collectivist burden of Zionism and Israeli reality. Drugs, again, provided a way.

The founders of the Israeli psytrance scene were recently discharged male soldiers.[50] Many of them were disappointed with their experiences in the Israeli military and felt a strong need to revolt. The reception of trance culture into Israeli society was facilitated because it contained many cultural components that resonate with Zionistic youth movements and military life—camping in nature, navigation, and male camaraderie. Trance founders repurposed practices acquired during their army service toward participation in the new psytrance culture.[51]

By the mid-1990s, Israel was becoming a psytrance powerhouse. Artists like Astral Projection, Infected Mushroom, Skazi, Sandman, Chakra, and Oforia became major names in the psytrance world. Israel was becoming not just an importer, but also an exporter of psychedelic culture.

"It would be hard to overstate the extent of the 'trance' phenomenon in Israel," wrote Sagiv. "In the last few years, this country of six million has become a major focus of the global rave culture."[52] The prominence of psy-trance in Israel society, he argued, is without parallel. "Trance has taken over the streets. It bubbles out from passing vehicles, is heard in the kiosks and grocery stores and deafens us in the boutiques. It is in television commercials, fashion shows, malls, half-time shows at football and basketball games, at bar and bat mitzva celebrations, circumcision rites and weddings . . . Its sound is now localized and familiar," wrote Nissan Shor.[53]

If the 1960s and 1970s psychedelic wave in Israel was confined to bohemian circles, the 1990s brought the democratization of psychedelia, as it spread across many sectors of Israeli society. "Trance cuts across ethnic and economic classes. . . . Druggies from India and greasers from the sub-urbs, girls from development towns with their tank tops and platform shoes dancing alongside buttoned-up BA students," reported the Tel Aviv weekly *Ha'ir*.[54] The Israeli Drug-War Authority, established in 1988, soon turned its attention to this new psychedelic underground.

The drug sociologist Hagit Boni-Noah describes a moral panic cam-paign launched against the psytrance movement, culminating in 1995 with public warnings that "thousands of Israelis getting stoned on the coasts of Goa are an immediate moral threat to Israeli society."[55] The prospect of ex-soldiers ingesting psychedelics was recast as a security threat. The newspapers warned that thousands of young Israelis will drug themselves at Goa's New Year's celebrations, and the head of the Drug-War Authority urged Israeli parents to organize a charter flight and bring their kids back home. The flight never took off, however (no parents signed up). Boni-Noah links the moral panic around backpacker drug use with the November 1995 assassination of Israeli prime minister Yitzhak Rabin, which had occurred a month earlier, creating moral confusion and fomenting a search for a scapegoat.[56] Ironi-cally, the trance scholar Elinor Carmi convincingly shows that the entire media drama was orchestrated by the Drug-War Authority itself to secure funds in upcoming parliament discussions.[57]

Confrontations between the authorities and the raging trance scene continued throughout the mid-to-late-1990s. Police routinely raided psy-trance parties, and even the homes of psytrance DJs and party producers.[58]

Newspapers reported horror stories of soldiers driving 160 kph on the freeway while on acid and elite IDF pilots tripping on LSD.[59] Israeli media, meanwhile, referred to psytrance parties as "acid parties." In 1996, a judge was asked to decide whether psytrance parties should be banned categorically. The judge rejected the equation of psytrance and drugs, declaring that "drugs can be taken in a rock concert, listening to oriental music and possibly even while listening to classical music."[60] Then, in July 1998, 40,000 Israelis attended a massive rally in Tel Aviv's Rabin Square, protesting the repression of the Israeli trance scene. The event was viewed as an impressive triumph for the local scene that led to its wider acceptance.[61]

The Israeli trance scene has continued to thrive in the past two decades, with the theme of escapism to an alternate psychedelic reality pervading scholarly accounts of the subject.[62] Alongside its attraction to the global, Israeli trance is firmly rooted in local culture.[63] Scholars note the ubiquity of Jewish-Zionist motifs in psytrance parties (incandescent Hanukkah candelabras, Day-Glo fluorescent stars of David) and that despite the inclusive Peace-Love-Unity-Respect (PLUR) rhetoric of trance culture, the social structures of trance parties often end up replicating deep-seated divisions within Israeli society.[64] The anthropologists Schmidt and Navon conclude that Israeli psytrance culture presents essentially different features than its overseas counterparts that have been associated by researchers with "insubordination," "dissent," and "cultural subversion."[65] This is perhaps to be expected in a country where thousands of soldiers go on psychoactive adventures each weekend, only to then return to their military units and fulfill their mandated roles. Either way, Israel remains a unique and intriguing test case for thinking about the political and social context of psytrance and psychedelic use.

THE ISRAELI PSYCHEDELIC SCENE SINCE THE MILLENNIUM

During the early 2000s, rumors of ayahuasca and peyote rituals from the West started to hit the beaches of Goa and the ashrams in Puna, a three-hour drive southeast of Mumbai. Israelis who were a dominant part of the international trance scene started participating in psychedelic medicine circles there and in Europe. Initially inviting South American musicians to conduct rituals in Israel, by 2002 some Israelis were leading the rituals themselves, adjusting them to fit Israeli and Jewish sensitivities while keeping the original cultural frameworks. These pioneers were again shifting the Israeli context for psychedelic experiences from the rowdy, high beat-per-minute, hardcore trance environment, known in Hebrew as *Karahana*, to a framework for healing and sacred medicine. While the ayahuasca crowd was at first predominantly from secular, liberal backgrounds, the movement soon generated surprising social mixtures involving both Palestinians and orthodox populations.[66]

The 2010s saw the growth of an integrated and committed Israeli psychedelic community. If previous local movements involving psychedelics repeatedly distanced themselves from drug associations, the new movement declared clearly: it *is* about the drugs. In 2009, the first Hebrew book *Techno-mystica* dedicated to psychedelic culture and ideology was published,[67] and in 2013, the Israeli psychedelic magazine *LaPsychonaut* appeared. Attempting to provide "a home for the psychedelic community," the crowdfunded magazine includes stories about harm reduction, psychedelic integration, and coming out of the psychedelic closet. Several psychedelic harm-reduction services emulating the practices of international organizations such as Zendo and Cosmicare (Anashim Tovim, Hof Mivtachim, Safezone [Israeli]) began operating at psytrance parties.[68] The first Israeli psychedelic conference Altered Minds (Meshanim Toda'a) took place in the American Zionist House in 2017. The event sold out, attracting over 500 individuals and featuring a cadre of Israeli and international speakers.

In 2017, the international organization Students for Sensible Drug Policy (SSDP) launched an Israeli chapter, and an Israeli psychedelic podcast called "Todaa Raba" started featuring local guests. The prominent daily *Haaretz* began covering the subject with surprising tenacity, sometimes publishing two or three items on the subject on the same weekend, and even featuring a regular column about it. A growing number of local books and movies on the subject have also appeared, as well as several social media groups counting dozens of thousands of members, suggesting that psychedelics have moved into the mainstream.

Professional work in psychedelic spaces has developed rapidly. In 2007, psychedelic research returned to Israel. The Be'er Ya'akov Mental Health Center became one of a few international sites for the Phase I MDMA trials conducted by the Multidisciplinary Association for Psychedelic Studies (MAPS). During the 2010s, Israeli researchers became regular speakers in the international psychedelic conference scene, universities began offering courses, and the first Israeli program training psychedelic therapists launched. Twenty-first-century Israel prides itself on being a *Start-Up Nation.*[69] In the early 2020s, as international psychedelic corporations began making headlines, Israel too generated its first batch of psychedelic start-ups, including Nextage, PsyRx, and Pharmocann, capitalizing on the success of the local cannabis industry.

CONCLUSION

The story of psychedelics in Israel was shaped by the country's culture and history, reflecting both its local conditions and its outward-facing stance. Throughout the decades, psychedelics have been repeatedly used by Israelis as cosmic escape routes out of the oppressive reality of a geographically isolated, ideologically charged country under constant security threat. They played a role in cultural movements that challenged Israeli social norms, leading to scandal (and outward getaways) at times, but mostly staying within bounds, conversing with local culture, and eventually gaining growing acceptance. Over the past thirty years, as Israel grew increasingly assimilated into global markets and discourses, Israel's relationship with these drugs has been shaped by growing inward and outward flows of individuals, culture, knowledge, and capital, leading the country to become a psytrance powerhouse and a significant psychedelic research center. Finally, building on a local culture of entrepreneurship and the country's growing reputation as a start-up hub, this has led to the emergence of a local psychedelic industry. Today, the influence of psychedelics crosses social and cultural boundaries, as the drugs spread across diverse groups in Israeli society to include liberals, West Bank settlers, ultra-Orthodox Jews, and Palestinians, acquiring diverse meanings and reflecting the disparate faces of contemporary Israeli identity.

NOTES

1. Rachel Elboim-Dror, "'He's Coming from Our Midst, the New Hebrew': The Youth Culture of the First Alyiahs" (in Hebrew), *Alpaim* 12 (1996): 104–135; Tammy Razi, "On the Margins: Youth Subculture in Tel Aviv during the British Mandate Period" (in Hebrew), *Zmanim: A Historical Quarterly*, no. 106 (2009): 64–75.

2. Tom Segev, *Elvis in Jerusalem: Post-Zionism and the Americanization of Israel*, trans. Haim Watzman (New York: Metropolitan Books, 2002); Oz Almog, *Goodbye to Shrulik: Changes in the Values of Israeli Elites [Hebrew]* (Haifa, Israel: Haifa Univesity & Zmora Bitan, 2004).

3. Benjamin R. Barber, *Jihad vs McWorld* (Random House, 2010); Mike Featherstone, *Undoing Culture: Globalization, Postmodernism and Identity* (Sage, 1995); Uri Ram, *The Globalization of Israel: McWorld in Tel Aviv, Jihad in Jerusalem* (Routledge, 2013).

4. H. Wijsenbeek and R. Landau, "A Review on the Use of Lysergic Acid Diethylamide in Psychiatry" (in Hebrew), *Harefuah* 58 (1960): 281–286.

5. Ido Hartogsohn, *American Trip: Set, Setting, and the Psychedelic Experience in the Twentieth Century* (Cambridge, MA: MIT Press, 2020), chap. 1.

6. David Karislovsky, "Clinical Observations on the Effects of LSD-25" (in Hebrew), *Dapim Refueeim* 19, no. 1 (May 1960): 28–39.

7. Hartogsohn, *American Trip*, 40–43.

8. Yigal Sarna, *Yonnah Wallach* (in Hebrew) (Jerusalem: Keter, 1993).

9. Yair Qedar, *The Seven Tapes*, Documentary, 2012.

10. Sarna, *Yonnah Wallach*.

11. Qedar, *The Seven Tapes*.

12. Assaf Inbari, "New Age: The Fall of the Secular State," 1999, accessed August 21, 2011, Http://Inbari.Co.Il/En_hilonim.Htm.

13. David Avidan, *LSD Trip—Personal Report* (in Hebrew) (Tel Aviv: The 30th Century, 1968).

14. Nadav Neuman, "If You Go Tripping on LSD: On the Forgotten Place of Psychedelics in Israeli Poetry [Hebrew]," *Moznaim* (October 2016), 26–36.

15. Anita Shapira, *Israel: A History* (UPNE, 2012).

16. Yehonatan Geffen, *Good Dope* (in Hebrew) (Kineret-Zmora Bitan, 2001), 72.

17. Haggai Ram, *Intoxicating Zion: A Social History of Hashish in Mandatory Palestine and Israel* (Stanford, CA: Stanford University Press, 2020).

18. Quoted in Ram, *Intoxicating Zion*, 153.

19. Oz Almog, *The Sabra: The Creation of the New Jew* (University of California Press, 2000).

20. Geffen, *Good Dope*, 117.

21. Geffen, *Good Dope*, 80.

22. Ori Drumer, *Jacque Katmor Is Wishing You a Good Death* (Nahum Gutman Museum, 2012).

23. Drumer, *Jacque Katmor Is Wishing You a Good Death*, 46.

24. Drumer, *Jacque Katmor Is Wishing You a Good Death*, 46.

25. Etti Avramov, "Ann Legend" (in Hebrew), *Tel Aviv Newspaper*, April 6, 2004, 57.

26. Drumer, *Jacque Katmor Is Wishing You a Good Death*, 41.

27. Drumer, *Jacque Katmor Is Wishing You a Good Death*, 88.

28. While this chapter focuses on the prominent Tel Aviv scene, psychedelic use was also happening in other parts of Israel. In the early 1970s, an early Zionist settlement called Rosh Pina, in northern Israel, became inhabited by hippies living an off-the-grid lifestyle and making frequent use of drugs, including psychedelics. (See Mariana Ruah-Midbar and Tali Aluhav, "The Hippie Colonie in Rosh Pina," *Ofakim Begeografia* 97 (2019): 107–135. The northern city of Haifa also had a psychedelic scene, with dozens of youth reportedly tripping together every weekend on the Rotschild House lawn (some of these people later became figures of cultural prominence). (Interview with Amit Daniel).

29. Drumer, *Jacque Katmor Is Wishing You a Good Death*, 89.

30. Gabi Zohar, *Happiness Has No End: On Mystical Sects, New Groups and Psychological Marathons in Israel* (in Hebrew) (Tel Aviv: Sahar, 1992), 44.

31. Zohar, *Happiness Has No End*, 43.

32. "Israeli Police Report on Sects," 1982, https://web.archive.org/web/20060707015551 /http://www.katot.org/Files/KatotPage.asp?katotpage=36#RinaShani.

33. Noya Kochavi, "Rina Shani Is Not a Friend" (in Hebrew) *Haaretz*, August 9, 2008, https:// www.haaretz.co.il/gallery/1.3361009.

34. Yakov Rotblit, December 10, 2020.

35. Oded Heilbronner, "'Resistance through Rituals'—Urban Subcultures of Israeli Youth from the Late 1950s to the 1980s," *Israel Studies* 16 (October 1, 2011): 28–50, https://doi.org/10 .1353/is.2011.0027; Nissan Shor, "Dancing with Tears in Our Eyes: History of Club and Discotheque Culture in Israel," *Tel Aviv: Resling* (in Hebrew), 2008.

36. Stephen Snelders, "The LSD Therapy Career of Jan Bastiaans," MD Multidisciplinary Association for Psychedelic Studies Bulletin 8 (1998): 18–20.

37. "KaZetnik Code E.D'M.A," *HaOlam Haze*, June 10, 1987.

38. Udi Meller, "'It Wasn't the Devil Who Created Auschwitz but Man': Twenty Years since KaZetnik's Death [Hebrew]," *Makkor Rishon*, July 14, 2021, https://www.makorrishon.co .il/news/374439/.

39. For readings about De-Nur's LSD experiences, see Erika Dyck and Chris Elcock, "Reframing Bummer Trips: Scientific and Cultural Explanations to Adverse Reactions to Psychedelic Drug Use," *Social History of Alcohol and Drugs* 34, no. 2 (2020): 271–296; and Iris

Robeling-Grau, "How to Understand Shivitti?" in *Holocaust History and the Readings of Ka-Tzetnik* (Bloomsbury Publishing, 2018).

40. Nasia Shafran, "From Palmach Travels to the Mochileros" (in Hebrew), *Panim: Quarterly Journal for Culture, Society and Education* 35 (2006).

41. Elinor Carmi, *TransMission: The Psytrance Culture in Israel 1989–1999* (in Hebrew) (Tel Aviv: Resling, 2013); Daria Maoz, "Drug Use among Young Israeli Backpackers in India" (in Hebrew), in *Backpackers and Drugs*, ed. Hagit Boni-Noah (Jerusalem: Israeli Anti-Drug Authority, 2008), 169–89.

42. Maoz, "Drug Use among Young Israeli Backpackers in India."

43. *Flipping Out—Israel's Drug Generation*, 2017, https://www.bbc.co.uk/programmes/b00bbxqt.

44. Joshua Schmidt, "Full Penetration: The Integration of Psychedelic Electronic Dance Music and Culture into the Israeli Mainstream," *Dancecult: Journal of Electronic Dance Music Culture* 4, no. 1 (2012): 39.

45. Tamir Leon, "Israeli Travelers in India and Drugs" (in Hebrew), in *Backpackers and Drugs*, ed. Hagit Boni-Noah (Jerusalem: Israeli Anti-Drug Authority, 2008), 190–226.

46. Segev, *Elvis in Jerusalem*; Almog, *Goodbye to Shrulik*.

47. Almog, *Goodbye to Shrulik*, 21–23.

48. Assaf Sagiv, "Dionysus in Zion," *Azure: Ideas for the Jewish Nation* 9 (2000): 155–178, 170.

49. Sagiv, "Dionysus in Zion," 173.

50. Carmi, *TransMission*, 36.

51. Carmi, *TransMission*, 92–93.

52. Sagiv, "Dionysus in Zion," 167.

53. Quoted in Joshua Schmidt and Liora Navon, "'In Dance We Trust': Comparing Trance-Dance Parties among Secular and Orthodox Israeli Youth," *Israel Affairs* 23, no. 6 (2017): 1127.

54. Quoted in Sagiv, "Dionysus in Zion," 167.

55. Hagit Boni-Noah, "The Construction of a Social Problem among Drug Using Backpackers: The Development of Advocacy, Prevention and Treatment of Backpacker Drug Casualties in Israel" (in Hebrew), in *Backpackers and Drugs*, ed. Hagit Boni-Noah (Jerusalem: Israeli Anti-Drug Authority, 2008), 18.

56. Boni-Noah, "The Construction of a Social Problem."

57. Carmi, *TransMission*, 154.

58. Carmi, *TransMission*, 56.

59. Lior Elhai, "We Drove 160 Kph High on Acid," *Yediot Ahronot*, October 19, 1997; Yoram Yarkoni, "In the Acid Parties I Met Combat Pilots and Other Officers," *Yediot Ahronot*, July 7, 1993.

60. Dorit Gabay, "It's Official: An Acid Party Is Not Necessarily a Drug Party," *Maariv*, July 21, 1996.

61. Carmi, *TransMission*.

62. Schmidt and Navon, "'In Dance We Trust,'" 1128.

63. Schmidt and Navon, "'In Dance We Trust.'"

64. Schmidt, "Full Penetration."

65. Schmidt and Navon, "'In Dance We Trust,'" 1141.

66. Mishor reports on ultra-Orthodox (Haredi) ayahuasca circles operating in northern Israel. See Zevic Mishor, "Digging the Well Deep: The Jewish 'Ultra-Orthodox' Relationship with the Divine Explored through the Lifeworld of the Breslov Chasidic Community in Safed," 2015. Roseman and colleagues tell of the intricacies of binational ayahuasca rituals bringing together Israeli and Palestinian participants and including icaros in both Hebrew and Arabic. Leor Roseman et al., "Relational Processes in Ayahuasca Groups of Palestinians and Israelis," *Frontiers in Pharmacology* 12 (2021), https://doi.org/10.3389/fphar.2021.607529.

67. Ido Hartogsohn, *Technomysica: Consciousness in the Digital Age* (Givatayim, Israel: Madaf, 2009).

68. Yahav Erez, "Safe Zones in Recreational Settings in Israel: The Emergence of Psychedelics Expertise" (Master's thesis, Bar Ilan University, 2020).

69. Dan Senor and Saul Singer, *Start-up Nation: The Story of Israel's Economic Miracle* (New York: Random House Digital, 2011).

BIBLIOGRAPHY

Primary Sources

Avramov, Etti. "Ann Legend (Hebrew)." *Tel Aviv Newspaper*, April 6, 2004, 57.

Elhai, Lior. "We Drove 160 Kph High on Acid." *Yediot Ahronot*, October 19, 1997.

Flipping Out—Israel's Drug Generation, 2017. https://www.bbc.co.uk/programmes/b00bbxqt.

Gabay, Dorit. "It's Official: An Acid Party Is Not Necessarily a Drug Party." *Maariv* (July, 1996).

Geffen, Yehonatan. *Good Dope* (in Hebrew). Kineret-Zmora Bitan, 2001.

Hartogsohn, Ido. *Technomysica: Consciousness in the Digital Age*. Givatayim, Israel: Madaf, 2009.

"Israeli Police Report on Sects, 1982." https://web.archive.org/web/20060707015551/http://www.katot.org/Files/KatotPage.asp?katotpage=36#RinaShani.

Karislovsky, David. "Clinical Observations on the Effects of LSD-25" (in Hebrew). *Dapim Refueeim* 19, no. 1 (May 1960): 28–39.

"KaZetnik Code E.D'M.A." *HaOlam Haze*, June 10, 1987.

Kochavi, Noya. "Rina Shani Is Not a Friend [Hebrew]." *Haaretz*, August 9, 2008. https://www
.haaretz.co.il/gallery/1.3361009.

Wijsenbeek, H., and R. Landau. "A Review on the Use of Lysergic Acid Diethylamide in Psychiatry"
(in Hebrew). *Harefuah* 58 (1960): 281–286.

Yakov Rotblit, interview with author, December 10, 2020.

Yarkoni, Yoram. "In the Acid Parties I Met Combat Pilots and Other Officers." *Yediot Ahronot*
(July 1993).

Secondary Sources

Almog, Oz. *Goodbye to Shrulik: Changes in the Values of Israeli Elites* (in Hebrew). Haifa, Israel:
Haifa Univesity and Zmora Bitan, 2004.

Almog, Oz. *The Sabra: The Creation of the New Jew*. Berkeley: University of California Press, 2000.

Avidan, David. *LSD Trip—Personal Report* (in Hebrew). Tel Aviv: The 30th Century, 1968.

Barber, Benjamin R. *Jihad vs. McWorld*. New York: Random House, 2010.

Boni-Noah, Hagit. "The Construction of a Social Problem among Drug Using Backpackers: The
Development of Advocacy, Prevention and Treatment of Backpacker Drug Casualties in Israel"
(in Hebrew). In *Backpackers and Drugs*, edited by Hagit Boni-Noah, 18. Jerusalem: Israeli Anti-
Drug Authority, 2008.

Carmi, Elinor. *TransMission: The Psytrance Culture in Israel 1989–1999* (in Hebrew). Tel Aviv:
Resling, 2013.

Dromer, Uri. "Jacque Katmor Is Wishing You a Good Death." Nahum Gutman Museum, 2012.

Dyck, Erika, and Chris Elcock. "Reframing Bummer Trips: Scientific and Cultural Explanations
to Adverse Reactions to Psychedelic Drug Use." *Social History of Alcohol and Drugs* 34, no. 2
(2020): 271–296.

Elboim-Dror, Rachel. "'He's Coming from Our Midst, the New Hebrew': The Youth Culture of
the First Alyiahs" (in Hebrew). *Alpaim* 12 (1996): 104–135.

Erez, Yahav. "Safe Zones in Recreational Settings in Israel: The Emergence of Psychedelics Expertise." Master's thesis, Bar Ilan University, 2020.

Featherstone, Mike. *Undoing Culture: Globalization, Postmodernism and Identity*. London: Sage,
1995.

Hartogsohn, Ido. *American Trip: Set, Setting, and the Psychedelic Experience in the Twentieth Century*.
Cambridge, MA: MIT Press, 2020.

Heilbronner, Oded. "'Resistance through Rituals'—Urban Subcultures of Israeli Youth from the
Late 1950s to the 1980s." *Israel Studies* 16 (October 2011): 28–50. https://doi.org/10.1353/is
.2011.002.

Inbari, Assaf. "New Age: The Fall of the Secular State." Accessed on August 12, 2011. http://inbari
.co.il/en_hilonim.htm.

Leon, Tamir. "Israeli Travelers in India and Drugs" (in Hebrew). In *Backpackers and Drugs*, edited by Hagit Boni-Noah, 190–226. Jerusalem: Israeli Anti-Drug Authority, 2008.

Maoz, Daria. "Drug Use among Young Israeli Backpackers in India" (in Hebrew). In *Backpackers and Drugs*, edited by Hagit Boni-Noah, 169–189. Jerusalem: The Israeli Anti-Drug Authority, 2008.

Mishor, Zevic. "Digging the Well Deep: The Jewish 'Ultra-Orthodox' Relationship with the Divine Explored through the Lifeworld of the Breslov Chasidic Community in Safed." Phd dissertation, University of Sydney, 2015.

Neuman, Nadav. "If You Go Tripping on LSD: On the Forgotten Place of Psychedelics in Israeli Poetry" (in Hebrew). *Moznaim* (October 2016): 26–36.

Qedar, Yair. *The Seven Tapes*. Documentary, 2012. Studio: Ha'ivrim. https://www.youtube.com /watch?v=JWKd84JHkR8&ab_channel=yairqedar.

Ram, Haggai. *Intoxicating Zion: A Social History of Hashish in Mandatory Palestine and Israel*. Stanford, CA: Stanford University Press, 2020.

Ram, Uri. *The Globalization of Israel: McWorld in Tel Aviv, Jihad in Jerusalem*. Routledge, 2013.

Razi, Tammy. "On the Margins: Youth Subculture in Tel Aviv during the British Mandate Period" (in Hebrew). *Zmanim: A Historical Quarterly*, no. 106 (2009): 64–75.

Robeling-Grau, Iris. "How to Understand Shivitti?" In *Holocaust History and the Readings of Ka-Tzetnik*. New York: Bloomsbury Publishing, 2018.

Roseman, Leor, Yiftach Ron, Antwan Saca, Natalie Ginsberg, Lisa Luan, Nadeem Karkabi, Rick Doblin, and Robin Carhart-Harris. "Relational Processes in Ayahuasca Groups of Palestinians and Israelis." *Frontiers in Pharmacology* 12 (2021): 1–18.

Ruah-Midbar, Mariana, and Tali Aluhav. "The Hippie Colonie in Rosh Pina." *Ofakim Begeografia* 97 (2019): 107–135.

Sagiv, Assaf. "Dionysus in Zion." *Azure: Ideas for the Jewish Nation* 9, no. 155–178 (2000): 38–64.

Sarna, Yiga. *Yonnah Wallach* (in Hebrew). Jerusalem: Keter, 1993.

Schmidt, Joshua. "Full Penetration: The Integration of Psychedelic Electronic Dance Music and Culture into the Israeli Mainstream." *Dancecult: Journal of Electronic Dance Music Culture* 4, no. 1 (2012): 1127–1147.

Schmidt, Joshua, and Liora Navon. "'In Dance We Trust': Comparing Trance-Dance Parties among Secular and Orthodox Israeli Youth." *Israel Affairs* 23, no. 6 (2017): 1127.

Segev, Tom. *Elvis in Jerusalem: Post-Zionism and the Americanization of Israel*. Translated by Haim Watzman. New York: Metropolitan Books, 2002.

Senor, Dan, and Saul Singer. *Start-up Nation: The Story of Israel's Economic Miracle*. New York: Random House Digital, 2011.

Shafran, Nasia. "From Palmach Travels to the Mochileros" (in Hebrew). *Panim: Quarterly Journal for Culture, Society and Education* 35 (2006).

Shapira, Anita. *Israel: A History*. The Schusterman Series in Israel Studies. Waltham, MA: Brandeis University Press, 2012.

Shor, Nissan. "Dancing with Tears in Our Eyes: History of Club and Discotheque Culture in Israel." In *Tel Aviv: Resling* (in Hebrew), 2008.

Snelders, Stephen. "The LSD Therapy Career of Jan Bastiaans." *MD Multidisciplinary Association for Psychedelic Studies Bulletin* 8 (1998): 18–20.

Zohar, Gabi. *Happiness Has No End: On Mystical Sects, New Groups and Psychological Marathons in Israel* (in Hebrew). Tel Aviv: Sahar, 1992.

Mark Gallagher

INTRODUCTION

When LSD-25 reached Britain, it first passed through rarefied channels of asylums, universities, research institutes, day hospitals, and night clinics, before percolating into British cultural life. The key players in the birth of its medical career in the UK are still relative unknowns compared to figures prominently associated with the emergence of LSD in North America. Most famously, perhaps, the Scottish psychiatrist R. D. Laing (1927–1989) used LSD in his psychoanalytic practice and at the experimental community that he formed at Kingsley Hall, in the east end of London, in the 1960s. LSD started as an experimental psychiatric treatment in Britain following the discovery of its profound mind-altering effects. By the mid-1960s, it was fueling experiments in living that often challenged traditional psychiatric authority. Soon after the pharmacological revolution of psychiatry in the 1950s, an "anti-psychiatric" resistance was beginning to take shape.[1]

Robin Farquharson (1930–1973), a prize-winning game theorist, former Oxbridge academic, and frequent detainee of mental hospitals, had been a resident of Kingsley Hall. He was inspired by Timothy Leary to "drop out," leading to him becoming a key figure in the early life of radical activist groups, including People Not Psychiatry (PNP) and the first mental patients' unions. Farquharson is a transitional figure through whom it is possible to explore the transformation of LSD from a therapeutic tool used by psychiatrists to a weapon of countercultural subversion turned against the psychiatric authorities. This chapter focuses on acid-inspired anarchism, shedding light on the trajectory of LSD in Britain between the 1950s and 1970s. Farquharson's story reveals links between countercultures, "anti-psychiatry," and the emergence of mental patient unionism in Britain. Did LSD play a part in attempts in Britain to challenge institutionalization, subvert psychiatric authority, and create alternative postasylum spaces of sanctuary and social experimentation?

As the historian Sarah Shortall suggested, "if the psychedelic drug culture has been deemed relatively insignificant, this suggests that historians have tended to accept dominant cultural narratives defining non-medical drug use as escapist or artificial, and therefore as historically and politically irrelevant." However, as Shortall recognized, "these substances tell us much about the operation of fundamental cultural distinctions—between truth and illusion, inside and outside—which organise discourses far beyond those specifically concerned with drugs."[2] Historians of mental patient unionism in Britain have not paid enough attention to Farquharson or his journey from academia to mental health activism. Through an exploration of the ideas and circumstances that propelled the radical trip of Robin Farquharson, his story opens a window onto a journey toward collective action with fellow psychiatric patients, via anti-psychiatry, from his time at Kingsley Hall, through his experiment in dropping out and taking LSD, to his involvement in early mental patient unionism.

"ACID COMMUNISM"

Before his untimely death in 2017, the British cultural theorist Mark Fisher was writing a book with the provisional title *Acid Communism*.[3] All that remains of it is an unpublished introduction, but its ideas have endured thanks to his interpreters.[4] Fisher was calling for a reappraisal of 1960s and 1970s countercultures, having previously been dismissive of "the hippies and all their works."[5] There, he identified a "conjugation" between a class consciousness achieved by workers, consciousness-raising activities of socialists and feminists, and the mind expansion and "aestheticization of everyday life" practiced by groups of largely middle-class psychedelic drug users.[6]

According to Fisher, when these forms of consciousness were raised and interrelated, people challenged conceptions of normality and tested the limits of what was socially acceptable by experimenting with new possibilities.

Through changes in consciousness, people experienced a denaturalization of conventional concepts and forms of conduct, they recognized the "plasticity of reality" and the possibility of change.[7] The "acid" in the term "acid communism" was described by Matt Colquhoun (2020) as "a corrosive and denaturalising multiplicity," an "ideological accelerator through which the new and previously unknown might be found in politics we mistakenly think we already know, reinstating a politics to come."[8] It seemed to offer experimental ways of combating what Fisher called "capitalist realism," the fatalistic acquiescence to the view that there is no alternative to capitalism.

Fisher first conceived of the term "acid communism" in opposition to capitalist realism after he heard the radical psychiatrist and countercultural icon R. D. Laing described as an "acid Marxist." In truth, Laing was never a Marxist, and his relationship to LSD was complicated. He certainly never saw it as a means of large-scale cultural transformation or revolutionary social and political struggle, though he evidently played to the gallery when it suited him. For Laing, it was more a matter of exploring "inner space," but there was an anarchistic dimension to how LSD was used at the experimental community that he formed at Kingsley Hall.[9]

Fisher and his sympathetic interpreters were not interested in Laing, the "anti-psychiatrists," or in acid per se, but their willingness to look again at this period raises questions about the unexplored histories of LSD. While Fisher's concept of acid communism was concerned with mid-twentieth-century attempts at "the liberation of human consciousness from the norms of capitalist society" and "the expression of a desire for an experimental (rather than prescriptively utopian) leftist politics," the concerns of radical psychiatrists and patient activists in the 1960s and 1970s were more specifically focused on matters of mental illness, patients' rights, and alternative forms of mutual aid and communal living.[10] But the reflections of Fisher and his interpreters on acid communism provoke fresh thought about the emergence of subcultures in Britain in the 1960s and 1970s and their formation in relation to psychiatry, the discipline through which LSD first found a home in the UK, as happened elsewhere.

"EXPERIENTIAL ANARCHY" AT KINGSLEY HALL

Following Adrian Chapman's polyhedral thematization of Kingsley Hall as "an inner spaceship," "an embattled middle-class countercultural plantation," "a site of spiritual renewal and development," "a single-building arts colony," and "a countercultural experiment," it can also be characterized as "an acid commune" or "a site of experiential anarchy."[11] Along with fellow psychiatrists, the South African David Cooper (1931–1986), the American Joseph Berke (1939–2021) and others, Laing founded the Philadelphia Association, through which the residential community was established at Kingsley Hall in 1965. Ostensibly, there were no doctor-patient relationships nor any formal hierarchy at the residence, where people lived together and where, at times, LSD flowed freely.[12] Later, he would refer to his philosophy as "experiential anarchy," meaning that he had "no designs on trying to stop and start how anyone experiences the world" and "no designs on controlling, manipulating or dominating that person, to lay down the law and say what is the case and what is not the case, then to re-enforce this with a system of rewards and punishments."[13]

Expressing his admiration for Buddhism, Laing later referred to how "the fresh free air" of experiential anarchy does not turn "our souls, our world of experience, our experience of the world, our state of consciousness into a police state."[14] He thought that "in the West, the state of our hearts, minds, souls, experience, is a totalitarian state."[15] In one sense, the residential community at Kingsley Hall was part of a broader transnational tendency toward deinstitutionalization and the growth of national and local mental health associations and small therapeutic communities run on democratic principles.[16] In another sense, it was a radical outlier in Britain, a place that staged a theatrical dramatization, a carnivalesque inversion of psychiatric authority, hosting lectures, conferences, exhibitions, and other happenings, facilitating the emergence of an "anti-university" from within an "anti-hospital."[17] Intended to be a noncoercive place of refuge for the disturbed and the disturbing, people were allowed, even encouraged, to go through madness without medical intervention.

One resident of Kingsley Hall who was evicted for going too far was Farquharson. As he remembered it, "I had been evicted by Ronnie Laing from his 'household' for psychotics at Kingsley Hall, for use and abuse of the telephone—40 minutes to Canada at five in the morning he didn't find funny."[18] Farquharson was a self-confessed "telephone head" and "communications freak," known by many to be in the habit of making long-duration and long-distance international phone calls. According to him, Laing never grasped that he "had made the call only because no one in all the Hall was willing to wake up and talk with me."[19] Laing recalled that Farquharson "was about sixteen stone, he didn't like walls, so he went on a rampage, smashing and ripping everything, trying to knock doors and walls down—what are you going to do with someone like that?"[20] Laing later recounted how Farquharson had an idea to relocate the Kingsley Hall community to Addis Ababa, commenting that he was "a very strange guy . . . very intelligent and totally out of his fucking mind."[21]

ROBIN FARQUHARSON: "REVOLUTIONARY ANARCHIST"

Following his eviction from Kingsley Hall, Farquharson was inspired by Leary's call to drop out and experiment with LSD, and within a few years, he joined the first mental patients' unions, playing a key role creating communal spaces for former mental patients and those who would otherwise be hospitalized. While living at a commune flat in London in the early 1970s, Farquharson was interviewed for a Communes Research Project conducted by the academic Andrew Rigby.[22] He described himself politically as a "revolutionary anarchist, with a preference for non-violent methods."[23] He told Rigby that he aimed "to replace the present system by a new system in which coercion won't be relevant."[24] Rigby asked, "Do you feel that turning to drugs holds any revolutionary potential?" "That's right," replied Farquharson. "If you want to make converts, give them some acid first."[25]

Farquharson was born into a rich and respectable family in Pretoria, South Africa. He came to Oxford University in 1950 to study politics, philosophy, and economics, and he went in and out of mental hospitals through most of his adult life. In the 1950s, he considered Rupert Murdoch a close friend, with whom he ran the Oxford student magazine *Cherwell* and cofounded the philosophical Voltaire Society.[26] In the 1950s, he was a Laming Travelling Fellow, which enabled him to study in Paris, and then a Research Fellow at Nuffield College, Oxford, before attaining his DPhil. His 1958 DPhil thesis, *An Approach to Pure Theory of Voting Procedure,* earned the Monograph Prize of the American Academy of Arts and Sciences in social sciences in 1961, and it was later published as a book. In 1963, Farquharson used his substantial inheritance to recruit a guerrilla army to secretly set up a revolutionary struggle against apartheid in South Africa, but he was conned out of his money by a group of shrewd, hard-drinking Irishmen, who promised they could procure guns, grenades, and explosives for him.[27]

He was dismissed from his final academic post as a Senior Research Fellow at Cambridge in 1964, and the following year, he had his South African passport withdrawn for his part in lobbying on behalf of the South African Non-Racial Olympic Committee for South Africa to be excluded from the 1964 Olympic Games in Tokyo. Following his stay at Kingsley Hall sometime between 1966 and 1967, Farquharson became a British citizen in 1968, and in the same year, a book on his "social experiment" in "dropping out" in London was published. In the preface to his book *Drop Out!* he wrote, "I am a manic-depressive. When I'm up, I have no judgement, but fantastic drive; when I'm down, I have judgement, but no drive at all. In between I pass for normal well enough."[28] He revealed that he had "a history over twelve years of intermittent psychosis, mania, cyclothymia."[29]

According to the philosopher Sir Michael Dummett, who coauthored scholarly journal articles with Farquharson, he was an "exceptionally brilliant young man," but "his psychosis prevented him from accomplishing any more research."[30] The description of Farquharson as "exceptionally brilliant and extremely intelligent" was repeated by a string of colleagues and friends from his Oxford days.[31] Before he plunged into a world of squatter communes and crash pads in the mid-1960s, Farquharson had shared a flat with John Searle, later a professor of philosophy at the University of Berkeley, and Nigel Lawson, who became Chancellor of the Exchequer in Margaret

Thatcher's Conservative government.[32] Dummett remarked, "[H]ad it not been for the illness that afflicted him, he would doubtedly have become a very famous man, and probably have led a happy life," but "his early pioneering work was forgotten by almost everyone."[33]

"BREAK ON THROUGH": FROM PSYCHIATRY TO THE OTHER SIDE

The supposed emancipatory potential of LSD in the context of the psychiatric system was most clearly articulated in Britain through the "acid anarchism" of Farquharson. To understand why LSD was so politically subversive for him and why he thought and acted as he did, it is important to consider the psychiatric and countercultural contexts in which this acid anarchism emerged. On the face of it, the history of LSD in Britain is a conventional tale of a promising new drug that was initially kept under strict scientific and medical control, but which escaped the lab and clinic and was taken up by much less responsible parties, prompting its prohibition. Before 1952, when Ronald Sandison (1916–2010) became the first psychiatrist in Britain to treat patients with LSD, he was already making some markedly proto-Laingian moves.

In 1950, just two years after the inception of the National Health Service, Sandison remarked that "if we value wisdom and integration of the personality we must find a way for making something out of psychosis."[34] His suggestion, he said, "controversial though it may be, is that the maintenance of mental hospital culture rests on valuing psychosis and wisdom as all variants of one process."[35] Shortly afterward, however, Sandison, like others, was eager to disentangle the association of drugs such as LSD with psychotic symptoms or hallucinations by providing a new name that would not possess the negative connotations of a term like "hallucinogenic" or "psychotomimetic." Whereas Humphry Osmond coined the word "psychedelic," meaning "mind-manifesting," Sandison coined the term "psycholytic," meaning "mind-loosening." In Britain in the mid-1960s, Laing and his associates broke free from the rigid hierarchies of the hospital system and valued LSD and madness as potentially leading to a liberating voyage through inner space, if not to revolution.

Along with Sandison, the first investigators to work with LSD in 1950s Britain were psychiatrists and a psychopharmacologist. Wilhelm Mayer-Gross (1889–1961) carried out the earliest experiments with volunteer subjects, mainly his psychiatric colleagues at Crichton Royal Hospital in Dumfries, Scotland.[36] Joel Elkes (1913–2015), a psychopharmacologist who headed up the first department of experimental psychiatry at the University of Birmingham, undertook LSD research in his labs, advised British intelligence on the drug, and secured support for the first purpose-built LSD clinic in the world, at Powick Hospital, Worcestershire.[37] There, Sandison pioneered the use of LSD psychotherapy at the 100-year-old Victorian asylum.[38] Despite the marginality of psychoanalysis in British mental hospitals at this time, Sandison was a committed Jungian who steadfastly held that LSD could give access, not only to the depths of the personal unconscious, but to the universal archetypes of the collective unconscious.

Elsewhere, an experiment using LSD at a "psychiatric night hospital" on the premises of Marlborough Day Hospital was directed by Joshua Bierer.[39] Research with LSD in the 1950s took place against the backdrop of profound shifts in psychiatry, with far-reaching developments in psychopharmacology and new mental health legislation in the UK. Powick was the major center of LSD therapy in Britain between 1952 and 1972, treating hundreds of patients, but for the first ten years, it remained relatively low-key, arousing limited public interest beyond professional circles. An American author of a book on LSD therapy who visited Powick Hospital in 1963 was astonished to find that LSD was so little known among the general public: "this work which I hardly dared mention in the States was technical trivia in England, little known and less worth discussing."[40] Yet, within a few years of his visit, public awareness of LSD in Britain had grown as the chemical moved out of the clinic and along the highways and byways of countless trippers.

In 1962, BBC television showed a documentary in which LSD was publicized as a promising new therapeutic tool that supported psychoanalytic theory and practice. By 1967, Granada television had captured the cultural appeal of psychedelics beyond medicine on its program *It's So Far Out It's Straight Down*, about the London counterculture, featuring a defense of "psychedelia" by the Beatles' Paul McCartney. Television was pivotal in carrying the acid evangelism of Leary far and wide. This was largely owing to the advice of the Canadian media theorist Marshall McLuhan, who suggested to Leary that a catchy jingle in the style of a Pepsi television commercial would be a good way of broadcasting and promoting LSD.[41] That was how Leary's infamous 1965-mantra "Turn on, tune in, drop out" was born.

The growing mass media played a significant role in shaping public perceptions of LSD, as would famous British musicians like the Beatles and emerging "underground" bands like Pink Floyd. But to access news and information on acid subcultures at that time, it was necessary to consult underground newspapers, where drugs were often discussed and where US counterculture made inroads into the UK. From 1966, *International Times* or *IT*, intended to be London's equivalent of New York's *Village Voice,* the radical weekly newspaper covering art, literature, and leftist politics, or the more countercultural *East Village Other*, was a major source of information and means of international transmission of ideas on LSD, communal living, ways of exploring consciousness, and alternatives to psychiatry.[42] Underground newspapers like *IT*, funded by Paul McCartney and John Lennon, reprinted stories from papers around the world that were also part of the US-based Underground Press Syndicate.

Mimeograph technology facilitated the flourishing of the underground press and emerging youth cultures in the UK. Television contributed to the creation of what McLuhan called a "global village," demanding involvement in and stimulating a heightened and instantaneous awareness of events in distant places, and also helping LSD to become a global chemical messenger.[43] In 1967, after Leary appeared on television, Farquharson claimed that, "remembering his live voice more clearly than all the written words I had read on the same subject, I acted."[44] Here was an early embodiment of McLuhan's conjecture that while in the electronic age awareness of others was heightened, there would also be a retribalization of humanity. R. D. Laing first met Leary in 1964 and was later asked by *IT* if he "recommended a different form of dissemination" of LSD from Leary's popularization of the drug through the mass media.[45] In response to the interviewer's suggestion that Leary "felt this urgency to turn on as many people as quickly as possible, and blow the consequences," he said that he "respected that position," but that was not his "own style."[46]

In the early days of LSD research, the drug seemed to afford psychiatrists insight into psychotic illnesses if they took it themselves. Laing took this psychiatric approach further by suggesting that under LSD one may "experience a period of super-sanity" and that the aim of therapy is to "enhance consciousness rather than diminish it."[47] For Laing, the drugs used in therapy would have to be "consciousness expanding drugs, rather than consciousness constrictors—the psychic energisers, not the tranquillisers."[48] He thought that psychosis could be "a natural way of healing our own appalling state of alienation called normality," and "true sanity entails in one way or another the dissolution of the normal ego, that false self competently adjusted to our alienated social reality."[49] Such realizations prompted at least some anti-psychiatrists to take action to address what they saw as the alienating effects of social institutions. David Cooper and Joseph Berke were principal organizers of the Anti-University of London, which started in 1968. Cooper saw the Anti-University, like anti-psychiatry, as part of a revolt against the "institutionalisation of experience and action in this society."[50] He introduced the term "anti-psychiatry" as analogous with the idea of "anti-art" of the Dadaist movement in France, to imply opposition to certain psychiatric practices, "above all, the social violence that was done in the institutionalising process."[51] The short-lived Anti-University provided courses and seminars on various subjects, including "Anti-Institutions" and "Psychiatry of Revolution."[52]

By 1974, Cooper came to believe that "LSD, taken by certain people at the right time and in the right context, can more deeply mobilize revolutionary potential."[53] He thought that "as we revolutionize our 'psycho-chemistry' and our lives, substances like LSD will become superfluous," but that "for the time being, in pre-revolutionary society, the careful use of such substances by certain persons under strictly observed conditions may facilitate personal revolution, which can be integrated into the wider context of liberation of the society."[54] Just as psychosis had been valued by Sandison, and then arguably weaponized by Laing, LSD was seen by Cooper as a tool to prepare the revolutionary activist. If it were possible for radical psychiatrists to employ such tools in the service of transformative or revolutionary ends, why not their patients, thought Farquharson.

DROPPING OUT AND ACID ANARCHISM

On one occasion, when Farquharson was living in a basement commune in 1970, he announced to his companions that he could get some liquid acid if everyone put some money in—he collected £5. He came back with a jar of orange juice that he said contained the LSD. According to one participant, Richard Lancaster, Farquharson was clearly in a manic state and "laying fairly heavy/speedy vibes on everyone," causing Lancaster to become "very anxious about tripping in these circumstances."[55] But, after a while, no-one had come on and Farquharson "announced the failure of an experiment to induce tripping in a group of people by suggestion alone, with a placebo— there was no acid in the orange juice."[56] Later that evening, Farquharson appeared on a television programme on Alternative Society organisations. Lancaster recalled that

> Robin suddenly came up to the camera looking quite freaky, pulled out a fiver, announced that no one needed cash ("we need housing and food, not money"), and tried to rip the note to pieces. It wouldn't rip properly, so he borrowed a match and set light to it. It was the £5 we had given him earlier.[57]

Soon after, Farquharson found himself detained once again in his favourite "bin," Horton Hospital, for several months.

It was three years earlier, in 1967, following his exclusion from Kingsley Hall, that Farquharson "dropped out" and first experimented with LSD. In the opening chapter of *Drop Out!* he explained that he "had often heard the slogan 'Turn on, tune in, drop out'." But it was Leary himself who sparked his interest. Leary, he remarked, "had been, as I had been, a university don and the author of learned works and whose academic career, like mine, though for different reasons, had collapsed in ruins."[58] Yet, unlike him, Leary "had carved an existence and a name for himself almost from scratch, in the non-academic world."[59] He did not recall Leary's exact words, but for Farquharson, in essence he was saying:

> Rid yourself of responsibility, quit the rat-race. Don't obey society's paralysing conventions, you have a simple road to escape them. Leave your job, leave the acquisitive society, you can still inhabit its cities physically while nevertheless becoming totally insulated from the ulcer-generating pressures of its oppressive system of employee and of boss, of high salaries never overtaking rising costs and rising standards of living. Step out of the trap; the door is open. 'Drop out!'[60]

Farquharson stressed that he did not encourage abandoning constructive activity. On the contrary, he believed that "dropping out is a highly creative act," that it "means the opportunity to explore, in freedom, your own true potentialities."[61] In the early 1970s, after its original structure was dismantled, Farquharson convened his own Anti-University courses on what he called the "Alternative Society."[62] An *IT* advertisement urged prospective students to contact the course leader at his temporary residence, Horton Hospital, a massive mental institution in Surrey.[63] For Farquharson, "the Alternative Society is about a transformation that takes place first in the minds of individual human beings [and] the essence of the transformation that takes place is the lifting, temporary or permanent, partial or complete, of the barrier which divides the conscious from the unconscious mind."[64] The continuities from the LSD psychotherapy of Ronald Sandison to Farquharson's Alternative Society are evident, but so are the links with Laing's preference for transcendental journeying through inner space.

Farquharson suggested that the barrier lifting took different forms: "[I]t may occur in, or be taken as, various forms of mental illness, diversely diagnosed."[65] It may happen "as the result of taking 'soft drugs,' particularly LSD or cannabis," and "it may arise as a result of a lengthy period of psychoanalysis."[66] "Typically," he asserted, "its initial advent causes great confusion of mind; confusion which, once the individual has adjusted to the change, gives way to clarity and calm."[67] In *Drop Out!* he reported that acid "had profoundly changed [his] life attitudes and situation."[68] The LSD insight, he said, had enabled him "to make sense of what before had seemed like a purposeless affliction":

Not only is it much clearer to me what is happening when my mania rages; I am also now in a position to accept the fact of the psychosis as something validly and perhaps valuably deflecting my life from its previous direction, and able to apply my energies to finding exactly what that direction should be and following it. . . .

LSD affects not only perception, but motivation. After LSD, one is likely to be much less attracted by money and luxuries and material success; much less concerned about the requirements and taboos of convention; more sensitive to, and to value much more highly, perceptual experience and personal relationships. The detachment from worldly considerations is closely similar to the effect of many religious conversions.[69]

It was clear to Farquharson that the religious experience, the psychotic experience, and the LSD experience were "simply sights on the same landscape through different windows."[70] He saw these experiences as "variants of a single phenomenon."[71] He claimed that the lifting of the barrier constituted "the opening of the gate in the soul," producing "a reorientation of the subject's ethical attitudes from concern for self to concern for others; from Right to Left," and "a freshening of perception, so that the whole world is seen anew."[72] As a result, "very powerful creative forces are unleashed in the mind," the effects of which "may be felt in many fruitful ways," including "the ability to organise on a large scale."[73] For Farquharson, a personal voyage and spiritual transformation led him to take part in activities of anarchistic social determination, including forms of practical self-organization with fellow psychiatric patients.

Farquharson claimed that he was "divinely inspired" and "a servant of God," but he "did not feel any kinship with the Church."[74] He thought that "communes are the microcosms of the form of government of the future, and the Federation of Communes is the archetypal future state."[75] It was direct participation in the deliberative democracy of voluntary associations that attracted him. For Farquharson, "the basic theoretical problem is to devise a proper large scale decision-making procedure which does not have the disadvantage of the voting system."[76] The disadvantages of voting, according to him, were that it led to "a gross over-simplification of the nation's will," "most alternatives cannot be discussed," and it "leads to the party system."[77] When asked if he saw society in terms of social classes, Farquharson was adamant that he did not. Instead, he thought that "there are different levels, different kinds of schools, different kinds of incomes, different kinds of speech."[78] He insisted that if he did "think in terms of classes it is in terms of A, B, C, D—not antagonistic groups."[79]

He sought "a system in which there was much more frequent consultation and a much richer range of alternatives available, in which the decision was taken directly by the electorate and not indirectly through the parliamentary system."[80] He typically had a copy of *IT* on hand, as he did at a Pretoria mental hospital in 1969, when he first read about a new group, PNP.[81] On his return to London, he joined the group, with whom he sought "a real people's alternative to objective and objectifying psychiatry," endeavoring to set up a household like Kingsley Hall, which would have people in it who were "not currently agonizing" and could "act as helpers," but where there would be "no rigid frontier" between helpers and agonizers.[82]

Farquharson vowed that he "would obviously be on both sides of whatever frontier there was."[83] After his drop-out experiment in 1967, he searched for a place where he and others could let go—"geographies of licence, places pervaded by a feeling of relaxation and self-determination"—which were sometimes present, but only rarely, in mental hospitals.[84] Farquharson sought to reproduce the sanctuary that mental hospitals were supposed to provide, but in a setting beyond the reach of the tentacles of psychiatry and the state. Michael Barnett, the founder of PNP, remarked that Farquharson "saw such an environment as providing the support he would need when he was freaking out, so that he could go through it, which hospitals did not allow, but blocked."[85]

According to Barnett, "society, normal society refused to allow him to experiment like this, but a group of people committed to finding out whatever there was to discover would surely allow him full scope to explore his own mystery and chance."[86] PNP aimed to provide "a program not of interference but of extended liberty, not of manipulation but of nurture and growth."[87] For PNP, "psychiatry is politics," and "the blatant aim of current politics is to keep things more or less as they are," so "people who break down because they cannot find a way to live sanely in an insane society are shattered forces for change."[88] Under the auspices of the Situationist Housing Association formed by Farquharson, PNP found its first house. LSD was not central to PNP, although members "frequently helped those suffering from the effects of bad acid trips," and "later it even had 'specialists' in this work."[89]

Farquharson once said, "I don't like going to mental hospital because it stops me getting my psychotherapy—LET US MAKE A WEAPON OF OUR SICKNESS—Socialist Patients Kollective."[90] He had a knack for making international connections, and he put this ethos of the Heidelberg-based radical mental health organization Das Sozialistische Patientenkollektiv (SPK) into practice in the service of all the emerging radical mental health associations in Britain, including PNP, the Scottish Union of Mental Patients (SUMP), and the Mental Patients Union (MPU).[91] He offered a squatted building to MPU shortly before his tragic death in 1973, and the subsequent MPU headquarters in London were named Robin Farquharson House in his memory. Farquharson died on April 1 from injuries sustained in a fire at a derelict terrace house where he was squatting; two Irish laborers who lived at the house with him were later convicted of unlawful killing. Did the psychiatrists' tools dismantle the psychiatrists' house? Did mental patients make a weapon of their illness? It is clear that a leading pioneer of the UK mental patient movement was fundamentally shaped by the ideas of anti-psychiatry, his direct experience of the Kingsley Hall experiment, and the varied psychedelic radicalism of Laing, Cooper, and Leary, not to mention his own theory of voting and his forays into the London alternative scene.

Farquharson's acid anarchism should be understood in light of Laing's facilitation of trips through inner space, when he, a psychiatrist, became convinced of the need for "a place where people who have travelled further and, consequently, may be more lost than psychiatrists and other sane people, can find their way *further* into inner space and time and back again."[92] Laing sought an "*initiation* ceremonial," and psychiatrically, he said, "this would appear as ex-patients helping future patients go mad."[93] It has been argued by the Survivors History Group, a community history project led by former patients, or survivors, of psychiatry, that the link between professional-led anti-psychiatry and patient-led mental patient unionism was not strong. However, it is incontrovertible that Farquharson drew on his own direct involvement with the Kingsley Hall experiment in the course of his transition from academic dropout to mental health activist.[94]

LSD acted as a communal catalyst and conduit for Farquharson as he moved from Kingsley Hall, via inspiration from Timothy Leary, into other experiments for communal living and alternatives to the university, psychiatry, and mental hospitals. The fruits of Farquharson's acid anarchism were diverse, including the Community Organisation for Psychiatric Emergencies (COPE). COPE "set up houses (the true asylums) for people so that they could 'work through' this madness as a healing process."[95] It helped people who had "freaked out" and "need[ed] space to try and work things out without getting a lot laid on them, and would otherwise be sent to the bin."[96] They linked with "encounter (therapy) consciousness-raising groups of a self-help nature in London."[97]

As a member of the White Panther Party, an antiracist, far-left group originally founded in the US with chapters across Britain, Farquharson tore down the perimeter fences at the Isle of Wight Festival in 1970, declaring the festival free. These events inspired another acid anarchist, Bill "Ubi" Dwyer, to initiate the free festival movement in Britain. In Dwyer, acid anarchism was most clearly articulated in "The Acid Issue" of the periodical *Anarchy*, where he stated that LSD assisted one in self-discovery, raising "awareness of one's own dignity, sovereignty and sacredness," supporting the rejection of authority and the "espousal of a society organised without authority."[98] Dwyer argued, "It is the mental attitude of voluntary servitude, which is the greatest support of authority . . . [and] it is exactly this psychological slavery, this surrender to the personality of others, that LSD attacks."[99] For these men, LSD was "a holy sacrament," but also "a potential deadly enemy" to the power and position of the authorities.[100]

While psychedelic science, techno-utopian microdosing, and lysergic legitimation through randomized controlled trials dominate the discourse of the psychedelic renaissance today, if the acid anarchist past is anything to go by, the new wave could yet take a more antiestablishment turn. For MPU, anti-psychiatry was not "the antithesis of psychiatry—'Patients' Control' was the antithesis of psychiatry.[101] In the early 1970s, the MPU envisaged "that patients will begin to mimic psychiatry to such an extent that psychiatry will lose its professional gleam, it will become a joke."[102] While it is true that by and large, collective action by mental patients in Britain emerged independent of the activities of Laing, Cooper, Berke, and associates, the direct link to that group, in the person of Robin Farquharson, illuminates the context in which psychiatry became the target of subversive subcultures of activism and how ideas of anti-psychiatry, the anti-university and the alternative society led Farquharson to participate in practical self-organization and mutual aid with fellow mental patients.

NOTES

1. Nick Crossley, "R.D. Laing and the British Anti-Psychiatry Movement: A Socio-Historical Analysis," *Social Science and Medicine* 47 (1998): 877–889; Nick Crossley, "Mental Health, Resistance and Social Movements: The Collective-Confrontational Dimension," *Health Education Journal* 61 (2002): 138–152; Nick Crossley, *Contesting Psychiatry: Social Movements in Mental Health* (Abingdon, UK: Routledge, 2006); Adrian Chapman, "Re-Coopering Anti-Psychiatry: David Cooper, Revolutionary Critic of Psychiatry," *Critical and Radical Social Work* 4, no. 3 (2016): 421–432; Oisin Wall, *The British Anti-Psychiatrists: From Institutional Psychiatry to the Counter-Culture, 1960–1971* (Abingdon, UK: Routledge, 2017).

2. Sarah Shortall, "Psychedelic Drugs and the Problem of Experience," *Past and Present* 222, Supplement 9 (2014): 206.

3. Mark Fisher, "Acid Communism (unfinished introduction)," *Blackout* (blog), https://my -blackout.com/2019/04/25/mark-fisher-acid-communism-unfinished- introduction/.

4. See especially Jeremy Gilbert, "Psychedelic Socialism," *Open Democracy*, December 22, 2017. https://www.opendemocracy.net/en/psychedelic-socialism/. Fisher's acid communism ideas have been developed in an ongoing UK podcast series, *ACFM*.

5. "Acid Communism, Labour, and the Counterculture with Jeremy Gilbert," on the podcast *Politics Theory Other*, https://soundcloud.com/poltheoryother/63-acid-communism-labour -and-the-counterculture-w-jeremy-gilbert.

6. Fisher, "Acid Communism."

7. Mark Fisher, talk on capitalism and consciousness given at "All of this is temporary" event at Rich Mix, London, February 23rd 2016, https://www.youtube.com/watch?v =deZgzw0YHQI.

8. Matt Colquhoun, *Acid Communism* (Pattern Books, Anti-Copyright 2020).

9. R. D. Laing, *The Politics of Experience and The Bird of Paradise* (London: Penguin, 1990), 105.

10. Colquhoun, *Acid Communism*.

11. Adrian Chapman, "Dwelling in Strangeness: Accounts of the Kingsley Hall Community, London (1965–1970), Established by R. D. Laing," *Medical Humanities* (2020). https://link .springer.com/article/10.1007%2Fs10912-020-09656-0.

12. Dominic Harris, *The Residents: Stories of Kingsley Hall, East London, 1965–1970 and the Experimental Community of RD Laing* (London: Dominic Harris, 2012).

13. R. D. Laing, "Psychotherapy as Celebration," *Wellspring* 1 (1984): 6–10; transcript of a talk delivered in October 1983 at the Queen's Hall, Edinburgh, under the sponsorship of Wellspring; University of Glasgow Library, Special Collections, Papers of Ronald David Laing, MS Laing A1.

14. R. D. Laing, "Hatred of Health," *Journal of Contemplative Psychotherapy* 1 (1987): 85.

15. Laing, "Hatred of Health."

16. Catherine Fussinger, "'Therapeutic Community', Psychiatry's Reformers and Antipsychiatrists: Reconsidering Changes in the Field of Psychiatry after World War II," *History of Psychiatry* 22 (2011): 146–163; Helen Spandler, *Asylum to Action: Paddington Day Hospital, Therapeutic Communities and Beyond* (London: Jessica Kingsley, 2006); Helen Spandler, "Spaces of Psychiatric Contention: A Case Study of a Therapeutic Community," *Health & Place* 15 (2009): 672–678; Claire Baron, *Asylum to Anarchy* (London: Free Association Press, 1987).

17. Colin Jones, "Raising the Anti: Jan Foudraine, Ronald Laing and Anti-Psychiatry," in *Cultures of Psychiatry and Mental Health Care in Postwar Britain and the Netherlands*, ed. Marijke Gijswijt-Hofstra and Roy Porter (Amsterdam: Rodopi, 1998), 283–294.

18. Robin Farquharson, *Drop Out!* (London: Penguin, 1971), 54.

19. Farquharson, *Drop Out!* 54.

20. Bob Mullan, *Mad to be Normal: Conversations with R. D. Laing* (London: Free Association Books, 1995), 181.

21. Mullan, *Mad to be Normal*, 189.

22. This Communes Research Project was the basis of Rigby's book *Communes in Britain* (London: Routledge and Kegan Paul, 1974).

23. *Bitman* no. 6, "Ex-Bitman Robin Special Issue," May 8, 1973, 5. https://content.wisconsinhistory.org/digital/collection/p15932coll8/id/12044. *Bitman* was an inexpensive magazine produced by BIT, a 24-hour free information and help service in London involved in creating "free spaces" and supporting communes with funds by publishing and selling expensive travel magazines.

24. *Bitman* no. 6, "Ex-Bitman Robin Special Issue."

25. *Bitman* no. 6, "Ex-Bitman Robin Special Issue."

26. Neil Chenoweth, *Virtual Murdoch: Reality Wars on the Information Highway* (London: Vintage, 2002), 17–19.

27. *Bitman* No. 6, 2, https://content.wisconsinhistory.org/digital/collection/p15932coll8/id/12041.

28. Farquharson, *Drop Out!* 7.

29. Farquharson, *Drop Out!* 51–52.

30. Michael Dummett, "The Work and Life of Robin Farquharson," *Social Choice and Welfare* 25 (2005): 475.

31. Chenoweth, *Virtual Murdoch*, 15–21.

32. Chenoweth, *Virtual Murdoch*, 16–17.

33. Dummett, "The Work and Life of Robin Farquharson," 82–83.

34. Ronald Sandison, "The Re-socialization of the Psychiatric Case," *Mental Health* (London) 10, no. 4 (1951): 88.

35. Sandison, "The Re-socialization of the Psychiatric Case."

36. W. Mayer-Gross, W. McAdam, and J. Walker, "Psychological and Biochemical Effects of Lysergic Acid Diethylamide," *Nature* 16 (1951): 827–828.

37. P. B. Bradley, C. Elkes, and J. Elkes, "On Some Effects of Lysergic Acid Diethylamide (L.S.D. 25) in Normal Volunteers," *Journal of Physiology* 121, no. 2 (1953): 50–51.

38. R. A. Sandison, A. M. Spencer, and J.D.A. Whitelaw, "The Therapeutic Value of Lysergic Acid Diethylamide in Mental Illness," *Journal of Mental Science* 100 (1954): 491–507; R. A. Sandison, "Psychological Aspects of the LSD Treatment of the Neuroses," *Journal of Mental Science* 100 (1954): 508–515.

39. Joshua Bierer and Ivor W. Browne, "An Experiment with a Psychiatric Night Hospital," *Proceedings of the Royal Society of Medicine* 53, no. 11 (1960): 930–934.

40. W. V. Caldwell, *LSD Psychotherapy: An Exploration of Psychedelic and Psycholytic Therapy* (New York: Grove Press, 1968), 92.

41. Neil Strauss, *Everyone Loves You When You're Dead: Journeys into Fame and Madness* (New York: HarperCollins, 2011), 337–338; Tim Wu, *The Attention Merchants: The Epic Scramble to Get inside Our Heads* (New York: Knopf, 2016), 152–154.

42. Barry Miles, "The Underground Press," British Library, https://www.bl.uk/20th-century-literature/articles/the-underground-press.

43. Marshall McLuhan, *The Gutenberg Galaxy: The Making of Typographic Man* (Toronto: University of Toronto Press, 1962), 21.

44. Farquharson, *Drop Out!* 14.

45. R. D. Laing, "Dr Ronald Laing Talks with Felix Scorpio," *International Times* 59 (1969): 6.

46. Laing, "Dr Ronald Laing Talks with Felix Scorpio."

47. R.D. Laing quoted in Adrian Laing, *R.D. Laing: A Biography* (London: Peter Owen, 1994), 121.

48. Ibid.

49. Laing, *The Politics of Experience*, 119.

50. David Cooper, "Beyond Words," in *The Dialectics of Liberation*, ed. David Cooper (Harmondsworth, UK: Penguin, 1968), 197.

51. David Cooper, "David Cooper: Interview by Ron Lacey," *Openmind* 3 (1983): 8.

52. "Anti-University Announces Courses," *International Times* 24, January 19–February 1 (1968): 3, 49; David Cooper, *The Grammar of Living* (New York: Pantheon, 1974), 35.

53. Cooper, *The Grammar of Living*, 35.

54. Cooper, *The Grammar of Living*.

55. *Bitman* no. 6, "Ex-Bitman Robin Special Issue," May 8, 1973, 5. https://content .wisconsinhistory.org/digital/collection/p15932coll8/id/12044.

56. *Bitman* No. 6, "Ex-Bitman Robin Special Issue," May 8, 1973, 4. https://content .wisconsinhistory.org/digital/collection/p15932coll8/id/12043/rec/1.

57. *Bitman* No. 6, "Ex-Bitman Robin Special Issue," May 8, 1973, 4. https://content .wisconsinhistory.org/digital/collection/p15932coll8/id/12043/rec/1.

58. Farquharson, *Drop Out!* 13.

59. Farquharson, *Drop Out!*

60. Farquharson, *Drop Out!* 14.

61. Farquharson, *Drop Out!* 30.

62. *International Times*, 121, January 13–27 (1972), 3; See also Jakob Jakobsen, "Antiuniversity of London—An Introduction to Deinstitutionalisation," in *Antiuniversity of London—Antihistory Tabloid*, ed. Jakob Jakobsen (London: MayDay Rooms, 2012), 9–12 (also accessible at https://antihistory.org/deinsti).

63. *International Times*, 121, January 13–27 (1972), 3.

64. Farquharson, "The Alternative Society," in *Bitman* no. 6, "Ex-Bitman Robin Special Issue," 3.

65. Farquharson, "The Alternative Society," in *Bitman* no. 6, "Ex-Bitman Robin Special Issue," 3.

66. Farquharson, "The Alternative Society," in *Bitman* no. 6, "Ex-Bitman Robin Special Issue," 3.

67. Farquharson, "The Alternative Society," in *Bitman* no. 6, "Ex-Bitman Robin Special Issue," 3.

68. Farquharson, *Drop Out!* 111.

69. Farquharson, *Drop Out!* 110–111.

70. Farquharson, *Drop Out!* 110.

71. Farquharson, *Drop Out!*

72. Farquharson, "The Alternative Society," in *Bitman* no. 6, "Ex-Bitman Robin Special Issue," 3. <https://content.wisconsinhistory.org/digital/collection/p15932coll8/id/12042>

73. Farquharson, "The Alternative Society."

74. *Bitman* no. 6, 4. <https://content.wisconsinhistory.org/digital/collection/p15932coll8/id/12043>

75. *Bitman* no. 6, 5. <https://content.wisconsinhistory.org/digital/collection/p15932coll8/id/12044>

76. *Bitman* no. 6.

77. *Bitman* no. 6.

78. *Bitman* no. 6.

79. *Bitman* no. 6.

80. *Bitman* no. 6.

81. Michael Barnett, *People Not Psychiatry: A Human Alternative to Psychotherapy* (London: Allen & Unwin, 1973), 191.

82. Barnett, *People Not Psychiatry*, 110; 75; 191–192.

83. Barnett, *People Not Psychiatry*, 191–192.

84. Erving Goffman, *Asylums: Essays on the Social Situation of Mental Patients and Other Inmates* (New York: Anchor Books, 1961), 230–231.

85. Barnett, *People Not Psychiatry*, 192.

86. Barnett, *People Not Psychiatry*.

87. "The Sick Scene," *International Times*, 59, July 4–17 (1969): 3.

88. "The Sick Scene."

89. Barnett, *People Not Psychiatry*, 126; 129.

90. *Bitman* No. 6, 8. https://content.wisconsinhistory.org/digital/collection/p15932coll8/id/12047; See also Wolfgang Huber, *Turn Illness into a Weapon: For Agitation by the Socialist Patients' Collective at the University of Heidelberg* (English translation) (Heidelberg, Germany: KRRIM, 1993).

91. Mark Gallagher, "From Asylum to Action in Scotland: The Emergence of the Scottish Union of Mental Patients, 1971–1972," *History of Psychiatry* 28, no. 1 (2017): 101–114.

92. Laing, *The Politics of Experience*, 105–106. Emphasis in original.

93. Laing, *The Politics of Experience*, 106. Emphasis in original.

94. Survivors History Group, "Survivors History Group Take a Critical Look at Historians," in *Critical Perspectives on User Involvement*, ed. Marian Barnes and Phil Cotterell (Bristol: Policy Press, 2011), 7–18.

95. "COPE," *Bittersweet* 14 (1975), 28.

96. "COPE," *Maya Free Nation News* 2, October (1974): 2.

97. "COPE," *Bittersweet* 14 (1975): 28.

98. Bill Dwyer, "Feed the Head. LSD The Magic Acid," *Anarchy* 3 (1970): 5, 11.

99. Dwyer, "Feed the Head," 11.

100. Letter from Bill Dwyer, *International Times* 121, January 13–27 (1972): 3.

101. MPU, *Maya Free Nation News*.

102. MPU, *Maya Free Nation News*.

BIBLIOGRAPHY

Primary Sources

"Anti-University Announces Courses." *International Times*, 24, January 19–February 1 (1968), 3, 49.

"COPE." *Bittersweet* 14 (1975), 28.

"COPE." *Maya Free Nation News*, 2, October (1974), 2.

Bitman No. 6. "Ex-Bitman Robin Special Issue," May 8, 1973, 5.

Cooper, David. "David Cooper: Interview by Ron Lacey." *Openmind* 3, June/July (1983): 8.

Dwyer, Bill. "Feed the Head. LSD The Magic Acid," *Anarchy*, 3 (1970), 5, 11.

Farquharson, Robin. "The Alternative Society," unpublished introductory chapter of manuscript "I AM GOD," in *Bitman* no. 6, "Ex-Bitman Robin Special Issue," May 8, 1973, 3.

Huber, Wolfgang. *Turn Illness into a Weapon: For Agitation by the Socialist Patients' Collective at the University of Heidelberg* (English translation), Heidelberg: KRRIM, 1993.

International Times, 121, January 13–27, 1972, 3.

Letter from Bill Dwyer, *International Times*, 121, January 13–27, 1972, 3.

MPU, *Maya Free Nation News*, October 2, 1974, 3.

"The Sick Scene," *International Times*, 59, July 4–17, 1969, 3.

Transcript of a talk delivered in October 1983 at the Queen's Hall, Edinburgh, under the sponsorship of Wellspring. Printed text, with pencil emendations by R. D. Laing; University of Glasgow Library, Special Collections, Papers of Ronald David Laing, MS Laing A1.

Secondary Sources

Barnett, Michael. *People Not Psychiatry: A Human Alternative to Psychotherapy*. London: Allen & Unwin, 1973.

Baron, Claire. *Asylum to Anarchy*. London: Free Association Press, 1987.

Bierer, Joshua, and Ivor W. Browne. "An Experiment with a Psychiatric Night Hospital." *Proceedings of the Royal Society of Medicine* 53, no. 11 (1960): 930–934.

Bradley, P. B., C. Elkes, and J. Elkes. "On Some Effects of Lysergic Acid Diethylamide (L.S.D. 25) in Normal Volunteers." *Journal of Physiology* 121, no. 2 (1953): 50–51.

Caldwell, W. V. *LSD Psychotherapy: An Exploration of Psychedelic and Psycholytic Therapy*. New York: Grove Press, 1968.

Chapman, Adrian. "Dwelling in Strangeness: Accounts of the Kingsley Hall Community, London (1965–1970), Established by R. D. Laing." *Medical Humanities* (2020). https://link.springer.com /article/10.1007/s10912-020-09656-0.

Chapman, Adrian. "Re-Coopering Anti-Psychiatry: David Cooper, Revolutionary Critic of Psychiatry." *Critical and Radical Social Work* 4, no. 3 (2016): 421–432.

Chenoweth, Neil. *Virtual Murdoch: Reality Wars on the Information Highway*. London: Vintage, 2002.

Colquhoun, Matt. *Acid Communism*. Pattern Books, Anti-Copyright 2020.

Cooper, David. "Beyond Words." In *The Dialectics of Liberation*, edited by David Cooper, 197. Harmondsworth, UK: Penguin, 1968.

Cooper, David. *The Grammar of Living*. New York: Pantheon, 1974.

Crossley, Nick. *Contesting Psychiatry: Social Movements in Mental Health*. Abingdon, UK: Routledge, 2006.

Crossley, Nick. "Mental Health, Resistance and Social Movements: The Collective-Confrontational Dimension." *Health Education Journal* 61 (2002): 138–152.

Crossley, Nick. "R. D. Laing and the British Anti-Psychiatry Movement: A Socio-Historical Analysis." *Social Science and Medicine* 47 (1998): 877–889.

Dummett, Michael. "The Work and Life of Robin Farquharson." *Social Choice and Welfare* 25, no. 2–3 (2005): 475–483.

Farquharson, Robin. *Drop Out!* London: Penguin, 1971.

Fisher, Mark. Talk on capitalism and consciousness given at "All of this is temporary" event at Rich Mix, London, February 23, 2016. https://www.youtube.com/watch?v=deZgzw0YHQI.

Fisher, Mark. "Acid Communism (Unfinished Introduction)." *Blackout* (Poetry and Politics) 25 (2019).

Fussinger, Catherine. "'Therapeutic Community,' Psychiatry's Reformers and Antipsychiatrists: Reconsidering Changes in the Field of Psychiatry after World War II." *History of Psychiatry* 22 (2011): 146–163.

Gallagher, Mark. "'From Asylum to Action in Scotland: The Emergence of the Scottish Union of Mental Patients, 1971–1972'." *History of Psychiatry* 28, no. 1 (2017): 101–114.

Gilbert, Jeremy. "Acid Communism, Labour, and the Counterculture." On the podcast Politics Theory Other. https://soundcloud.com/poltheoryother/63-acid-communism-labour-and-the -counterculture-w-jeremy-gilbert.

Gilbert, Jeremy. "Psychedelic Socialism." Open Democracy, December 22, 2017. https://www.opendemocracy.net/en/psychedelic-socialism/.

Goffman, Erving. *Asylums: Essays on the Social Situation of Mental Patients and Other Inmates.* New York: Anchor Books, 1961.

Jakobsen, Jakob. "Antiuniversity of London—An Introduction to Deinstitutionalisation." In *Antiuniversity of London—Antihistory Tabloid*, ed. Jakob Jakobsen. London: MayDay Rooms, 2012. https://antihistory.org/deinsti.

Jones, Colin. "Raising the Anti: Jan Foudraine, Ronald Laing and Anti-Psychiatry." In *Cultures of Psychiatry and Mental Health Care in Postwar Britain and the Netherlands*, edited by Marijke Gijswijt-Hofstra and Roy Porter, 284–294. Amsterdam: Rodopi, 1998.

Laing, Adrian. *R.D. Laing: A Biography.* London: Peter Owen, 1994.

Laing, R. D. "Hatred of Health." *Journal of Contemplative Psychotherapy* (1987): 77–86.

Laing, R. D. "Dr Ronald Laing Talks with Felix Scorpio." *International Times* 59 (1969): 6.

Laing, R. D. *The Politics of Experience and The Bird of Paradise.* London: Penguin, 1990.

Laing, R. D. "Psychotherapy as Celebration." *Wellspring*, no. 1 (1984): 6–10.

Mayer-Gross, W., W. McAdam, and J. Walker. "Psychological and Biochemical Effects of Lysergic Acid Diethylamide." *Nature* 16 (1951): 827–828.

McLuhan, Marshall. *The Gutenberg Galaxy: The Making of Typographic Man.* University of Toronto Press, 1962.

Miles, Barry. "The Underground Press." British Library, May 25, 2016. https://www.bl.uk/20th-century-literature/articles/the-underground-press.

Mullan, Bob. *Mad to Be Normal: Conversations with R. D. Laing.* London: Free Association Books, 1995.

Rigby, Andrew. *Communes in Britain.* London: Routledge and Kegan Paul, 1974.

Sandison, R. A. "Psychological Aspects of the LSD Treatment of the Neuroses." *Journal of Mental Science* 100 (1954): 508–515.

Sandison, Ronald. "The Re-socialization of the Psychiatric Case." *Mental Health* (London) 10, no. 4 (1951): 87–96.

Sandison, Ronald A., A. M. Spencer, and J. D. A. Whitelaw. "The Therapeutic Value of Lysergic Acid Diethylamide in Mental Illness." *Journal of Mental Science* 100, no. 419 (1954): 491–507.

Shortall, Sarah. "Psychedelic Drugs and the Problem of Experience." *Past and Present* 222, Supplement 9 (2014): 187–206.

Spandler, Helen. *Asylum to Action: Paddington Day Hospital, Therapeutic Communities and Beyond.* London: Jessica Kingsley, 2006.

Spandler, Helen. "Spaces of Psychiatric Contention: A Case Study of a Therapeutic Community." *Health & Place* 15 (2009): 672–678.

Strauss, Neil. *Everyone Loves You When You're Dead: Journeys into Fame and Madness*. New York: HarperCollins, 2011.

Survivors History Group, "'Survivors History Group Take a Critical Look at Historians." In *Critical Perspectives on User Involvement*, edited by Marian Barnes and Phil Cotterell, 7–18. Bristol, UK: Policy Press, 2011.

Wall, Oisin. *The British Anti-Psychiatrists: From Institutional Psychiatry to the Counter-Culture, 1960–1971*. Abingdon, UK: Routledge, 2017.

Wu, Tim. *The Attention Merchants: The Epic Scramble to Get inside Our Heads*. New York: Knopf, 2016.

19 BECOMING MODERN IN CHINA WITH AN INDIGENOUS AMAZONIAN PSYCHEDELIC BREW

Alex K. Gearin

Ayahuasca is a psychoactive brew that originated among Indigenous Amazonian groups[1] and recently became popular among fringe spirituality and healing networks across much of the Western world.[2] Eager to experience a deeper connection to nature, relief from mental afflictions, and vivid mental imagery, ayahuasca drinkers across the globe have helped revive and transform Indigenous shamanism in Peru, Brazil, and Colombia and spawned a range of religions and New Age or neo-shamanic approaches across Europe, North America, Australia, and elsewhere. While the Indigenous, religious, and neo-shamanic types of ayahuasca use have gained considerable attention from researchers, the psychoactive brew has recently emerged in mainland China and is at the center of a nominally secular and remarkably original style of use. This chapter provides an ethnographic sketch of this new phenomenon. It examines how ayahuasca is used in a major city (Tier 1) in mainland China by young Chinese professionals searching for holistic wellness, self-cultivation, and a competitive edge in capitalist environments. To protect the identities of the people who organized and attended the ayahuasca retreats in mainland China, I refrain from describing the cities where the events were typically occurring.

Attempting to explain why ayahuasca has become so popular across the globe, researchers have suggested that the brew helps to spiritually recuperate individuals who are disenchanted by modern society.[3] In doing so, they pit ayahuasca against the secularizing teleologies that define a key strand of modernization theory. Social theorists have illustrated how historical processes of modern rationalism, materialism, and capitalism provided a remarkable mastery of the world, but at the grave expense of eroding spiritual and existential meaning. In his tome *A Secular Age* (2007), Charles Taylor suggests the modern erasure of enchantment has buffered and dislodged the self from wider cosmic orders, leaving it subject to a historically distinct malaise. The inability of spirits, gods, or the supernatural to compel the self is accompanied by a wider vacuum of meaning, he argues, in which "our actions, goals, achievements, and the like, have a lack of weight, gravity, thickness, substance."[4] In Max Weber's terms, individuals living under industrial capitalism are progressively disenchanted and transformed into cogs in the machinery of rational pursuits aimed at precision, steadiness, and speed, becoming "specialists without spirit, sensualists without heart."[5] Considering what was lost to such an instrumental modernity, Stephen Kalberg suggests that religion entrenched the premodern world with ethical foundations and "coherent constellations of values that address fundamental questions concerning the ultimate meaning of life."[6] The notion of recovering aspects of a premodern world animates much of the global revival of ayahuasca drinking, and certainly its popular neo-shamanic strand, which enacts a therapeutic primitivism.[7] Tracing ayahuasca to the spiritual and Indigenous depths of the Amazon rainforest, neo-shamanic practitioners bring to lived experience a meaningful and porous cosmos perceived as coming from far beyond the existential vacuum of modernity.

Ayahuasca has engaged such crises of meaning through a unique infusion of the cultural with the chemical. According to Ido Hartogsohn and others, the ingestion of psychedelic alkaloids, such as those in ayahuasca, can result in an enhanced perception of meaning or "cause things to appear dramatically more meaningful than they would otherwise seem to be."[8] When the drink meets the primitivist imaginaries of neo-shamanic cosmology, such an enrichment of meaning tends to have existential import. The psychologist and early psychedelic researcher Ralph Metzner explained that "the real beauty of the teachings of ayahuasca spirits is that they can help provide meaning, purpose and direction to one's life."[9] In response to philosophers who have warned of the impoverishment of meaning in industrialized societies, Hartogsohn situates the meaning-enhancing function of ayahuasca and other psychedelics "in the broader cultural context of late modernity's struggle to make sense and meaning of life in increasingly atomized, individualized, and stress-ridden societies."[10] Ayahuasca is popularly consumed in neo-shamanic circles in an attempt to reenchant a capitalist world that has been disenchanted,[11] which can also be observed in how neo-shamanic ayahuasca cosmology pits a toxic society against a healing nature.[12] The ayahuasca plant-spirit has become popular across the globe as a shamanic medicine ascribed to a spiritual nature beyond the disenchantment of society.

Modern Chinese society would appear particularly ripe for reenchantment, given that it experienced one of the most profound histories of rampant secularization. Laying out a brief history of Chinese religiosity and modernization can help us understand the wider context and fertile grounds upon which a hyper-modern form of ayahuasca use emerged there. Chinese society was the subject of dramatic political and cultural reforms and revolutions during much of the twentieth century. The religious-type activities that permeated premodern China and its social institutions became dramatically singled out, categorized, and under assault by nationalist elites who placed "religion"—a newly appropriated institutional category—in opposition to political, economic, and cultural efforts.[13] The result included a sometimes brutal and often "relentless disenchantment of social life,"[14] accompanied by the sacralization of the Maoist secular state. After Mao Zedong's death in 1976, an era of intense governmental repression toward religiosity receded. The revival of Daoism, Buddhism, Christianity, and spiritual sects during the 1980s coincided with widespread capitalist reforms, economic opening-up to global interests, and the proliferation of local consumer markets. Today, religious and spiritual activities exist within a fast-paced and highly technological society saturated by capitalistic demands, consumeristic desires, and materialistic impulses. With a nod to Weber, Arthur Kleinman (2011) suggests that this new context of commercial and capitalistic materialism was a leading source of disenchantment in contemporary China. He explains that the "quest for religious meaning" and the "popular hunger for religious values and sentiments are sought after to confront a secular world that is increasingly seen to be hyper materialistic and wildly commercial . . . The hyperpragmatism of everyday political life is also a stimulus for this quest."[15]

Yet the quest for spirituality in China has been stimulated not only as a reaction against a secular and commercial world, but through practices that spectacularly absorb a modern capitalist environment. As Adam Chau has explained, the classic disenchantment thesis is too simple an explanation in China, given the widespread practices of performing magical rituals, offerings, and prayers to help with everyday commercial, economic, and social challenges.[16] In instrumental fashion, worshipers may call upon deities to miraculously get them a new job, resolve a business dilemma, cause clouds to release rain, diagnose an illness, or reveal the winning numbers of a lottery. The thirst for spirituality in contemporary China is popularly quenched by the magical achievement of modern world mastery, not simply from a divine fountain of meaning outside or lost to modernity.

The utilitarian ethos of ayahuasca use that I examined in mainland China shares a general attitude with this wider context of Chinese religiosity. Here, ayahuasca is drunk by individuals not to overcome a malaise of modern meaning and discover the purpose of life, but to help execute a greater mastery over worldly affairs. Ayahuasca is animated less by a crisis of meaning than an instrumental and pragmatic modernity. Those who drink ayahuasca measure the value of the practice instrumentally by its capacity to inspire actionable changes to workplace and corporate contexts, and this pragmatism shapes their ayahuasca visions and otherworldly experiences. Such a mundane and instrumental use of ayahuasca would likely come as a surprise to many Euro-American ayahuasca enthusiasts. But utilitarian applications of the brew have long been observed in South America too. Among Indigenous Amazonian groups, specialists have drunk ayahuasca to find lost objects, discover the plans of enemies,[17] cleanse the body for enhancing sensory acuity when hunting,[18] study astronomical and ecological correspondences,[19] and inspire artistic creations.[20] Aligned with research on the myth or social construction of disenchantment,[21] this wider view suggests that the neo-shamanic idea of ayahuasca reenchanting a meaning crisis of modern life should be understood as a provincial perspective grounded in a largely Euro-American social and cultural history.

The ability of ayahuasca use to be compatible with radically different pursuits—whether for therapeutic intervention, mystical experience, corporate inspiration, or hunting prowess—appears to be due to its remarkable sensitivity to the intention and background beliefs of the participants and to the social context and style of the consumption. These variables of influence have been described by early psychedelic researchers as the individual's psychological "set" and the social and environmental "setting" in which their experience takes place.[22] This chapter explores how capitalist dynamics and Chinese modernization influence the inner experiences and nominally secular cosmology of ayahuasca drinkers in a major city in mainland China. In their approach to ayahuasca, modern life is not the pathological antithesis of enchantment. The situation is inverted. Disenchantment is cured by an ecstatic capitalist attitude, practice, and sensibility.

AYAHUASCA IN A CHINESE METROPOLIS

Ayahuasca is typically translated in Chinese as "dead, vine, water" (*si teng shui* 死藤水), which is somewhat reminiscent of the Indigenous Quechua terminology of *aya*, meaning "spirit," "soul," and "deceased ancestors," and *huasca*, meaning "vine" and "woody rope." It is difficult to ascertain when ayahuasca was first introduced to Chinese society. Françoise Barbira Freedman (2014) notes that Indigenous ayahuasca shamans were traveling to Beijing at the turn of the twenty-first century, although it is not clear if they were operating ayahuasca sessions in China then.[23] Part of the difficulty in mapping a history of ayahuasca in China is that the society's strict drug laws and risks of punishment have generated a strict code of privacy among users. The ayahuasca brew is prohibited in China, and it recently became a topic of concern in official government social media news accounts. In early 2021, a Beijing police article on Weibo, the largest microblogging platform in China, describes a person being arrested for possessing ayahuasca in China.[24] The article includes a propaganda infographic with skeleton hands reaching over the heading "New Drug: Dead Vine Water is Coming!" (*xin xing du pin, si teng shui lai le*). The Quechua meaning of ayahuasca as "spirit" and "ancestors" is turned into a creepy image of death. Underneath is an illustration of a Mazatec Indian dancing and wearing a large, feathered headdress, accompanied by the text: "Ayahuasca is a medicinal plant from the Amazon rain forest. It has been used for hallucinogenic activity in religious rituals." The police described the arrested person as "addicted to the illusion created by the ayahuasca," "out of touch with reality," "similar to autism," and with a reference to the American science fiction film, it says that the person "confessed to living in a world like *Inception* . . . sometimes he can't distinguish between dreams and reality and is worried he will do extreme behaviors." It finishes by stating, "But now he faces the severe punishment of the law!" Around the same time, a pattern of similar articles about ayahuasca appeared across China on more than a dozen social media accounts of local police stations.

Ayahuasca drinking in mainland China overlaps with the *shen xin ling* (身心灵) or Body-Heart-Soul milieu and its reinvention of New Age spirituality.[25] Some of the Chinese ayahuasca drinkers that I studied regularly attend *shen xin ling* workshops and activities in search of holistic wellness and spiritual inspiration. Given the sensitive nature of writing about ayahuasca therapies in a society with very strict drug prohibition, the following ethnographic writing requires a very delicate approach. I have minimized or anonymized some important details, such as specifics of the retreat location, life histories of participants and organizers, and the workplaces of the participants. But, to my surprise, such concerns were not shared by many of the ayahuasca drinkers that I spoke with in mainland China. When speaking with Zhang, an executive at a large multinational firm, I was struck by his lack of interest regarding the risks when he said that "technically, it is not illegal, because it's just natural plants," and "if you're a good person, helping society, I believe you will be okay." He, like many others, was not very interested in my response that alkaloids in the ayahuasca brew were in fact illegal in China. By contrast, Ting Ting, a manager at a large technology firm, spent fifteen minutes at the beginning of our interview in raw hesitation, questioning me about my intentions and research methods. She asked how long the data would be kept, exactly where I intended to publish, and how I planned to protect her identity. She wanted to contribute to the research, adding, "It's important to share these stories. Ayahuasca has helped me. It's helped many people here." But the dangers that she sensed were real, and even though we spoke mostly about how ayahuasca had helped her career, she was reluctant to identify the company that employs her. Our conversation hovered at a much more abstract level, suspended above a fearful cloud of persecution. Her words, like the ayahuasca visions she described, were only partially able to integrate into mundane discourse. Such an ineffability was not only spiritual or phenomenological in nature, but veritably punitive and constituted by the constraints of China's drug policies.

What appears to have been the only ongoing commercial ayahuasca business operating in China was largely cultivated by one person. Luke, a young and energetic ayahuasca specialist from Europe, has conducted almost weekly ayahuasca retreats in mainland China for six years, involving hundreds of participants, most of whom are Chinese participants. In the beginning, mainly foreigners attended, and then over time, Chinese nationals increasingly came too. Transnational flows of knowledge and practice that draw from the heterogenous South American traditions of ayahuasca drinking are visible in Luke's use of ritualistic music, aromatics, and paraphernalia. To help gather knowledge and training in the craft of serving ayahuasca, Luke has been on more than ten visits to Brazil and Peru to learn from Indigenous Shipibo healers, urban Daimistas, and Uniao do Vegetal ayahuasca specialists. Yet, setting himself against such traditions, Luke describes his approach as secular. "I have great respect for the different ayahuasca traditions," he tells the fifteen mainly Chinese attendees at a retreat shortly before everyone drinks the brew. "We have our own way. It's not the shamanic approach, or religious approach, but the therapeutic approach, the secular approach." Luke describes the events specifically as "sessions" and "processes" rather than ceremonies or rituals.

The sanitization of ayahuasca into a secular framework is remarkably novel. It aims, in theory, at weakening the enchantment of ayahuasca or even creating a disenchanted modality. However, in practice, such sanitization appears merely cosmetic. For instance, Luke describes personally drinking ayahuasca to seek counsel from the inner intelligence of "the plants" when needing to make a crucial decision in his business or personal life. Furthermore, there is no strict codification of secular belief at these retreats. Participants describe encountering spirits, gods, and other worlds in their ayahuasca visions, and Luke makes no effort to correct them along secular lines. Spiritual practitioners are often obliged to justify themselves in modernist contexts,[26] and describing ayahuasca drinking as secular and therapeutic gives it a modernist bent, which is Luke's explicit intention. He told me:

> To bring the plants [ayahuasca] to the modern world, sometimes it needs to be translated. If you start talking to a manager from a company who is very square-minded about power animals and *mariri*, he is going to think you are crazy. My background is more aligned with companies and corporate mindsets. I talk more in terms of anxiety, depression, purpose, mission, conflict . . . When they don't see you wearing feathers, when you speak in a language they understand, the outcome is better.

As demonstrated next, claiming that the practice is secular also helps separate it from an association with religious communities or consensual moral universes and makes it more individualistic, pragmatic, and instrumental. In allopathic or modern medicine, therapy is typically not designed to reveal the moral truth and meaning of the cosmos; rather it is based upon a deficit model aimed at returning a patient to a livable and functional state.

When I began researching Luke's networks in 2019, he was developing a "portfolio" of retreats in Beijing, Shanghai, and Shenzhen, which included mainly Chinese "customers" and "clients." "We have different packages and services, all designed to help people transform," he explained. Luke's ayahuasca business includes a core product, entitled "Bridging the Gap," which aims to take clients beyond a functional state and enhance their vocational abilities. It is a leadership program designed specifically to help corporate managers, entrepreneurs, and chief executive officers to advance their careers and live happy and fuller lives. The program typically includes workshops, coaching sessions, a workbook with "weekly assignments," and two or three ayahuasca sessions spread across three months. It costs each client RMB 60,000 (approximately 9,000 USD). Clients are supported by Luke and retreat helpers in the overall goal of Bridging the Gap, where they seek to align an internal self, called "the Monk," with an external self, called "the Suit." The Monk refers to "an authentic self, spirit, heart, purpose, and intuition," and the Suit refers to "external success, occupation, material belongings, ego, and mind." Group sessions of drinking ayahuasca, which are called the "Amazonian Emotional Process," help individuals perceive and understand the gaps between their two selves. Such gaps are shaped by "emotional blockages and familiar conflicts," "fear and anxiety," and "addiction problems." Coaching sessions and knowledge seminars supplement the ayahuasca drinking retreats to help the client "take action" to close the gap between the two inner selves and "implement change" in their workplace environment or domestic life.

Chinese ayahuasca consumers pursue happiness and integrity by aligning the Monk and the Suit. The objective is both personal and vocational, and the coaching and workshop activities help clients "integrate what they experience in the session with ayahuasca to their companies," Luke explained to me. "Ayahuasca creates a powerful inner awareness, and this has a high premium for managers constantly trying to overcome blind spots," he added. Switching conveniently between secular and spiritual language, the program includes references to Daoism, Buddhism, and other "ancient techniques made practical," which are defined precisely in relation to the objectives of Bridging the Gap. In doing so, the approach reflects broader religious practices in China that "create new compositions out of selected elements of tradition—elements often selected for their perceived compatibility with modern, secular values."[27] The Monk is attuned to an intuitive and ecstatic "flow" of the Dao, which ultimately needs to be unified with the mundane and rational decisions of the Suit in domestic and workplace life.

AN ETHNOGRAPHIC SKETCH OF THE AYAHUASCA SESSION

As I arrived to the ayahuasca event, I was surprised by the large walls that surrounded the housing estate. Two security officers watched over the small entry. Inside are elaborate and perfectly detailed gardens, multistory villas, and remarkably clean and new streets that project a video game–like quality. A shining Porsche drives past. Gardeners are busy working. For those not enrolled in the larger Bridging the Gap program, the one-evening ayahuasca retreat costs RMB 2,000 (300 USD). These individuals usually attend the retreats for personal healing, curiosity, or spiritual exploration, and share the event with the Bridging the Gap participants. Most participants are upper-middle-class Chinese working professionals between twenty to thirty-five years of age. People arrive to the retreat on Saturday during the early afternoon. Everyone is instructed to turn off their phones and "unplug ourselves" for the duration of the retreat. Sitting in the "process room"—where the ayahuasca drinking will take place after dark—everyone draws with colored pencils graphic illustrations of their personal "intention for the process" on pieces of paper, which are then arranged on the walls. Luke's sharp analytic mind is on full display as he shares with the group the latest science on the therapeutic properties of ayahuasca. "Ayahuasca is a tool. It can help you know yourself better. That is all," he tells the group in English. Everyone at the retreats has been prescreened as having "appropriate intentions" during an initial phone call with Luke and by signing an elaborate agreement indicating their medical background, along with confidentiality and personal responsibility clauses.

Before the ayahuasca-drinking session, everyone is taken to a neighboring park for group activities designed to "let go of the stresses of work and life." This included hugging a stranger in the group for two minutes, followed by talking with this person about how that made you feel. Each person looks into the eyes of a stranger for two minutes, and finally pairs up with another person and takes turns being blindfolded while being led for ten minutes through winding paths, descending stairs, and across roads. Luke later told me that these exercises are good for creating a sense of trust and support among the group, which helps participants learn to "let go" when drinking ayahuasca, given that the "visions appear from darkness and are guided by music and what feels like an outside source." Returning to the process room as the sun sets, the group dons white clothing and closely lines the walls sitting on yoga mats, each with a pillow, a bucket, and eye shades. As the group sits in a large circle, a rope is passed around, and each participant speaks of their "intention for the process" while tying a knot in the rope. Shortly afterward, everyone drinks the brew, including all attendees and facilitators.

In the middle of the session room is a large, glowing salt crystal, surrounded by sage leaves, *palo santo* fragrant wood, a piece of ayahuasca vine, and a pine cone. One wall of the room is decorated with a large Indigenous

Amazonian Shipibo fabric, a large Chinese script for driving away ghosts (next to a figure of the Daoist deity, *guan yu*), and an image of a Tibetan buddha, which are all above the place where Luke sits and observes the group while controlling musical equipment. After everyone drinks the brew, there are forty minutes of silent meditation. The lighting is very low. Then the music begins. The ayahuasca sessions last for a period of four to six hours, and the music included Indigenous Amazonian healing songs or *icaros*, high-energy Italian opera performances by male and female singers, 1980s Chinese pop music about friendship and family, South American folk ayahuasca music about sacred plants, Persian and Middle Eastern religious chants, and classical Indian music. The music is very loud. Over the course of the evening, three cups of ayahuasca are offered. Everyone drinks the first cup; most people have the second cup as well; and few have the third. Most participants lie down and explore inner visions. When someone purges, vomiting into the bucket, Luke moves over to them and smudges them with aromatic sage smoke, or sometimes the Amazonian fragrant wood *palo santo*. Sometimes he massages people's backs in an attempt to make them purge more. He also uses a range of aromatic liquids that Peruvian shamans use, including Agua de Florida. He circles the group, rubs the strong aroma on the participants' hands, and tells them to apply it to their faces and necks. During the session, some people cry, and some vomit, but most of the time, the participants are silent and still.

Part of the way that participants "bridge the gap" between their inner Monk and outer Suit is through surrendering to the challenging bodily processes and otherworldly visions of ayahuasca drinking. Imbibing ayahuasca is often a challenging experience for people, and the directed goal of "letting go" is tested physically and existentially. By learning to surrender to the ayahuasca visions and trust the process, participants release "traumatic blocks stored in their bodies"—typically through vomiting, crying, or sweating. Issues related to participants' childhood, and especially their relations with parents and family, are common blocks that are recognized and purged during the ayahuasca sessions. The ayahuasca drinkers find themselves navigating inner scenes and worlds that are spectacular and otherworldly, but also scenes that are very mundane, ordinary, and secular, often concerning family and friends or oriented squarely toward obstacles and conflicts in their every-day jobs. In the most general sense, for the dozen Chinese entrepreneurs and corporate leaders whom I spoke with about their ayahuasca practice, the process of drinking ayahuasca is directed at personal healing. Purifying the body through purging and visionary awareness opens the psyche to an enduring state of "flow," in which the inner self and outer self—the Monk and the Suit—operate as one. Such an ideal state is marked by less stress, enhanced creativity, workplace success, and overall happiness and satisfaction in professional and personal life.

At the end of the session, the effects of the brew are largely finished for most people, and after Luke concludes the session with a ritualistic statement about peace, well-being, and happiness, some people congregate in the kitchen sharing stories about their visions and talking about mundane life events. Others stay in the process space, resting, sleeping, meditating, or conversing quietly. Most people are asleep by 3 a.m.

The morning after the ayahuasca session, everyone meets at 8 a.m. in the process room for a one-hour ecstatic dance session designed to integrate into the body the healing transformations from the previous night. Afterward, everyone lies on the ground and follows a guided mediation that culminates with visualizing throwing fears, hatred, and pains into an imaginary fire in a cave, embracing their ambitions, and breathing light and awareness into the body. After a quick breakfast, everyone joins together for a three-hour "integration circle," which is the final part of the retreat. The "intention" rope is passed to the last person who had made a knot the previous night. That person then undoes the knot and verbally shares with the group what happened in the ayahuasca experience and how the person feels now. Some speak in English, and others in Chinese. Many people describe gratitude for the experience, feelings of elation, and shared insights or convictions about changes they now want to make in their lives. After the three-hour integration sharing session, the participants eat a small lunch together, and then everyone leaves and the event finishes by early Sunday afternoon. Luke encourages participants to receive an included yet optional one-hour coaching session with him approximately one week after the event to help them better integrate the retreat into daily life.

CASE STUDY 1: TING TING

Ting Ting, a Chinese woman in her early thirties, started drinking ayahuasca in 2018 for personal and professional reasons. She explained to me how ayahuasca had helped her overcome family trauma and advance her career. She grew up in a large city in China, and after completing university studies in her early twenties, she moved to Shanghai with the hope of making a successful career in the information technology (IT) sector. But this dream was not the only thing drawing her to the large metropolis. Before she left home, her father had been diagnosed with a terminal disease and given less than two years to live. "I went to Shanghai for work. Deep down I knew I was leaving because I couldn't bare the situation."

A decade after her father died, she drank ayahuasca in a group setting in mainland China, trying to heal what she described as deeply embodied guilt, shame, and sadness caused by neglecting her father's death and failing to support her mother and brother. During her first ayahuasca sessions, she had many otherworldly visions, cried for several hours, and vomited a few times. "My body had been carrying a massive emotional burden," she explained. "After all the crying and the insights during the process [of drinking ayahuasca], I felt so light in my jaw and neck and that's usually where the stress is centered." She kept returning to the ayahuasca retreats because she ultimately felt that the sessions helped her forgive herself and this had positive repercussions in her life, including at her job as a manager at an IT firm. "What I learned from my father's death is that you will not feel shame if you try your best to take care of someone or do something good," she explained. Reflecting on her ayahuasca sessions, she added: "After releasing the pain from my body, I became more comfortable with myself. My colleagues appeared more open to my ideas because I can manage my body language and expectations better now." She describes her company culture as fast-paced, competitive, and challenging. Her goal is to increase her salary and advance her career by doing good work and getting noticed by busy senior colleagues. She explained that this requires a social tact that her ayahuasca visionary experiences helped her to cultivate.

Ting Ting had many visionary experiences the first few times she drank ayahuasca. Some of them included worldly figures, places, and scenes—including visions of her family members and her workplace colleagues—and other visions were more surreal and otherworldly. She related to the worldly and otherworldly visions in a similar way. They all provided psychological insight. In one telling vision, she witnessed her coworkers. She describes a kind of enchanted vision of workplace rationality that is not dull or lifeless, but rather magical, energetic, and scary:

> After I cried for two or three hours [about her father and family trauma], I then puked a little bit. I was working on my own journey. I started seeing snakes and my coworkers. So, if you open a watch, you will see how it works on the inside. You will see all those wheels working in an organized way, working at a fixed pace. I was seeing this, but it was not metal wheels. They were snakes, turning around, in fixed rotation. All of them are moving in a clockwise direction and there is one in particular on top of all of it, and it's looking at me. Sometimes it gets really close to my face and then it goes back to the workings. It was black and yellow, and the snake is my least favourite animal. So, it was scary, but I wasn't too afraid. The snake would let me know that it's watching me with its tongue, then it would return to the clock's workings.

By witnessing her colleagues and a clock turning with snakes but not feeling terribly afraid, Ting Ting described confidently encountering a scary, otherworldly scene that entangled workplace environments, mechanical time, and animal sentience. In this case, ayahuasca made her porous to an invisible cosmic realm that spins to the cogs of workplace life. Such a porosity lends psychological insight to Ting Ting. She explained, "The vision of the snakes reminded me that I am sometimes as alert as a snake. I am very quiet, usually, but I am very sensitive to changes, sound, or any disturbance to my life. So, that's what I got from that experience." In a different vision, she saw dozens of red lanterns floating up to the sky, each with a face on it of someone she loved or someone she despised, including her workplace colleagues and her new and old friends. The vision taught her to "let go of other people's opinions easier." She explained:

> When I saw the lantern, I thought, it's not their hope to make me sad, but I choose to be sad. It's all on me. So, as the lanterns floated away, I was able to

let some of my frustration and anger or unsatisfied feelings go with those people. Some of those people are in my company, working with me every day, or some are friends I sometimes see during the weekend . . . People who don't believe in me, I now don't see them as a threat to blocking me from progressing in my company, and I don't let their opinion bother me as much now. The ayahuasca helped me feel it's not personal anymore. I realized their advice is not always compatible with my expertise and development.

By unifying an inner and outer self through otherworldly ayahuasca experiences of releasing "negative energies" from her body, Ting Ting described improving her management techniques and exceling in her career ambitions. Following the "Bridging the Gap" method, she purged a series of afflictions ascribed to her family history and to her perceptions of workplace relations. This purging and visionary experience brought a sense of embodied grace and confidence to her workplace life. By encountering ayahuasca visions as personal psychological material requiring interpretation, she pursues happiness and attempts to simultaneously heal family trauma and gain success as a manager at a technology company.

CASE STUDY 2: WANG

Wang, a thirty-four-year-old, spent the first half of his life in California, as a Chinese American, and then moved to China after college to study business management at a leading university. Shortly after his studies, he married a local Chinese woman, had a child with her, and began working as a manager for a Chinese company in a large city near Shanghai. After living in China for twelve years, he began drinking ayahuasca for personal and professional reasons. His reasons included a desire to become less angry at home and in the workplace. He had become increasingly stressed as an executive manager at a fast-food franchise. The business was excelling quickly, partly based on the success of his management efforts, and he was finding it difficult to cope with the new challenges and levels of responsibility that came with opening more stores. Business language and thinking permeated his approach to ayahuasca. He described the group-bonding activities at the beginning of the retreat as being like a good job interview where the hiring committee takes you out of the office into a park and the group can "network together" and "informally exchange." Wang told me that he keeps attending ayahuasca retreats because they provide him with a lasting sense of calmness and peace that helps him be more tender and perceptive as a father and husband and more successful as a manager and business coach.

His intentions for drinking ayahuasca have been primarily to deal with the stress of work and to control his temper. His inner experiences of drinking ayahuasca follow a pattern that intersects with the Bridging the Gap philosophy. He described how the beginning of the session is usually mentally challenging, disorienting, and otherworldly, but eventually he "reaches a certain level" or experiences a "new ego death," and then the rest of the session involves graceful periods of exploring worldly affairs. He narrated a violent and otherworldly ayahuasca experience that eventually gave way to a period of visionary grace:

> I was just an observer, like an audience member, watching. I wasn't scared. I wasn't worried or anxious. Physically, I did feel sick. I was seeing the same thing if I opened or closed my eyes. It was violent. Small and large creatures were climbing the walls, kicking and punching each other, and flying around. There was blood and water in the air. Ancient symbols were glowing on the walls, and trees and plants were growing out of them. The sensation, the smells, it was very real. The ceiling I remember vividly. It was open to outer space, and there was no sun, but I could feel a warmth like the sun.

During this visionary experience, he then vomited. Shortly afterward, he achieved a state of visionary peace and "flow," in which he felt confident to tackle challenges and, he explained, "turn the positive energy into something applicable." In a state of visionary grace, he realized that his pride had been affecting his management skills in negative ways that made the business operate less efficiently. He was failing to address performance issues with key managers and HR staff. Rather than expecting them to simply follow his orders, he now desired to manage his staff with less pride and be a better listener. He visualized the designs of the planned new restaurants. He could navigate around the space "like in a video game," whereby he realized that the "customer experience" was dull and needed more investment in the short term. Ayahuasca helped Wang appreciate a potential lack of meaning, a dullness, that should be improved with more natural light, colored furniture, and a more pleasing design to attract repeat customers. He explained, "I visualize some of my challenges, and think, okay, tomorrow morning I want to make this decision and I want to start rolling out this execution. It's very detailed and very clear." Wang describes his otherworldly ayahuasca visions as "strange" and "entertaining," and he had a lot more to say about the worldly aspects of his visions. Following the Bridging the Gap model, his ayahuasca sessions involved a release of negative emotion, followed by a unity of grace and reasoning, intuition and rationality, spirit and success. The stress of the workplace was discharged in the form of strange and violent otherworldly visions that enabled a renewed spirit to permeate his workplace decisions and attitude.

ENCHANTED RATIONALITY IN MODERN CHINA

If Weber was around today and aware of all this, he would have been puzzled. He had never closely studied the phenomenological basis of mysticism and generally conceived of it as antithetical to rationalization (in the bureaucratic or efficiency "means to ends" type). He suggested that mystical experience, in its "orgiastic" and "ecstatic" forms, led away from rationality, given its ineffability and excessive otherworldly orientation.[28] Yet ayahuasca use in mainland China involves ecstatic visionary experiences where everyday action is rationalized through the integration of the spiritual and the mundane, or the Monk and the Suit.

By cloaking a business model in a spiritual experience, the Bridging the Gap practice shapes the visionary exaltation of ayahuasca to the demands of capitalist competition. The inner forms and acts of the ecstatic experience are harnessed to inspire attitudes and perceptions that are compatible with worldly business affairs. Describing the benefits in a corporate context, Luke explained that Bridging the Gap "changes the quality of your decision making in alignment with your unified self." In contrast to neo-shamanic ayahuasca practices in Western societies, which focus on otherworldly primitivist visions associated with nature and Indigenous spirituality to confront a crisis of modern life, this practice of drinking ayahuasca in mainland China is nominally secular and overtly embraces modern life in the pursuit of worldly visionary experiences and pragmatic workplace mastery. While some have argued that ayahuasca has become globally popular by liberating modern souls from the disenchanted iron cage of instrumental rationality, a novel, inverted scenario exists in mainland China, in which entrepreneurs and executive managers rationalize ayahuasca experiences in the hope of achieving a competitive edge in capitalistic environments.

The practice of unifying the Monk and the Suit and Bridging the Gap with the help of ayahuasca drinking disturbs classic theories of modern disenchantment. The overcoming of disenchantment with ayahuasca—if such terms are even appropriate in this new context—is an ideal pursued not in the service of religious revival, but in the service of corporate goals and the overcoming of business challenges. For instance, ayahuasca has provided Wang with an inner visionary environment to develop his management skills and workshop his customer service ideas. Self-discovery and existential questions such as who or what he is are less important than the pragmatic questions of how to be better at what he is doing. In this case, the consequence of disenchantment is not a malaise of modern rationality but rather a weakness in conducting business. More precisely, the secular sphere requires a synthesis with the intuitive and visionary grace of the Monk to generate a happy and successful life in capitalistic environments that extend to the existential depths of the self. When Ting Ting makes meaning from her visions, such meaning orients a rational way of life in which attitudes and embodied comportment are adjusted to improve her leadership and management skills.

The Bridging the Gap approach in mainland China represents a remarkably pragmatic and instrumental style to drinking ayahuasca. But unlike the popular Chinese religious practices described by Adam Chau (2006) and others, it is stripped of the capacity for miraculous intervention or magical efficacy and approached as a somewhat humanistic endeavor. The emphasis on integrating ayahuasca visions into daily life downplays the enchantment of ayahuasca by placing the agency squarely upon the individual. The value of the otherworldly visionary experience is measured or celebrated by its capacity to inspire actionable changes in everyday life, including in workplace and/or corporate contexts. Such an inspiration is materialized only through the person making conscious decisions and taking conscious actions after drinking ayahuasca. Participants are ultimately responsible for achieving worldly affairs, and they draw upon the otherworldly ayahuasca visions as experiences for cultivating the self in mundane contexts or ordinary life.

By ascribing the vistas of ayahuasca to the inner workings of the psyche, the Bridging the Gap practice of drinking ayahuasca is made particularly amenable to a liquid modernity that pivots upon individual flexibility, responsibility, and desires. The rise of individualism in modern China presents a psychological problem in which the liberated psyche faces new sets of challenges that manifest as particular structures of feeling.[29] The visionary use of ayahuasca in mainland China by a young, corporate professional class raises such new challenges to ecstatic heights. Stresses of Chinese modernity manifest in the afflictive experiences that the ayahuasca drinkers aim to purge, purify, and release from their bodies. Participants cleanse the psyche of stress and afflictions that were inhibiting a grace in the rational pursuit of self-interest in workplace contexts. A religious telos is pursued not against the hyperpragmatism of everyday, but within it, in a unification of the Monk and the Suit. The ecstatic, ineffable other worlds of ayahuasca visions are made useful to the mundane, secular challenges and conflicts of corporate life. The Monk and the Suit are not opposites but two sides of the same capitalist coin. They provide the grounds for integrating religious sensibilities and rational action into a coherent image of the modern self.

NOTES

1. B. Brabec de Mori, "Tracing Hallucinations: Contributing to a Critical Ethnohistory of Ayahuasca Usage in the Peruvian Amazon," in *The Internationalisation of Ayahuasca*, ed. B. C. Labate and H. Jungaberle (Zurich: Lit Verlag, 2011), 23–47.

2. K. Tupper, "The Globalization of Ayahuasca: Harm Reduction or Benefit Maximization?" *International Journal of Drug Policy* 19, no. 4 (2008): 297–303; E. Fotiou, "The Globalization of Ayahuasca Shamanism and the Erasure of Indigenous Shamanism," *Anthropology of Consciousness* 27, no. 2 (2016):151–179; B. C. Labate, C. Cavnar, and A. Gearin, *The World Ayahuasca Diaspora: Reinventions and Controversies* (New York: Routledge, 2017).

3. C. Kaplan, "Forward: Ayahuasca and the Coming Transformation of the International Drug Control System," in *The Internationalisation of Ayahuasca*, ed. B. C. Labate and H. Jungaberle (Zürich: Lit Verlag, 2011), 131–144; K. Tupper, "Ayahuasca Healing Beyond the Amazon: The Globalization of a Traditional Indigenous Entheogenic Practice" *Global Networks* (2009): 120; C. Partridge, *The Re-enchantment of the West*, vol. 2 (New York: T&T Clark International, 2005), 96.

4. C. Taylor, *A Secular Age* (Cambridge, MA: Harvard University Press. 2007), 303–307.

5. M. Weber, *The Protestant Ethic and the Spirit of Capitalism* (New York: Routledge, 1992 [1905])

6. S. Kelberg, "Introduction: Max Weber: The Confrontation with Modernity," in *Max Weber Readings and Commentary on Modernity*, ed. S. Kelberg (Oxford, UK: Blackwell Publishing, 2005), 29.

7. A. K. Gearin, "Primitivist Medicine and Capitalist Anxieties in Ayahuasca Tourism Peru," *Journal of the Royal Anthropological Institute* 28, no. 2 (forthcoming/2022).

8. I. Hartogsohn, "The Meaning-Enhancing Properties of Psychedelics and Their Mediator Role in Psychedelic Therapy, Spirituality, and Creativity," *Frontiers in Neuroscience* 12 (2018): 3.

9. R. Metzner, *Ayahuasca: Human Consciousness and the Spirits of Nature* (Philadelphia: Running Press, 1999), 97.

10. Hartogsohn, "The Meaning-Enhancing Properties of Psychedelics," 3.

11. Kaplan, "Forward: Ayahuasca and the Coming Transformation," 19.

12. A. K. Gearin, "Ayahuasca Neoshamanism as Cultural Critique in Australia," in *The World Ayahuasca Diaspora: Controversies and Reinventions*, ed. in B. Labate, C. Cavnar, and A. Gearin (New York: Routledge, 2017), 123–141.

13. V. Goossaert and D. Palmer, *The Religious Question in Modern China* (Chicago: University of Chicago Press 2011).

14. M. Yang, "Introduction," in *Chinese Religiosities: Afflictions of Modernity and State Formation*, ed. M. Yang (Berkeley: University of California Press, 2008), 8.

15. A. Kleinman, "Quests for Meaning," in *Deep China: The Moral Life of the Person*, ed. Arthur Kleinman et al. (Berkeley: University of California Press, 2011), 273.

16. A. Chau, *Miraculous Response: Doing Popular Religion in Contemporary China* (Stanford, CA: Stanford University Press, 2006), 2.

17. L. E. Luna, *Vegetalismo: Shamanism Among the Mestizo Population of the Peruvian Amazon* (PhD diss., Stockholm University, 1986), 60.

18. G. H. Shepard, "A Sensory Ecology of Medicinal Plant Therapy in Two Amazonian Societies," *American Anthropologist* 102, no. 2 (2004): 252–266.

19. R. Reichel-Dolmatoff, *Rainforest Shamans: Essays on the Tukano Indians of the Northwest Amazon* (London: Themis Books, 1997).

20. A. Gebhart-Sayer, "The Geometric Designs of the Shipibo-Conibo in Ritual Context," *Journal of Latin American Lore* 11, no. 2 (1985): 143–175.

21. J. Josephson-Storm, *The Myth of Disenchantment: Magic, Modernity and the Birth of the Human Sciences* (Chicago: Chicago University Press, 2017).

22. T. Leary, R. Metzner, and R. Alpert, *The Psychedelic Experience: A Manual Based on the Tibetan Book of the Dead* (New York: University Books, 1964).

23. B. F. Freedman, "'Shamans' Networks in Western Amazonia: The Iquitos-Nauta Road," in *Ayahuasca Shamanism in the Amazon and Beyond*, ed. B. C. Labate and C. Cavnar (New York: Oxford University Press, 2014), 130–158, 141.

24. Ping An Beijing (平安北京) 2020. Ayahuasca! Be alert to the invasion of new drugs. (死藤水！警惕新型毒品的入侵). https://weibo.com/ttarticle/p/show?id=2309404585326214513249, accessed online March 2021. Translation by author.

25. A. Iskra, "Navigating the Owl's Gaze: Mainland Chinese Body-Heart-Spirit Milieu and Circulations of New Age Teachings to the Sinosphere." *Nova Religio* 25, no. 4 (2022): 5–31.

26. Goossaert and Palmer, *The Religious Question in Modern China*, 304.

27. Goossaert and Palmer, *The Religious Question in Modern China*, 304.

28. M. Weber, "The Social Psychology of World Religion," in *From Max Weber: Essays in Sociology*, ed. C. W. Mills and H. Gerth (London: Routledge 2009), 290.

29. A. B. Kipnis, "Introduction: Chinese Modernity and the Individual Psyche," in *Chinese Modernity and the Individual Psyche*, ed. A. Kipnis (New York: Palgrave, 2012), 7.

BIBLIOGRAPHY

Brabec de Mori, B. "Tracing Hallucinations: Contributing to a Critical Ethnohistory of Ayahuasca Usage in the Peruvian Amazon." In *The Internationalisation of Ayahuasca*, edited by B. C. Labate and H. Jungaberle, 23–47. Zurich: Lit Verlag, 2011.

Chau, A. *Miraculous Response: Doing Popular Religion in Contemporary China*. Stanford, CA: Stanford University Press, 2006.

Fotiou, E. "The Globalization of Ayahuasca Shamanism and the Erasure of Indigenous Shamanism." *Anthropology of Consciousness* 27, no. 2 (2016): 151–179.

Freedman, Françoise Barbira. "'Shamans' Networks in Western Amazonia: The Iquitos-Nauta Road." In *Ayahuasca Shamanism in the Amazon and Beyond*, edited by B. C. Labate and Clancy Cavnar, 130–158. New York: Oxford University Press, 2014.

Gearin, A. K. "Ayahuasca Neoshamanism as Cultural Critique in Australia." In *The World Ayahuasca Diaspora: Controversies and Reinventions*, edited by B. C. Labate, C. Cavnar, and A. K. Gearin, 123–141. New York: Routledge, 2017.

Gearin, A. K. "Primitivist Medicine and Capitalist Anxieties in Ayahuasca Tourism Peru." *Journal of the Royal Anthropological Institute* 28, no. 2 (2022): 496–515.

Gearin, A. K., and Calavia Saez, O. "Altered Vision: Sensory Individualism and Ayahuasca Shamanism." *Current Anthropology* 62, no. 2 (2021):138–163.

Gebhart-Sayer, A. "The Geometric Designs of the Shipibo-Conibo in Ritual Context." *Journal of Latin American Lore* 11, no. 2 (1985): 143–175.

Goossaert, V., and D. Palmer. *The Religious Question in Modern China*. Chicago: University of Chicago Press, 2011.

Hartogsohn, I. "The Meaning-Enhancing Properties of Psychedelics and Their Mediator Role in Psychedelic Therapy, Spirituality, and Creativity." *Frontiers in Neuroscience* 12 (2018): 1–5.

Iskra, A. "Navigating the Owl's Gaze: Mainland Chinese Body-Heart-Spirit Milieu and Circulations of New Age Teachings to the Sinosphere." *Nova Religio* 25, no. 4 (2022): 5–31.

Josephson-Storm, J. *The Myth of Disenchantment: Magic, Modernity and the Birth of the Human Sciences*. Chicago: Chicago University Press, 2017.

Kaplan, C. "Forward: Ayahuasca and the Coming Transformation of the International Drug Control System." In *The Internationalization of Ayahuasca*, edited by B. C. Labate and H. Jungaberle, 131–144. Zurich: Lit Verlag, 2011.

Kelberg, S. "Introduction—Max Weber: The Confrontation with Modernity." In *Max Weber Readings and Commentary on Modernity*, edited by S. Kelberg. Oxford, UK: Blackwell Publishing, 2005.

Kipnis, A. B. "Introduction: Chinese Modernity and the Individual Psyche." In *Chinese Modernity and the Individual Psyche*, edited by A. Kipnis. New York: Palgrave, 2012.

Kleinman, A. "Quests for Meaning." In *Deep China: The Moral Life of the Person*, edited by A. Kleinman, Y. Yan, J. Jun, et al. Berkeley: University of California Press, 2011.

Labate, B., C. Cavnar, and A. Gearin. *The World Ayahuasca Diaspora: Reinventions and Controversies*. New York: Routledge, 2017.

Leary, T., R. Metzner, and R. Alpert. *The Psychedelic Experience: A Manual Based on the Tibetan Book of the Dead*. New York: University Books, 1964.

Luna, L. E. *Vegetalismo: Shamanism among the Mestizo Population of the Peruvian Amazon*. PhD diss., Stockholm University, 1986.

Metzner, R. *Ayahuasca: Human Consciousness and the Spirits of Nature*. Philadelphia: Running Press, 1999.

Partridge, C. *The Re-enchantment of the West*, vol. 2. New York: T&T Clark International, 2005.

Reichel-Dolmatoff, R. *Rainforest Shamans: Essays on the Tukano Indians of the Northwest Amazon*. London: Themis Books, 1997.

Shepard, G. H. "A Sensory Ecology of Medicinal Plant Therapy in Two Amazonian Societies." *American Anthropologist* 102, no. 2 (2004): 252–266.

Taylor, C. *A Secular Age*. Cambridge, MA: Harvard University Press, 2007.

Tupper, K. "The Globalization of Ayahuasca: Harm Reduction or Benefit Maximization?" *International Journal of Drug Policy* 19, no. 4 (2008): 297–303.

Weber, M. *The Protestant Ethic and the Spirit of Capitalism*. New York: Routledge, 1992 [1905].

Weber, M. "The Social Psychology of World Religion." In *From Max Weber: Essays in Sociology*, edited by C. W. Mills, B. S. Turner, and H. Gerth. London: Routledge, 2009.

Yang, M. "Introduction." In *Chinese Religiosities: Afflictions of Modernity and State Formation*, edited by M. Yang. Berkeley: University of California Press, 2008.

20 TRIPPING IN KARACHI: EXPLORING THE INTERSECTION OF GENDER AND ITS FLUIDITY THROUGH PSYCHEDELIC SUBSTANCES

Manal Khan

A twenty-eight-year-old woman in Karachi, Pakistan—Dureja[1]—felt whole and complete in her body for the first time when she was on an acid trip, peacefully sitting on her apartment's balcony. A view of the setting sun, in a city full of skyscrapers, facing toward residential housing units, where *qawwali* (Sufi devotional music) echoes in the distance, can be had from her apartment. It was a small sanctuary that Dureja and her husband set up, each corner of it reminding them of the safety of "home." To be home and safe is often a rare experience for a lot of young women and nonbinary people in Pakistan, especially for those who want to experiment with gender and sexuality. On 150 μg of an acid tab, Dureja saw what a world without gender could be like—mystical. There was no need for gender and its specified roles, she said. Her trip sitter, Momin, also happened to be her husband. (A trip sitter is a caretaker, usually sober, who remains physically present with a person who decides to embark upon a psychedelic journey. They make sure that the experience of the tripper is comfortable until the substance wears off.)

"I'd see a field of vibrant flowers—breathing, swaying with the wind, just standing tall as humans. They tried to speak to me about letting myself go. Being fluid. Nothing more and nothing less," Dureja recalls from dreams that pushed her forward to experiment with her gender curiosity. Most of those images from her early teenage years did not stay with her, but the flowers always did. They were a recurring image in her memory from all those years that she felt incomplete.

On her first trip, she says, "acid got me," as if a nonbeing, a substance, had known what part of the equation needed solving. She says that she always had the mannerisms that defined someone as not "feminine" enough: "What comes beyond this, was something I didn't want my heart to acknowledge."

Dureja started taking small doses of acid, about 100–150 μg, every other month. With the assistance of a Facebook community, WhatsApp groups, and some private Instagram pages, the acquisition process for common psychedelics such as mushrooms and LSD isn't difficult. Dureja had a clear purpose for her recurring trips: to sit with the questions of self exploration that had surfaced during her first trip. "It helps me to have all cards on the table, to see with clarity: how can I explore into the depths of myself?" This is a devastating process that's been consuming her late twenties.

"I was in shambles when it began. It reminded me of the coward that I am."

Dureja is also a feminist activist, part of organizing the historic Working Women's March in Karachi in 2019, which was part of Pakistan's Aurat March movement held on International Women's Day (March 8). Karachi, the largest and most populous city, is the financial hub of Pakistan, contributing a staggering 25 percent of the national gross domestic product and housing 30 percent of its manufacturing sector. It is also Pakistan's most culturally heterogeneous city, with labor from all over the country, across genders, coming there to find work. This diverse cultural landscape means that patriarchal constraints on women's mobility, employment, political participation, and the performance of gender and sexuality vary significantly compared to that in other cities.[2] This is exacerbated by the fact that Karachi's geopolitical importance as the largest port city, handling 95 percent of the country's international trade, coupled with a history of ethnonationalist violence, has led to heavy militarization over the past four decades. Karachi's social and political landscape, thus, represents what the social scientist Laurent Gayer calls "ordered disorder," a phenomenon characterized by an entanglement of chaos and control.[3] The particular characteristics of Karachi's sociopolitical development have shrunk the space for women's movements to flourish as they have historically in cities like Lahore. In this context, the Aurat March was specifically significant for Karachi. Some of the demands of this protest were equal pay rights, bodily autonomy, the right to choose whom to love, safety for the transgender community, and a recognition of the earlier feminist movements of Pakistan. Gender has been a contested debate in the history of Pakistan, and Dureja is one of the people questioning it from the front lines. However, the issues that plague this resistance precede Pakistan itself and are very much rooted in South Asia's colonial experience in the nineteenth century.[4]

The British Crown established its official rule in India in the wake of the failed rebellion of 1857. Over the next half-century, Indian society went through drastic changes as the British executed their "civilizing mission." Indians were not passive observers throughout this process; in fact, British measures in the areas of law, education, and taxation were heavily contested by local politicians and intellectuals (predominantly men). However, the experience of subjugation also led to societal introspection among communities. Indian Muslim intellectuals like Sir Syed Ahmed Khan (1817–1898), whose writings on Muslim politics and work in education are considered to be the birth of Muslim nationalism (and thus the foundation of Pakistan), believed that this subjugation could be undone by emulating British values of progress and modernity, while also returning to the "true essence" of Islam. Thus, Khan and others who shared similar beliefs undertook reformist projects in their respective fields.

In the interest of returning to the "true essence of Islam," as well as appeasing the Victorian moral values that the colonial civilizing mission was rooted in, the fluidity that characterized the experience of gender and queerness in India increasingly came under attack. When the British introduced Section 377 into the Indian Penal Code, which outlawed "unnatural intercourse," they criminalized queer sexual activity, which had been a widely accepted phenomenon across India, as well as other parts of the Muslim world. However, Muslim reformists welcomed the initiative, arguing that Islam forbade such activity.[5]

In 1947, when Pakistan came into being, it inherited the colonial legal system in its entirety, and over the next many decades, increasingly Islamized it. Queerness in Pakistan, thus, is a highly surveilled and marginalized experience. For example, the Muslim Family Laws Ordinance of 1961, a seminal set of laws governing gender relations in Pakistan, did not recognize the rights of transgender people with the institutions of family and marriage. In fact, their status as "third gender" citizens was recognized only in 2019, being legally implemented from 2018 onward.[6] The complication within the dynamic of gender and sexuality as performed identities occurs when queerness cannot be physically identifiable. This can be seen in the responses to two Pride marches in Pakistan during the last decade. In 2011, the US embassy in Islamabad organized a Gay Pride march, where pride flags and subversive placards were displayed, expressing the visibility of a culture that could look beyond the gender binaries that have been the normative categories. The march was vehemently attacked and criticized in the local press for being un-Islamic. In the years since, there has not been an exclusive event to commemorate Gay Pride in Pakistan, and the yearly women's marches have been the only outlet of afforded visibility. In fact, in 2013, a local poll found that 83 percent of the population believes that there should be no place for homosexuality in Pakistan.[7]

In contrast to the opposition that the Gay Pride march of 2011 faced, the Trans Pride march organized in Lahore in 2018 by local trans activists was much more warmly received. In fact, the march was organized partly to demand the implementation of the Trans Rights Bill of 2018, as well as to introduce further legislation for the safety and inclusion of transgender people in society and protection against the violence that the sex workers in the community face. While cases of such violence are still common, there is a far more open conversation around them compared to the fluidity of gender that people experience in their personhood. In mainstream Pakistani culture, there has been no acknowledgment of LGBTQIA+ inclusion in life.

There have been similar conversations among the queer communities through private groups on Facebook, which started popping up in the virtual spaces around 2012. Haniya, who has been organizing to bring younger queer people together in online spaces for a moment of respite, says, "We have healing sessions, where we read together, have park and beach picnics and think about drugs that can provide us an alternate exploration of the mind, which is free-er than the reality." Dureja also took part in some of these online conversations, which helped attune her to the exploration of her mind. LSD tried to ask her: What within her body made her consistently unhappy with her physical form? Why did a fully functional and able-bodied woman not feel "complete"? She redirects me to a shared experience that psychedelic substances might lead to, which medical researchers have called "ego-dissolution."[8]

Historically, the connection between psychedelics and queer identity has been fraught. In North America, psychedelics were implicated in conversion therapies and used to treat the "disease" of homosexuality.[9] But some scholars have argued that this characterization privileges a medical encounter and does not sufficiently take personal use or private experimentation into consideration. Queer cultures have also embraced various drugs as part of carving out subcultures of queer identity.[10] These nonmedical encounters nonetheless sometimes borrowed medical concepts to explain the meanings behind the experiences.

On one end of the spectrum, ego-dissolution can result in gratifying mystical experiences, paired with spirituality and mindfulness. On the other hand, an individual can experience a "loss of self," as identified by the American philosopher William James. These experiences are characterized by a feeling of unity with one's surroundings, which is explicitly related to disturbed ego-boundaries, and thus ego-dissolution. Moreover, the mystical experience is likely to be therapeutic for most people.

Dureja has been struggling through most of her life: "I have always been hustling. For career, for money, for a better job. Questions of introspection did not stand a chance in my past life. I could not be in my head, asking who I was and why I felt so trapped in my own body."

She is five feet, eight inches tall, which is taller than the average South Asian woman. To be tall and broad is considered masculine, and in a conventionally heteronormative society, to be built differently puts one under a lot of bodily inspection and shame. Dureja says, "I did not like it when I was referred to as masculine, but at the same time, I was irked at how they tried to make me perform femininity."

Some of these observations are historically embedded in gendered expectations, which activists began disrupting in the 1960s, starting with women's rights.[11] Activist collectives such as All Pakistan Women's Association fought for the legal rights of child custody for women, the right to divorce, and the right to education for girls. Pakistan existed under a dictatorship during this period. Taking this movement to the streets and protesting for constitutional protections for women constituted a huge achievement, but challenging patriarchy did not extend to challenges to the state or military.

By the 1980s, these critiques changed and were no longer aligned with the state. Feminist demands shifted to criticisms of the patriarchy of the state, feudalism, and a forced religious identity as a national project. Groups of political organizers such as Women's Action Forum and Sindhiyani Tehreek spearheaded this era of feminist activism in Pakistan, which was agitating for a fair and democratic country. These political uprisings were largely rooted in a public sphere, from which the resistance within the homes of a Pakistani family began to sprout. Since these public demonstrations in the 1980s, public expressions of feminist activism have remained relatively dormant.

After three decades of no major uprising for the rights of women, in 2018, the first Women's March took place. Aided by new forms of media, the march took the Internet by storm. Women were once again out of the bounds of their homes and workspaces; they organized on the streets, holding offensive placards that advocated for the rights of women, demanding the right to their bodies and their sexuality. This demonstration was not just about the political rights of "women" as legislated; the new movement acknowledged trans and nonbinary people as significant participants in the resistance.[12]

* * *

The American psychedelic therapist and researcher Alexander Belser claims that the experiences of genderqueer people with psychedelics have yet not been documented beyond anecdotal evidence. He is a clinical research fellow, and in his psychotherapeutic practice, he focuses on preventing suicide among young gay and bisexual men. Dr. Belser emphasized the sociocultural, racial, and gender heteronormative privilege that affects the selection of subjects who become part of most psychedelic trials. This approach to psychedelic research has also been a deterrent in experimenting with psychedelic substances in an equitable manner. His vantage point as a queer cisgender man, working in the field of psychotherapy for more than twenty years, has helped him understand how genderqueer people who try to explore themselves through psychedelics are repeatedly put back in the closet. In the light of this ignorance within the medical research, Pakistan is not part of the conversation. No trials have been conducted within the communities of people located in marginalized geographies in this part of the world. The only mention of psychedelics as powerful hallucinogens came up in 2019, when *Herald Magazine*, a Pakistani, sociocultural, long-form publication, gave me the opportunity to explore altered states of consciousness, which led me to a booming psychedelic subculture in all of Pakistan. It also allowed me to explore intercity variations in substance-use patterns. As one of my interviewees in that story concluded: "In Karachi and Lahore, people want to incorporate psychedelic experiences into their daily lives. Peshawar has more of a 'burner culture'—revolving around ecstasy and meth. Islamabad is different. People there want to trip (on LSD and shrooms) all the time."[13]

Despite being a secretive initiative, stories from people like Dureja suggest that new subcultures are emerging. Dureja's case is encouraging, where her husband, Momin, is helping her explore the other side of the so-called closet: "We're on that wavelength where he knows when to offer care or love and when to give me space. He'll have water, fruit, and some snacks waiting for me, in case I feel the need to munch. If not, he'd be ready to step out with me, and having a car, and living close to the beach helps a lot."

* * *

Tripping for the first time on psilocybin mushrooms, twenty-eight-year-old Musfira, a resident physician from Karachi's Agha Khan University Hospital, had a different kind of awakening, one related to environmental justice. She said that the Earth has held human bodies in an embrace since we are born. She felt her body transcend its physical form to something greater, as an extension of the Earth.

She chose to trip with her husband, Rostam, as a trip sitter when they both traveled to Albany, New York, to continue their medical training. In a park close to her apartment, on a summer afternoon when she felt it was warm enough to put her at ease, while the breeze calmed her down, she decided to chew 2.5 g of dried psilocybin mushrooms. Musfira had planned for this trip, and she researched time and again about the clarity that psychedelic substances could bring to one's mind. This was not the impulsive decision that leads to the consumption of most drugs.

Ido Hartogsohn says in his book *American Trip* that it is difficult to think of many other concepts that are as fundamental and widely accepted in the study of psychedelics as "set and setting." The concept, most famously associated with the ideas of Timothy Leary, claims that the character of a psychedelic experience is determined by the user's character, expectations, and intentions (set), as well as the social and physical surroundings in which the drug experience takes place (setting). Leary went as far as to say that 99 percent of the specific response to LSD is determined by set and setting.

The young couple lay on their backs on the ground, the grassy fields cushioning them as Musfira gazed up into the sky. The sun shining from behind the clouds seemed like a perfect fractal to her, as her psilocybin broke down and settled into her bloodstream. She told Rostam how perfect the sky is if you imagine that you are the grass: "I pointed to the birds fluttering their way into the sky, marveling how majestic the nature of being is."

Rostam joked, "The birds are telling you: you go, girl!"

"I was still just swooned by nature. The sky, the trees, the sun, the warmth, and how all of these things around me, enabled me to exist, and I felt eternally grateful to the planet for this environment," said Musfira.

Rostam intervened just as her thoughts consumed her.

"There were some fungi where we lay, and I had spoken to Rostam in length about how they fit perfectly into the ecosystem of the forests."

"You go, girl!! said the Mycelium [fungi]," Rostam said.

"I broke out of my trance and asked him to repeat."

He repeated, explaining that he just meant it as a wish of encouragement.

"But I don't feel like a girl," Musfira retorted. "I felt like I was from the earth, staring at the sky, from the mere perspective of grass. I did not feel like a being separate from nature. I was a being that was beyond gender, but complete."

She distinctly remembers not feeling feminine or masculine until the sun went down and she peeled away from her husband while he made his way to pick up food.

"It was getting darker and my trip was fading off, as I walked back towards home, making my way through the park. I suddenly heard a man's footsteps following me, and the hypervigilance of being a woman brought me back to reality. Holy shit, gender still exists. . . . That was the first time that I was reminded that gender should just not be a thing anymore."

Musfira says that she was never curious about how she presents her gender besides being interested in men and women. She enjoys being feminine presenting and believes in the power that comes with it: "I wouldn't want to be a man, but I do believe that being without a defined gender might feel better to me. I have found myself double-checking my thoughts, when I feel nonbinary because there are people who experience it in the way they perform their gender and on the spectrum, it maybe isn't that difficult for me."

She still does not agree with the roles and expectations that are part of being traditionally feminine: "I have worked so hard and had difficult conversations with people around me, to be able to perform as much femininity as I feel comfortable with." Musfira comes from a traditionally Pukhtoon familial background, and wearing a hijab is often a mandatory part of this culture. Letting go of that, she says, has been a freeing experience for her.

Musfira also marveled at the thought of finding a safe outdoor spot to trip in when she was back home in Karachi. "In the city, we're always thinking about backup plans, safety, and having the right people around you." This equation can go wrong very easily.

The fear of having no space in Karachi to trip couldn't have been imagined absent the Soviet-Afghan war and the Khomeini revolution of Islam in Iran. The political unrest of these events discouraged incoming tourism from the West to the East, in the face of the Hippie Trail of the 1960s and 1970s. Hippies from Amsterdam, the US, Canada, Germany, London and more, would gather in Istanbul and head farther east, in big buses, to Tehran, Kabul, Herat, Peshawar, Lahore, Delhi, Kathmandu, Dhaka, Goa, Karachi, and Bangkok for their beaches. A forty-five-year-old Karachi broadcast journalist remembered his father recalling the "Americans" he met in the peak days of 1970s tourism in Karachi. He spoke of LSD as a substance that embarked upon a journey of thousands of miles, making its way to the beaches of Karachi. With its heightened sense of pop music and year-round tropical weather, the city made its mark on these explorers, who would plan further trips around India and Pakistan.

According to a friend of the unnamed person who runs the Pakistan-famous psychedelic Facebook community *Shroomwala* (which translates as "a person who owns shrooms"), until 2014 there were barely 100 people who might have experimented with psychedelics in Karachi, until they traveled to North America to go to college. It is common knowledge within the community that these students brought drugs back with them. I learned through my field research that LSD was the easiest of these to carry. Students and travelers would place the tabs between books and greeting cards to keep them safe from scanning by security, considering that the substance was yet not widely recognized.

"They were fascinated by the power of these substances and wanted to share that experience with their friends back home." An earlier story that I wrote about psychedelics in Pakistan also discusses the presence of a psychotherapist in Karachi who pairs psychedelics with her usual methods of therapy. She focuses on the importance of pairing therapy with a hallucinogen, however, uncertified and without the credentials of a psychedelic therapist, she believes it to be an alternative path to healing.

Despite being a signatory to the United Nations Convention for Psychotropic Drugs (1971), Pakistan lacks the regulatory scaffolding and funding to support research that might recognize the presence of psychedelic substances that are smuggled, imported, or grown as indigenous plants in the contrasting terrains of the country. These substances are far from being on the radar of the federal Anti-Narcotics Force. An LSD consumer in my earlier story confirms that the police are unaware of substances like LSD or shrooms, so they don't know what offense to charge users with. As a result, they end up persecuting psychedelic users in a manner similar to those using more familiar street drugs such as meth, heroin, and cocaine.

* * *

The second time that Musfira and Rostam decided to go on a trip together, they settled on a smaller one while traveling to Mexico. Rostam was taking 2.5 g of mushrooms while Musfira took up a lesser dose of 2g. She says, "In that particular trip, I had a sense of responsibility, where I automatically stepped into the role of a caretaker, considering this was Rostam's first time."

Musfira's only experience with psychedelic trips has been with Rostam. She felt safe with him. Also, having understood the role of a trip sitter, Rostam played his part in making her comfortable. According to Musfira, "He's a very soft, neutral, and comforting presence, who wouldn't guide my trip one way or the other, he was just listening, for the most part, making me expand more on the questions I already had spoken to him about earlier." He was also a partner who respected and supported Musfira's identity of being bisexual and exploring her sexuality through the times that she tripped with him, as her caretaker.

Stories of care work associated with psychedelics are not new. Erika Dyck, a Canadian historian of psychiatry at the University of Saskatchewan, explores the absence of women in the world of psychedelic research: "Women have provided support to the psychedelic experiences of their partners who have usually been men, in the role of a trip-sitter and that care work often gets undocumented." In her book *Psychedelic Prophets* (2018), she dives into the archive of a decade-long correspondence between Humphry Osmond, a British psychiatrist involved in early research into psychedelics and therapy, and Aldous Huxley, a proponent of psychedelics and the author of the seminal psychedelic work *The Doors of Perception* (1954). Both these brilliant minds were assisted by their wives, Jane Osmond and Maria Huxley and later Laura Huxley, in the lengths of their careers with psychedelics. Maria was a lover of the unknown, and as her curiosity took her forward, Huxley's interrogations with psychedelic trips were informed by her experiences. In addition, Alfred Hubbard, an enigmatic and tireless psychedelic evangelizer in the 1950s, would have been unable to mark his presence in the history of psychedelics if his wife, Ruth Hubbard, hadn't taken notes from his trips or curated the music that he was listening to while he tripped.

Dyck also spoke of the labor of women as wives that goes unrecognized, while medical workers such as nurses and facilitators at the historical psychedelic investigation trials were paid for their efforts: "The ignorance of women in psychedelics is nothing new because it traces back to the invisibility of women as researchers in science and STEM." She argues that preparing someone for an experience of psychedelic breakthrough takes a different kind of labor as an "empathetic observer," which was often taken for granted, and is followed by a period of integration that allows the person to process their trip. In the clinical trials and at home, most of these observers were women, mostly because of their assumed role as a nurturer.

* * *

A twenty-five-year-old, femme-presenting gender and sexually fluid resident of Karachi, Aiza Shakeel experienced her first LSD trip knowing the complications of her identity. Her relationship with self-actualization was only ever consolidated in her trips. She says, "I did not go on a trip wanting to explore myself or the gender and sexual identity of someone that I would like to be with, I reveled in the realization that I already knew my preferences."

According to her, it's also an "essentializing" of a queer person's experience of drugs when all life experiences that they have or perform are centered around their gender or sexual identity: "During my trip, I was surrounded by people who were swaying with the wind, dancing, and being intimate with their partners and friends. It was being at the Karachi beach, at night, under a full moon, untethered that really added to the freedom of a mind that comes with psychedelics."

Aiza is a researcher at Karachi Urban Labs, a think tank that explores infrastructure and urbanization in Karachi. In her everyday life, she dresses up in a *kameez* (tunic) and pants, heads to work, and commutes home. On weekends, she gathers with friends around a table with six cups of chai while they roll a few joints of hashish, mixed with tobacco, a blob of oiled "chars," heated up with a lighter flame, as someone tears up a Dunhill or a Marlboro Light, in order to make a blunt that is not too strong and not too light. It gives just the right amount of high that needs to kick in with a sip of black tea and a jolt of caffeine.

On one of these weekends, Aiza and her friends decided to pop 150 μg of LSD. At a *dhaba*, an open-air tea café in one of the more affluent neighborhoods of Karachi, closer to the sea, with coastal winds and a less polluted sky, Chota Bukhari has been a hangout spot for evening *baithaks*. The act of *baithak* is a tradition that has run through generations. The idea is to sit in communion after work or a long day of toiling in the city, where you can let off steam and have some snacks as the sun goes down and the very loud city comes close to collapsing in silence. As part of the *baithak*, Asad offered to share his 150 µg tab of acid with anyone who was willing to volunteer the split. Aiza agreed, even though she had always planned all her trips. But the prospect of this spontaneous choice seemed thrilling.

It's around 8 o'clock and the night gets quieter as Asad and Aiza begin their trip and head onto a journey that none of them can predict. There isn't an intended sitter or guide. Aiza gets up to go for a walk to a nearby store and to get some cigarettes for herself while some of her friends start bidding their farewells. "I'm just headed to a store that I have frequented a couple of times, but this time, I cannot stop laughing. I'm hysterical, their faces just seem different and funny. I also see the eyes of men on me. Just as the male bodies, omniscient around us at all times in Karachi. I got uncomfortable in my tiny second of joy. The freeness that LSD tried to bring me was occupied by men too."

For this experience, Aiza regrets not having a sitter who would make her feel safe if the trip went astray. After returning to the table where her friends were seated, she sees that Asad left without informing her, when she had depended on him to take her home. The mobility of women in Karachi is based on ride-hailing services like Uber or Careem, while men get to drive their family cars or bikes. Culturally, most women would not feel safe taking a long ride home in a taxi after 9 o'clock at night. It is 10 o'clock now, and Aiza had had a little jump scare, which added to the series of unfortunate events that had taken place during her trip.

Zainab Marvi, a human-centered design researcher at Bauhaus-Dessau, analyzes Karachi's gendered mobilities in her project "Feminist Practices as Urban Resistance." In Karachi, a metropolitan city, mobility is gendered. The free movement of men around the city impedes the mobility of other genders. Moreover, seen through an intersectional lens, these gendered mobilities are intertwined with other sociopolitical factors such as class, ethnicity, and violence. That is not to say that fear of violence among men does not exist. A male respondent shared that he is wary of political fighting between people of other ethnicities, religions, and political affiliations, which can escalate into physical violence.

According to the World Population Review, the current population of Karachi is at 16.8 million.[14] This makes the ever-so-chaotic New York City look small and orderly, with its 8.3 million population.[15] But New York City has a third of Karachi's total area of almost 700 square miles. Karachi has been a center of colonial and postcolonial violence based on ethnic and racial issues. Over the past three decades, as the country oscillated between military and democratic rule, land-grabbing and open gunfire have also been a customary occurrence in Karachi. Citizens of Karachi have had to find a way to navigate the danger and unpredictability of their lives around the disorder. Laurent Gayer calls Karachi an "Ordered Disorder" in his book exploring the intricate history of social and political struggles of the city: "For the residents of Karachi, including the barricaded city elites, violence has become part of the order of things. This is not to say that violence has become acceptable to Karachiites, but simply that they cannot imagine a future without it."

To engage in tripping and form a community, as an act of resistance, is a Karachi-centric experience. Dureja always felt that living in Karachi, having access to the beach and a close group of friends to go to for comfort, is one of her main reasons that she can take up psychedelics: "I have offered my friends to always feel welcome to my home as a setting for their psychedelic trip." Her husband, Momin, is also a companion in this endeavor. Momin would make sure to have a refrigerator stocked with fruits and snacks, juices, and ice water, as it's usually hot in Karachi. Dureja says, "If a friend schedules a psychedelic trip with us, helping to trip-sit them, we would request them to plan in advance, so we can be ready and home, to facilitate their experience from the start to its end."

Aiza, however, would disagree with this version of Karachi. Chaos is what she defines the city as: "My first-ever experience with LSD was only a success because we were away from the city. It was a curated experience."

Many who were part of this beach party that helped Aiza to be about thirty kilometers from the city speak of the distance from the concrete jungle that brought a lot of solace. A regular tripping experience for most women in Karachi looks like a thorough process of planning and mapping. In a culture where most adults live in nuclear families, interdependent on their parents, the material and moral implications of making life decisions individually are heavily laden with intrusive questions; "When will you be back?" "Who will you be hanging out with?" "How will you commute back home?"

Karachi and its experience change from person to person based on access to mobility in the city. Dureja's experience of tripping on a psychedelic substance for about twelve to sixteen hours is different from Aiza's experience of having to plan a beach visit weeks in advance. In a city that does not have a mass transit system, a car and driving skills become a necessity for people to commute from point A to point B, which layers in more precarity for women from the working class, who often cannot afford a car, or conservative homes, where women are not allowed to learn how to drive or go out alone, unchaperoned.

The fear of everyday violence is an underlying condition of existing and going about one's life in Karachi. A city that has not yet surrendered to the onslaught of political, social, and climate change unrest houses some of the most rebellious beings. People like Aiza, Dureja, Asad, and Momin, their friends, and the friends of their friends have grown up to see resistance within their homes. The attempt of bringing people together through psychedelics is their quest for freedom within their minds. Learning about the specificity or fluidity of gender is not only a home-grown resistance in Karachi; it also echoes the phenomenon of exploring gender euphoria in other tumultuous cities. Places like Rio de Janeiro, Cairo, Jerusalem, Kuta in Bali, and others, carrying their histories along with their role in psychedelic tourism and shamanism, strike a similar chord.

The evangelization of the therapeutic potential of psychedelic drugs is a shared sentiment among the young people of Karachi who speak about psychedelics. Just as Musfira got Rostam to try some and Dureja got Momin to as well, many people at the beach that Aiza tripped at were tripping for the first time ever. "If you have access to the beach, you might as well look towards a brighter horizon, assisted by the hallucinogens, of course," remarked Dureja.

NOTES

1. The conversations with all the people in this chapter come from interviews conducted by me over 2021–2022. All names have been changed for security reasons.

2. Natasha Ansari and Asad Sayeed, *Women's Mobility, Agency, and Labour Force Participation in the Megacity of Karachi* (London: London School of Economics, 2019).

3. For a detailed study of the relationship between violence and political development in Karachi, see Laurent Gayer, *Karachi: Ordered Disorder and the Struggle for the City* (New York: Oxford University Press, 2014). For how religion and ethnonationalism feature in the context of urban violence, see Oskar Verkaaik, *Migrants and Militants: Fun and Urban Violence in Pakistan* (Princeton, NJ: Princeton University Press, 2004).

4. For a detailed exploration of the continuities between women's activism in colonial South Asia and postcolonial Pakistan, see Ayesha Khan, *The Women's Movement in Pakistan Activism, Islam and Democracy* (London: I. B. Tauris, 2018).

5. Thomas Gugler, "Politics of Pleasure: Setting South Asia Straight," *South Asia Chronicle* 1 (2011): 355–392.

6. Zia Ur Rehman, "In Pakistan, a Leader in Trans Rights, Reality Is Slower to Change Than Law," *New York Times*, July 2, 2022, https://www.nytimes.com/2022/07/02/world/asia/pakistan-trans-rights.html.

7. Nick Duffy, "Transgender Pride March Takes Place in Pakistan," *Pink News*, December 31, 2018. https://www.pinknews.co.uk/2018/12/31/pakistan-transgender-pride/.

8. Timothy Leary, Richard Alpert, and Ralph Metzner, *The Psychedelic Experience*. This book is based on the writings of the *Tibetan Book of the Dead* and offers tips on how to handle the "ego death" that can occur on a high dose LSD trip. https://dash.harvard.edu/bitstream/handle/1/41647383/Timothy%20Leary%E2%80%99s%20Legacy%20and%20the%20Rebirth%20of%20Psychedelic%20Research.pdf?sequence=1

9. See Andrea Ens, *Wish I Would Be Normal": LSD and Homosexuality at Hollywood Hospital, 1955–1973*, MA thesis (University of Saskatchewan, 2019); Jesse Donaldson and Erika Dyck, *The Acid Room: The Psychedelic Trials and Tribulations of Hollywood Hospital* (Vancouver: Anvil Press, 2022).

10. Alex Belser, Clancy Cavnar, and Bia Labate, *Queering Psychedelics: From Oppression to Liberation in Psychedelic Medicine* (Santa Fe, NM: Synergetic Press, 2022).

11. Rubina Saigol, "The Past, Present and Future of Feminist Activism in Pakistan," *Herald*, July 15, 2019. https://herald.dawn.com/news/1398878/the-past-present-and-future-of-feminist-activism-in-pakistan.

12. Haseem uz Zaman, "Aurat March 2020: Women, Trans People, Non-binary Folks Rallying Stronger Than Ever!" *Geo News*, November 28, 2019. https://www.geo.tv/latest/258919-women-transgender-people-non-binary-folks-rallying-stronger-than-ever-for-aurat-march-2020.

13. Manal Khan, "In Pursuit of Altered States of Consciousness," *Herald*, December 1, 2018. https://herald.dawn.com/news/1398753.

14. The statistic for population is from https://worldpopulationreview.com/world-cities/karachi
-population

15. The statistic for population is from https://www.npr.org/sections/thetwo-way/2013/03/14
/174353179/new-york-city-hits-a-new-population-mark-topping-8-3-million.

BIBLIOGRAPHY

Ansari, Natasha, and Asad Sayeed. *Women's Mobility, Agency, and Labour Force Participation in the Megacity of Karachi*. London: London School of Economics, 2019.

Belser, Alex, Clancy Cavnar, and Bia Labate. *Queering Psychedelics: From Oppression to Liberation in Psychedelic Medicine*. Santa Fe, NM: Synergetic Press, 2022.

Donaldson, Jesse, and Erika Dyck. *The Acid Room: The Psychedelic Trials and Tribulations of Hollywood Hospital*. Vancouver, Canada: Anvil Press, 2022.

Duffy, Nick. "Transgender Pride March Takes Place in Pakistan." *Pink News*, December 31, 2018, https://www.pinknews.co.uk/2018/12/31/pakistan-transgender-pride/.

Ens, Andrea. "Wish I Would Be Normal": LSD and Homosexuality at Hollywood Hospital, 1955–1973. MA thesis, University of Saskatchewan, 2019.

Gayer, Laurent. *Karachi: Ordered Disorder and the Struggle for the City*. New York: Oxford University Press, 2014.

Gugler, Thomas. "Politics of Pleasure: Setting South Asia Straight." *South Asia Chronicle* 1 (2011): 355–392.

Khan, Ayesha. *The Women's Movement in Pakistan Activism, Islam and Democracy*. London: I. B. Tauris, 2018.

Khan, Manal. "In Pursuit of Altered States of Consciousness." *Herald*, December 1, 2018, https://herald.dawn.com/news/1398753.

Leary, Timothy, Richard Alpert, and Ralph Metzner, *The Psychedelic Experience*. Mexico, 1964.

Rehman, Zia Ur. "In Pakistan, a Leader in Trans Rights, Reality Is Slower to Change Than Law." *New York Times*, July 2, 2022, https://www.nytimes.com/2022/07/02/world/asia/pakistan-trans-rights.html.

Saigol, Rubina. "The Past, Present and Future of Feminist Activism in Pakistan." *Herald*, July 15, 2019, https://herald.dawn.com/news/1398878/the-past-present-and-future-of-feminist-activism-in-pakistan.

Verkaaik, Oskar. *Migrants and Militants: Fun and Urban Violence in Pakistan*. Princeton, NJ: Princeton University Press, 2004.

Zaman, Haseem uz. "Aurat March 2020: Women, Trans People, Non-binary Folks Rallying Stronger Than Ever!" *Geo News*, November 28, 2019, https://www.geo.tv/latest/258919-women-transgender-people-non-binary-folks-rallying-stronger-than-ever-for-aurat-march-2020.

CONCLUSION: THE FUTURE OF PSYCHEDELIC HISTORY

Erika Dyck and Chris Elcock

Canadian customs took no notice of a thirtysomething fisherman carrying his pole across the Washington State border on one September day in 1976. Had the agents interrogated him, however, they would have found him without a wallet and without ID. That man was Nick Sand, who had just lost his appeal of a fifteen-year prison sentence after being found guilty of conspiring to manufacture millions of doses of LSD and similar drugs.

By then, the fugitive Sand was already a legend in psychedelic lore. In the early 1960s, he favorably experimented with mescaline and peyote and concluded that he should dedicate his life to manufacturing psychedelics. Soon he was churning out hundreds of DMT hits out of his makeshift Brooklyn lab, and eventually he became Timothy Leary's official "alchemist." Subsequently, he met the chemist Tim Scully, and together they distributed their staples through an international trafficking network known as the Brotherhood of Eternal Love. By the early 1970s, their signature brand of acid—Orange Sunshine—had acquired a mythical status among transnational psychedelic communities.[1]

But Sand, it seemed, was just getting started. In November 1976, his partner, Judy Shaughnessy, joined him in rural British Columbia, where they began growing magic mushrooms for a living. A year later, they discovered the mystic teachings of Shree Rajneesh (later Osho) and were blown away. By spring 1978, their fungi scheme had yielded enough money for a trip to Rajneesh's ashram near Pune, India. Sand helped the ashramites by building them a hydroponic garden to grow fresh vegetables. He then identified a local source of ergotamine tartrate and bought a house in which he made huge amounts of LSD over the next three years.

In 2009, Sand claimed that over the course of his career, he had produced a staggering 14 kg of LSD (at 100 μg a dose, this would represent almost 140 million hits).[2] If this estimate is accurate, then this would mean that the number of acid tabs that he made while in India was likely in the millions. What happened to all that LSD? Could it have reached Mumbai's vibrant musical circles, and even the Bollywood industry?

By the time Sand's operation was underway, Indian musicians had already been experimenting with fuzz, delay, and reverb, whether in psychedelic funk bands like Atomic Forest or among the legendary soundtrack composers like Rahul Dev Burman and the brothers Virij Shah (better known by their duo name, Kalyanji-Anandji). At the turn of the 1970s, however, these artists started blending mind-bending synthesizers with more classic instruments,[3] just as the entire country was about to be swept away by an inimitable disco wave. They were joined by Bappi Lahiri, the composer whose name is almost synonymous with Indian disco. Lahiri had begun his Bollywood career in the mid-1970s, and he was immediately influenced by the psychedelic sounds of the time.[4]

The Bollywood disco scene in the 1980s received an important technological boost to further explore psychedelic sounds.[5] In 1982 a far less-known artist named Charanjit Singh became probably the first Indian musician to record an album using a synthesizer that Roland had just released in 1981, courtesy of the Japanese engineer Tadao Kikumoto. Kikumoto designed the TB-303 in an attempt to re-create the sound of a bass guitar, but his synthesizer was a total failure in that respect. Roland had to discontinue sales in 1984, having sold only a few thousand units; subsequently, others came to realize the unique potential of this new electronic bass line for use in a variety of fledgling electronic dance music scenes, and the TB-303 became immensely popular among techno, acid-house, and trance artists around the world.[6]

By that time, however, Singh had already released *Synthesizing: Ten Ragas to a Disco Beat*, which was much closer to Goa trance or acid house than to disco, while retaining Indian influences. Although *Synthesizing* became a cult album retrospectively, in large part because of its early use of the

TB-303, it was a commercial flop.[7] A year later, however, Lahiri himself used the bass line synth in *Wanted* (1984), a Western movie featuring the fast-paced and highly psychedelic disco song "Koi Lutera."

Could all these composers have experimented with Sand's Indian acid and come up with these sonic innovations, or was it just a matter of unadulterated artistic flair? Regardless, these stories about the emergence of Indian psychedelic disco seem to confirm what this book has illustrated: psychedelia was a rich cultural force that traveled freely around the world, with or without the psychoactive drugs commonly associated with this culture.

The twenty-first century has experienced a resurgence of interest in psychedelics, and that renewed cultural and medical fascination draws from this rich, if often hidden, mycelium network. In the third decade of this new century, several jurisdictions around the world are revisiting regulations governing the use of psychedelics as medicines, these histories and cultural associations continue to color the reputations of psychoactive substances as symbols of change, risk, curiosity, and experimentation. From the outset, psychedelics have walked a fine line between madness and insight, inspiring researchers to think outside the proverbial box when it comes to harnessing evidence and interpreting human behavior. Medicinal uses then created their own boxes. Spiritual guides and philosophers also used psychedelics to test commonplace boundaries of knowledge, questioning the rigidity of a system that distinguishes pathological states from enlightened ones.

In the twenty-first century, scientific research using psychedelics has accelerated, producing an ongoing resurgence of interest in these psychoactive substances as perhaps uniquely beneficial for treating human suffering. But this safe and reassuringly encouraging framing partially ignores some of the historical ways that psychedelics have seeped out of medical consultation rooms and into the cultural fabric of societies around the world, creating different kinds of attitudes, fashions, and critiques of convention. Historical reflection suggests that the psychedelic genie cannot be contained in a bottle. Whether approved as medicines or used for other purposes, psychedelics will continue to circulate, influencing culture, philosophy, medicine, art, and so on. How we come to know and understand psychedelics will depend on where we look to seek their influence and whose stories we tune into.

NOTES

1. Nicholas Schou, *Orange Sunshine: The Brotherhood of Eternal Love and Its Quest to Spread Peace, Love, and Acid to the World* (New York: Thomas Dunne Books, 2010).

2. Tim Scully, "Nick Sand: May 10, 1941–April 24, 2017," Erowid, May 4, 2017, https://www.erowid.org/culture/characters/sand_nick/sand_nick_biography2.shtml (accessed December 17, 2021). Scully also claims that it was Sand who secured a visa for Rajneesh to move to Oregon to start a commune there.

3. For instance, R. D. Burman wrote the upbeat "Dil Lena Khel Hai Dildar Ka" (from *Zamaane Ko Dikhana Hai*, 1981), replete with buzzing synths, psychedelic effects, and a transfixing dulcimer solo.

4. See, for instance, "Nothing Is Impossible," a fast-paced psychedelic freak-out from the movie *Zakhmee* (1974).

5. Tim Lawrence has likewise established a connection between disco and psychedelia in the US. See her *Love Saves the Day: A History of American Dance Music Culture, 1970–1979* (Durham, NC: Duke University Press, 2003).

6. Victor Branquart, "La grande histoire de la TB-303, la machine culte qui a plongé les lignes de basses dans un bain d'acide," *Trax*, September 15, 2021, https://www.traxmag.com/la-grande-histoire-de-la-tb-303-la-machine-culte-qui-a-plonge-les-lignes-de-basse-dans-un-bain-dacide/ (accessed March 22, 2022).

7. Stuart Aiken, "Charanjit Singh on How He Invented Acid House . . . by Mistake," *The Guardian*, May 10, 2011, https://www.theguardian.com/music/2011/may/10/charanjit-singh-acid-house-ten-ragas (accessed March 22, 2012).

BIBLIOGRAPHY

Aiken, Stuart. "Charanjit Singh on How He Invented Acid House . . . by Mistake." *The Guardian*, May 10, 2011, https://www.theguardian.com/music/2011/may/10/charanjit-singh-acid-house-ten-ragas (accessed March 22, 2012).

Branquart, Victor. "La grande histoire de la TB-303, la machine culte qui a plongé les lignes de basses dans un bain d'acide." *Trax*, September 15, 2021, https://www.traxmag.com/la-grande-histoire-de-la-tb-303-la-machine-culte-qui-a-plonge-les-lignes-de-basse-dans-un-bain-dacide/ (accessed March 22, 2022).

Lawrence, Tim. *Love Saves the Day: A History of American Dance Music Culture, 1970–1979*. Durham, NC: Duke University Press, 2003.

Schou, Nicholas. *Orange Sunshine: The Brotherhood of Eternal Love and Its Quest to Spread Peace, Love, and Acid to the World*. New York: Thomas Dunne Books, 2010.

Scully, Tim. "Nick Sand: May 10, 1941–April 24, 2017." Erowid, May 4, 2017, https://www.erowid.org/culture/characters/sand_nick/sand_nick_biography2.shtml (accessed December 17, 2021).

EPILOGUE: A GLOBAL HISTORY OF PSYCHEDELICS

Mike Jay

The word "psychedelic," coined in 1956 by the psychiatrist Humphry Osmond in correspondence with Aldous Huxley, turned out to be more than a new label for a family of mind-altering compounds represented primarily at that time by LSD and mescaline. It was an inflection point, after which a disparate group of plants, chemicals, and practices from across the globe were gathered together under a single rubric. It embodied a new understanding of the possibilities of drug use and communicated it to millions—and, thanks to the peculiar qualities of the drugs in question, even changed the states of consciousness that they produced.

This was, in part at least, Osmond and Huxley's intention. Psychiatrists had already coined various terms to describe these drugs—"psychotomimetic," "hallucinogen," "psychodysleptic"—but all connected their effects to mental illness, in particular the psychotic states associated with schizophrenia. Huxley wanted a word that implied an expansion and elevation of consciousness rather than an impairment or disorder, and one that connected the experience not to mental pathology, but to the life-changing epiphanies of saints and mystics. "The mental climate of our age is not favourable to visionaries," he observed;[1] the classifications developed by the doctors made such experiences into grounds for confinement in mental hospitals.

For the psychedelic experience to be reconceived in this way, it was not merely recent psychiatric coinages that needed to be overwritten, but the apparently neutral term that underpinned them: "drugs." Until the twentieth century, this was a name applied to all medications, in the sense that persists to this day in words such as "drugstore." From around 1900, however, it had acquired a secondary and parallel meaning, fraught with pejorative associations. In the first instances of its use, it was an abbreviated form of expressions such as "dangerous drugs," "drugs of pleasure," "addictive drugs," or "drugs of abuse"—intoxicants, typically opiates or cocaine, with a high risk of overdose or addiction that were to be administered only by medical professionals.[2] This abbreviated sense took on legal force during the "drug" prohibitions of the following decades, which loaded the word with shadow meanings of criminality and social deviance and associated it in particular with the problematic practices of ethnic minorities.

For the progressive thinkers of this era, "drugs" represented the worst of the disenchanted modern age: chemicals that dulled the mind and sapped the will, peddled by unscrupulous big business in industrial quantities and ever more potent and dangerous forms. They were viewed not as expanders of consciousness but social pacifiers, a notion captured most enduringly in Aldous Huxley's *Brave New World* (1932). Prior to his mescaline experience, Huxley had maintained a profound skepticism about the value of drugs for spiritual purposes. As late as 1952, he wrote in the epilogue of *The Devils of Loudun*, the book that preceded *The Doors of Perception*: "For the drug-taker, the moment of spiritual awareness (if it comes at all) gives place very soon to subhuman stupor, frenzy or hallucination, followed by dismal hangovers and, in the long run, by a permanent and fatal impairment of bodily health and mental power . . . What seems a liberation is in fact an enslavement."[3] His experience on mescaline, when he took it under Osmond's supervision in May 1954, demanded a new language that rescued it not merely from the taint implied by the new psychiatric terms, but from the framework of "drugs" in general.

The same conclusion was forced on the poet and classicist Robert Graves in January 1960, when he first took the compound psilocybin, recently isolated from the Mexican mushroom *Psilocybe mexicana*, with Gordon and Valentina Wasson in their New York apartment. As Sandoz's pink Indocybin pills took hold, Wasson played his tape recording of Maria Sabina, the Mazatec *curandera* who had guided him through his first mushroom encounter, invoking Christ in the form of Tlaloc, the pre-Hispanic deity of rain and fertility. For Graves, "it might have been the Goddess Aphrodite addressing her forward son Eros." He concluded that "the word 'drug', originally applied to all ingredients used in chemistry, pharmacy, dyeing and so on, has acquired a particular connotation in English, which cannot apply to *psilocybin*."[4]

The introduction of "psychedelic," with its positive associations of mind expansion, spiritual insight, and personal growth, was perfectly suited to its historical moment, in which psychiatry and pharmacology were both in a state of productive flux, and even more so to the extraordinary properties of the newly designated psychedelics themselves. By 1956, Osmond, together with collaborators such as Alfred Hubbard with his huge private stash of Sandoz LSD, had recognized that their effects were heavily dependent on the context in and attitude with which they were approached. They developed therapeutic models that abandoned the sterile medical atmosphere of the clinic in favor of warm, homely environments rich in sensory and aesthetic stimuli, such as comfortable sofas and sublime religious art. When Osmond administered mescaline to Huxley in his house in the Hollywood Hills, he made sure that his subject had vases of flowers and illustrated art history texts to absorb his attention and guide his experience.

"Set and setting," the phrase that came to denote these ideas and practices, emerged from the recognition that psychedelics rendered their subjects highly suggestible. The experience was readily directed and manipulated, and the insights that it generated were, in the term used by William James to characterize mystical experiences, "noetic": imbued with a sense of unquestionable truth that enabled therapists to imprint new beliefs and behaviors. This created a powerful self-reinforcing or looping effect: under the direction of a doctor, psychedelics were medicines; with a priest or shaman, they were sacraments; for the artist, they were agents that opened the mind to new forms of inspiration.

At the same time, the social determinants of psychoactive drug effects were dramatically illuminated by the sociologist Howard Becker, in a paper he published a few months before *The Doors of Perception*. Becker had been studying the use of marijuana by black jazz musicians in New York, a habit typically regarded by his professional colleagues as a symptom of deviance and criminality. He concluded, however, that within this subculture, it offered rewards that were not obtainable by other social groups. The average white American suburbanites of the 1950s, if they somehow found themselves high on marijuana, would experience its effects as alarming, alienating, and nightmarish; in the New York jazz scene, precisely the same drug effects would serve as a stimulus to pleasure, relaxation, sociability, and creativity. "Marihuana use," Becker concluded, "is a function of the individual's conception of marihuana and the uses to which it can be put."[5] Only once a desirable goal is recognized can the experience be appreciated and valued.

This insight proved supremely applicable to psychedelics. The "magic mushroom," as the editors of *LIFE* magazine christened it in 1957, was a striking example: once Wasson and Graves popularized their claim that mushroom intoxication was a sacred practice that long predated Christianity, the Mexican mushroom and the psychedelic compound derived from it became imbued with qualities that the stigmatizing term "drugs" was unable to encompass. Over the following two decades, it became clear that psilocybin-containing mushrooms grew widely across Europe and the US; there was no documented cultural or religious tradition for their use, but many examples of accidental ingestion have been recorded over the years by doctors, mycologists, and toxicologists. None of these experiences had been conceived as either mystical or therapeutic. Their subjects, on noticing the early onset of psilocybin's effects—dizziness, gastric disturbance, and odd and intrusive thoughts—had typically leaped to the conclusion that they had eaten poisonous fungi and were undergoing a toxic crisis, perhaps even a fatal one. Visual distortions were experienced as delirium or fever, and they often were rendered all the more disturbing by attendant physicians applying emergency medicine such as emetics or stomach pumps. Once the concept of a "psychedelic" became familiar, new frameworks for the experience were made available. The imprimatur of cutting-edge science, allied to the allure of an ancient lost religion, endowed the mushroom trip with medical and spiritual possibility.[6]

As the editors of this volume have shown, Aldous Huxley's books, essays, and broadcasts from the late 1950s, in which he energetically promoted the concept of "psychedelics" and made bold claims about their transformative potential for individuals and society at large, were translated into dozens of languages and formed the early basis for an international psychedelic culture. When the term established itself in mainstream discourse a decade later, it took on a widely understood complex of meanings and associations. "Psychedelic," as a philosophical idea, denoted a sense of cosmic wonder; as an aesthetic, it meant swirling colors, spirals, and decorative abstractions; as a musical style, it embraced distinctive tropes such as electrical pedal effects, polyphonic multitracking, or the use of the sitar; and as a lifestyle, it included the rejection of consumer values and dedication to spiritual questing or community living.

These associations shaped and defined psychedelics in the modern West for decades to come. By the same token, they obscured the disparate notions that Western science had evolved over the previous decades and the cultural niches that their plant sources had long inhabited in non-Western cultures, both of which this collection of studies has so vividly depicted. Prior to the inflection point of the mid-1950s, there were many very different lenses through which the experience could be viewed. As we learn from Magaly Tornay's eye-opening discussion in chapter 6 on the earliest days of LSD at Sandoz Pharmaceuticals, its first scientific researchers approached the new drug through a wide variety of frameworks, few of which found any resonance in the notion of "psychedelic" that emerged with Huxley. The compound's discoverer, Albert Hofmann, at first believed it to be a superpotent amphetamine; Werner Stoll, the son of Hofmann's boss, Arthur Stoll, and a psychiatrist at the Burghölzli clinic, interpreted its effects as a chemically induced psychosis. Some of the younger Stoll's psychiatric colleagues advanced it as a form of "psychic tuning" that could be used in ways analogous to shock treatment or insulin coma therapy, while others regarded it as a revealer of personality, the chemical equivalent of a Rorschach test. These models were frequently tested by giving LSD to both doctors and patients without their knowledge or consent.

In non-Western cultures, where what we now know as psychedelics have a considerably longer and richer history, the term remains effectively untranslatable. Attempts to paraphrase its meaning—for example, "plants that alter consciousness" or "plants that induce visionary experience"—are as likely to describe tobacco or fermented alcohol brews as the compounds that we now designate as psychedelic. As Ian Baker reveals in chapter 1, sacramental traditions of intoxication often involve ritual practices and plant brews that are not reducible to what pharmacology recognizes as their psychoactive components. And as Julien Bonhomme's transcultural study of iboga in chapter 8 demonstrates, these practices undergo subtle (and not so subtle) shifts once incorporated into the "psychedelic" paradigm: Indigenous African traditions of initiation and ancestor encounters are reconceived as healing quests that mirror the assumptions of Western psychotherapeutics. "Psychedelic," in these wider historical and global contexts, is a term that conceals as much as it reveals.

In the twenty-first century, the meaning of "psychedelic" has continued to evolve. Over the last two decades, the countercultural associations forged in the twentieth century have been challenged, and in many contexts supplanted, by a new understanding that has emerged from the confluence of clinical psychotherapy, the pharmaceutical industry, and the venture capitalists of Silicon Valley and beyond. Drugs that were until recently best known in the wider culture for inducing nervous breakdowns and causing their subjects to jump from tall buildings are now presented as miracles of modern science with the potential to revolutionise the treatment of mental illness and trauma. The Aldous Huxley of this psychedelic renaissance is Michael Pollan, who shares Huxley's winning talent for presenting himself simultaneously as insider and outsider: his mind-blowing trip descriptions and reports from the frontiers of neuroscience are accompanied by astonishment that "drugs," a category of experience that he had previously shunned, can generate such profound and transformative effects.

Yet the expansive rhetoric that accompanies psychedelics today can appear, in the longer view, as a shrinking of their possibilities. Redefining them as agents of science and medicine marginalizes the other uses described in this volume, in which they demonstrate equally striking potential as tools of creativity or social solidarity, ethnography or mass communication, philosophy or revolutionary politics. At the same time, it forces them into the Procrustean bed of institutional pharmacology, in which some of their properties are exaggerated and others truncated. The protocols of licensing and regulation by the US Food and Drug Administration demand the exclusion from drug trials of all extra-pharmacological variables—precisely the elements of "set and setting" now well established as crucial determinants of their efficacy. Psychedelic-assisted clinical therapy centers the medical professional, and thereby the power dynamics of the doctor-patient relationship; elsewhere, from the peyote meetings of the Native American Church to the radical psychiatry of the 1960s described in chapter 18 by Mark Gallagher, or the veterans' groups now treating their posttraumatic stress disorder with ayahuasca, non–medical group sessions have productively harnessed the ongoing mutual support offered by friends, kin, or fellow patients. The risk-averse modern clinic has steered its course away from the ceremonial ordeals or ecstatic group experiences that characterize Indigenous practice and the psychedelic counterculture alike; in their place, we are presented with the image of a solitary and passive patient, eye-mask and headphones screening the person from all external stimuli that might distract from the ministrations of a qualified psychotherapist.

In documenting the multiplicity of psychedelic histories—both those that unfolded before the term was coined and the distinctive forms that have since developed across the globe, from Israel to Latin America to the Netherlands—this volume both illuminates our current historical moment and glimpses fresh possibilities for a psychedelic future. The medicalization—and, not coincidentally, monetization—of psychedelics currently underway asserts a preeminent claim over the field through the authority of neuroscience and clinical trials; and yet this global history prompts us to ask whether, like the many other frameworks that preceded it, this is an act of meaning-making specific to its time and place. The landscape of novel psychedelic compounds continues to expand, and their protean, looping, and noetic qualities make the cultural forms and meanings that may accrete around them impossible to control or predict. Psychedelics have arrived in the cultural mainstream as a novel class of pharmaceutical medicines, but it may be that a very different set of meanings and practices will eventually emerge from this encounter. If the histories assembled in this volume have a lesson for the future, it is to expect the unexpected.

NOTES

1. Aldous Huxley, "Mescaline and the Other World," *Moksha* (1980): 62.

2. See John Parascandola, "The Drug Habit: The Association of the Word 'Drug' with 'Abuse' in American History," in *Drugs and Narcotics in History*, ed. Roy Porter and Mikuláš Teich (Cambridge University Press 1997), 156–167.

3. Huxley, "Mescaline and the Other World," 25; Aldous Huxley, *The Devils of Loudun* (London: Chatto and Windus, 1952), 363.

4. Robert Graves, *Oxford Addresses on Poetry* (Cassell, 1962), 138–139. Emphasis in original.

5. Howard Becker, "Becoming a Marihuana User," *American Journal of Sociology* 59, no. 3 (1953): 238.

6. See Mike Jay, "Fungi, Folklore and Fairyland," *Public Domain Review* (October 2020), https://publicdomainreview.org/essay/fungi-folklore-and-fairyland.

BIBLIOGRAPHY

Becker, Howard. "Becoming a Marihuana User." *American Journal of Sociology* 59, no. 3 (November 1953): 238.

Graves, Robert. *Oxford Addresses on Poetry*. Cassell, London: 1962.

Huxley, Aldous. *The Devils of Loudun*. London: Chatto and Windus, 1952.

Huxley, Aldous. "Mescaline and the Other World." Proceedings of the Round Table on Lysergic Acid Diethylamide and Mescaline in Experimental Psychiatry, held at the Annual Meeting of the American Psychiatric Association, Atlantic City, NJ, May 12 1955 (New York: Grune and Stratton, 1956), 46–50.

Jay, Mike. "Fungi, Folklore and Fairyland." *Public Domain Review* (October 2020), https://publicdomainreview.org/essay/fungi-folklore-and-fairyland.

Parascandola, John. "The Drug Habit: The Association of the Word 'Drug' with 'Abuse' in American History." In *Drugs and Narcotics in History*, edited by Roy Porter and Mikuláš Teich, 156–167. Cambridge: Cambridge University Press, 1997.

Acknowledgments

It has been an enormous privilege to work on this collection. The growing interest in psychedelics in the twenty-first century has opened up new lines of inquiry and encouraged us to play a role in updating this history by drawing attention to a more diverse set of stories and experiences outside North America. An undertaking such as this, however, could not be accomplished without the skillful work of many others behind the scenes.

We are particularly grateful to our translators, Amy Fletcher and Chris Elcock for translating chapters by Verroust, Dubus, and Dassonville; and to Amy Fletcher and Kali Carrigan for their translation of the chapter by Scholten and Salas. We also thank Patrick Farrell for his careful editorial work and the harmonizing of the prose in a book featuring such a wide range of contributors and with differing writing and citation styles. One of our reviewers recommended adding maps, and Patrick identified geographical flows for psychedelic substances, while Geoffrey Wallace produced colorful maps depicting the flows of psychedelics around the globe. In 1993, Michael Horowitz, Dana Reemes, and Kathleen Harrison created a historical map commemorating the fifty years since LSD's introduction. We have reproduced it here with their generous permission. Funding for the translations, editorial formatting, and maps was made possible thanks to the Canadian Social Sciences and Humanities Research Council funds (Dyck) and Julien Bonhomme's Collège de France funds for the translation of his chapter.

We found a great venue in the MIT Press, thanks to Matthew Browne, who immediately saw potential in the project and steered it through the peer review process. Three anonymous reviewers offered valuable feedback that strengthened this book in important ways and provided us with constructive recommendations on a large and diverse project spanning different geopolitical contexts. We have also benefited from scholarly advice and support from several people working in this field, including Nancy Campbell, Maziyar Ghiabi, David Herzberg, Osiris Romero González, Bia Labate, Nicolas Langlitz, Jim Mills, Lucas Richert, and Mat Savelli. We are grateful to members of the Alcohol and Drugs History Society for feedback on some of the individual chapters and the overall concept.

Erika gives special thanks to Felix and Amelia, who continue to expand her mind by asking why. And a big thank-you to her parents, Penny and Phil, who stepped up to help as she spent 2022 on crutches, but still tethered to the keyboard.

Contributors

Beat Bächi is a historian and author of *Vitamin C für alle!* (2009) and *LSD auf dem Land* (2020). He is currently researching farm animals in the Anthropocene—when he is not herding cows in the Swiss mountains.

Ian A. Baker is a historian and medical anthropologist. He is the author of seven books on Tibetan and Himalayan culture, including *Tibetan Yoga: Principles and Practices* and *The Heart of the World: A Journey to the Last Secret Place*. His PhD research investigated alchemy and cocaine in British colonial Burma.

Julien Bonhomme is a professor of anthropology at the École normale supérieure de Paris. He is the author of several books, including *Le Miroir et le Crâne: Parcours initiatique du Bwete Misoko* (2006), *The Sex Thieves. Anthropology of a Rumor* (2016), *Le Champion du quartier*, and *Se faire un nom dans la lutte sénégalaise* (2022).

Henrique Carneiro is a professor of modern history at the University of São Paulo, where he is the director of LEHDA-USP (Laboratório de Estudos Históricos das Drogas e da Alimentação [Laboratory of Historical Studies of Drugs and Food]). He is the author or coauthor of nine books, including *Drogas: A história do proibicionismo* (2018). He is also a founding member of the Interdisciplinary Group for Psychoactive Studies (NEIP-Núcleo de Estudos Interdisciplinares sobre Psicoativos).

Peter Sachs Collopy is a historian, archivist, and curator of American science, technology, and media. He serves as University Archivist at Caltech, edited the chapter "Video and the Self: Closed Circuit | Feedback | Narcissism" in *Video Theories: A Transdisciplinary Reader* (2022), and has published articles on video synthesizers, video as analog electronic photography, and white supremacy and its opponents in physical anthropology.

Ross Crockford, a former trial attorney, started his journalistic career in the early 1990s as a staff writer for *The Prague Post*. Currently based on Canada's west coast, he has written about the history of psychedelics for such publications as the *Vancouver Sun*, *Western Living*, *Reflex* (Czech Republic), and the *MAPS Bulletin*.

Gautier Dassonneville is a PhD in philosophy (Liege University and Lille-3 University) and a hypnotherapist in Liege, Belgium. He edited and introduced Jean-Paul Sartre's unpublished graduate thesis from 1927 on *L'Image dans la vie psychologique: Rôle et nature* (*Études sartriennes*, vol. 22, 2018). He also contributed to Michel Foucault's reading notes (French National Research Agency) project by describing and enriching the corpus of digitalised Foucault's archives, and by creating a digital exhibition on young Foucault as philosophy and psychology student during the 1940's and 1950's in Paris (https://eman-archives.org/Foucault-fiches/exhibits).

Júlio Delmanto was born and raised in São Paulo, Brazil. He is a journalist, with a master's and doctorate in social history from Universidade de São Paulo, and the author of *Camaradas caretas: Drogas e esquerda no Brasil* (2015) and *História social do LSD no Brasil: Os primeiros usos medicinais e o começo da repressão* (2020).

Zoë Dubus completed her PhD in contemporary history at the University of Aix-Marseille, France in 2022. Her research deals with the transformation of medical practices and health policies related to the use of psychotropic drugs from the nineteenth century to the present day in France. She has published several articles on this subject.

Erika Dyck is a professor and Canada research chair in the history of health and social justice at the University of Saskatchewan. She is the author or coauthor of several books, including *Psychedelic Psychiatry* (2008); *A*

Culture's Catalyst: Historical Encounters with Peyote and the Native American Church in Canada (2016); *Psychedelic Prophets: The Letters of Aldous Huxley and Humphry Osmond* (2018); and *The Acid Room: The Psychedelic Trials and Tribulations of Hollywood Hospital* (2022). She is the guest editor of the Chacruna Institute for Psychedelic Medicine series on women and psychedelics.

Chris Elcock holds a PhD in medical history from the University of Saskatchewan. He has published several peer-reviewed articles on the history of psychedelics, including an award-winning paper on the American psychedelic movement. He is the author of *Psychedelic New York: LSD and the Long Sixties in a Global Metropolis* (2023).

Mark Gallagher has published articles on the history of collective action by psychiatric patients and the birth of LSD therapy in the UK. He is a lecturer at Queen Margaret University, Edinburgh.

Alex K. Gearin is an assistant professor of medical humanities at the LKS Faculty of Medicine, the University of Hong Kong. He has conducted ethnographic research on ayahuasca-drinking communities in Australia, Peru, and China, and his work is featured in *Current Anthropology, Social Science and Medicine*, and *Journal of the Royal Anthropological Institute*. He is currently finishing a book entitled *Global Ayahuasca*.

Ido Hartogsohn is an assistant professor in the Graduate Program for Science Technology and Society at Bar Ilan University. His research focuses on the role of set and setting (context) in shaping the effects of psychedelic drugs. Hartogsohn's book *American Trip: Set, Setting, and the Psychedelic Experience in the Twentieth Century* was published by MIT Press (2020).

Mike Jay is an author and independent scholar who has written widely on the history of medicine, the mind sciences, and psychoactive drugs. His books include *The Atmosphere of Heaven* (2009), on the discovery of nitrous oxide; *High Society: Mind-Altering Drugs in History and Culture* (2010); and *Mescaline: A Global History of the First Psychedelic* (2019). He writes regularly for the *London Review of Books* and the *Wall Street Journal*, among other publications, and is an Honorary Research Fellow at University College London.

Andrew Jones is a PhD candidate in the Institute for the History and Philosophy of Science and Technology at the University of Toronto. His dissertation explores how LSD was used as a normalizing tool in child psychiatry in the 1960s in the US. He is also working on uncovering more about the history of LSD therapy in Ontario, Canada.

Manal Zahid Khan is a Falak Sufi Fellow in the Near Eastern studies department at New York University. She is a journalist based in New York whose beat covers the intersection of gender, culture, cinema, and psychedelics. Her work in the exploration of hallucinogens began in 2018, with the first-ever investigative, long-form story about the subculture of psychedelic substances in a postdrug-war Pakistan. Her recent work examines the relationship between queer identities and psyhedelics in the megacity of Karachi.

Wendy Kline is the Dema G. Seelye Chair in the History of Medicine at Purdue University. She is the author of three books: *Coming Home: How Midwives Changed Birth* (Oxford University Press, 2019); *Bodies of Knowledge: Sexuality, Reproduction, and Women's Health in the Second Wave* (University of Chicago Press, 2010); and *Building a Better Race: Gender, Sexuality, and Eugenics from the Turn of the Century to the Baby Boom* (University of California Press, 2001). Her current research on psychedelic medicine in the US and UK has been supported by both a Fulbright Distinguished Fellowship and British Academy Fellowship.

Hallam Roffey is a PhD candidate in the department of history at the University of Sheffield. His thesis examined debates around what constituted "obscenity" in 1970s and 1980s England. His current research focuses on countercultures, political radicalism, and psychedelics in Britain after the 1960s.

Gonzalo Salas is an adjunct professor of psychology in the Universidad Católica del Maule, Chile. He is the author or coauthor of several books, including *History of Psychology in Chile 1889–1981* (2009), *History of Psychology in South America* (2014), and *History of Psychology in Latin America:*

A Cultural Approach (2021). He is a founding member of the Chilean Society for the History of Psychology and the director of a grant about Amanda Labarca, a prominent Chilean feminist of the twentieth century.

Hernán Scholten is a lecturer, research assistant, and PhD candidate in the department of psychology at the Universidad de Buenos Aires (Argentina). He is the author or coauthor of several books, including *History of Psychology in Latin America* (2021), *Freudisms of Gregorio Bermann* (2018), and *Oscar Masotta and Phenomenology* (2001). He is also the cofounder and administrator of El Seminario www.elseminario.com.ar, a website dedicated to the history of psychology and related disciplines since 2000.

Stephen Snelders is a research fellow in the history and philosophy of science at the Faculty of Science, Utrecht University. His PhD thesis dealt with the history of LSD and psychiatry in the Netherlands. His latest book, *Drug Smuggler Nation: Narcotics and the Netherlands, 1920–1995* (Manchester University Press, 2021), includes the history of the illegal production and trade of LSD, XTC, and other psychedelics.

Magaly Tornay is a historian and postdoc at the University of Bern, Switzerland. She has written books on the history of psychoactive drugs (*Zugriffe auf das Ich*, 2016), on clinical trials in a rural psychiatric clinic (*Testfall Münsterlingen*, 2019, with Marietta Meier and Mario König),), and on the psychoanalysis of nurses' dreams (*Träumende Schwestern*, 2020). She is currently coleading a research project on the history of bioethics.

Vincent Verroust is a doctoral student in philosophy, history of science and epistemology at the Université Picardie Jules Vernes, France. He is the founder of the French Psychedelic Society, which is at once a hub for researchers working on psychedelics, a community for users, and an association for scientific mediation. He is also employed as the scientific coordinator in charge of the work on psychedelics at the Network of Health Establishments for the Prevention of Addictions (RESPADD) in collaboration with the Psychiatry - Commorbidities - Addictions team of the Paul Brousse Hospital in Paris.

Timothy Vilgiate is a PhD student at the University of Texas at Austin. He received his MA in history at the University of Colorado, Colorado Springs. His current project looks at the history of psychedelic plant research in Mexico during the twentieth century.

Itamar Zadoff is a PhD candidate in the department of Asian Studies, University of Haifa. His dissertation deals with "The Psychedelic Communities in Israel and Japan and Their Cultural Footprints." He is the head of the Wadokan Dojo, Aikido, and Kobudo and an expert in Japanese language and culture.

Index

Lotsof, Howard, 190, 192–194, 196, 204
LSD, 1–2, 7, 8–9, 11, 59, 63, 103, 193,
    215–217, 222–223, 226, 262–263,
    480, 495, 497
  and British anarchism, 309–324, 423–427,
    429, 433–439
  in British psychiatry, 122, 126–135,
    424–425, 429–430, 432
  in "clinical theology," 288–289, 293,
    295–298, 300–302
  and creativity, 339–342, 380, 382–387,
    402–406
  in Czech psychiatry, 99–115
  in Dutch psychiatry, 358–364, 366, 370,
    409
  in French psychiatry, 75–77, 78, 80–84,
    86–93
  in Israeli psychiatry, 400–402
  in Latin American psychiatry, 3, 241–253,
    379–283
  as model psychosis, 101, 144–148,
    153–155, 239–253, 380, 394, 400–401
    (see also psychotomimetic)
  and mystical experience, 285, 296–298,
    321, 340, 366, 367, 394, 408 (see also
    parapsychology)
  in Pakistan, 473–474, 477, 479, 482,
    484–487
  in Swiss psychiatry, 141–142, 144–155
  and technology, 333, 336–338, 340–348
Lysergamid, 102, 103, 104, 107, 110

MacDonald, Andrew, 25
Maillart-Garg, Meena, 28
Manson, Charles, 1
Marvi, Zainab, 485
Multidisciplinary Association for Psychedelic
    Studies (MAPS), 315
Marcuse, Herbert, 319
Marie-Janot, Maurice, 173
Marijuana, 2, 365, 385, 387, 497–498. See also
    cannabis

Marins, José Mojica, 386
Marks, Sarah, 80, 100
Martins, Clovis, 381–382
Mas de Ayala, Isidro, 250
Matus, Don Juan, 171
Mayer-Gross, Wilhelm, 61, 430
Mazatec, 168, 170, 230, 266–267, 271, 453,
    493. See also Mexico, mushrooms in
McKenna, Terence, 168, 170
McLuhan, Marshall, 334–337, 338, 342,
    347, 431
  Understanding Media (1964), 335–336
MDMA, 393, 394
Merck, 60, 61
Merleau-Ponty, Maurice, 61
Mescaline, 2, 5, 7, 8, 194, 270, 335,
    341–342, 345, 369, 405, 491, 495, 496,
    497. See also peyote
  in psychiatry, 51–66, 69n35, 130, 145,
    150, 194, 251, 263
Methamphetamine, 144, 223, 340, 341, 360,
    482
Metzner, Ralph, 366, 450
Mexico, 10, 169–170, 193, 195
  mushrooms in, 261–262, 265–271, 276,
    483
Michaux, Henri, 270, 405
Minkowski, Eugene, 244
Moliterno, Angelino, 390, 391
Monoamine oxidase inhibitor (MAOI), 26,
    43n21, 251
Montoya, Enrique Gonzalez Rubio, 170
Morales, Francisco Pérez, 382
Moreau, Jacques-Joseph, 59–60
Moreira, Juliano, 240
Mourgue, Raoul, 61
Mozambique, 175
Murdoch, Rupert, 428
Murguía, Daniel, 250
Mushrooms, 10, 24–26, 28, 59, 168–169,
    206, 228–229, 261–278, 479, 482.
    See also psilocybin

Naranjo, Claudio, 194, 253
Naranjo Vargas, Plutarco, 250–251
Narby, Jeremy, 195, 203, 206
Narcoanalysis, 193–194, 360, 361
Native American Church, 501
Netherlands, 3, 11, 167, 193, 196–198, 203, 204, 408
   and LSD, 357–371, 409
   and psilocybin, 359, 361, 369
Neuman, Nadav, 402
Neville, Richard, 367
New Age, 194–196, 203–204, 206, 449, 454
Nichols, Florence, 10, 285–288, 290–293, 298–302
Nickles, David, 324
Nightshade (solanaceae), 33, 59
Nizan, Paul, 57
Nol, Onno, 357, 365, 370–371
Novartis, 216, 217
Ntewusu, Samuel, 172
Nunes Filho, Eustachio Portella, 380–382

Oliveira, André Luiz de, 385
Ololiuqui, 2
Onorato, Amelia C. de, 243–244
Opium, 25, 33, 365, 369
   morphine, 251
Osmond, Humphry, 251, 262–263, 273, 340, 429, 483, 496
   coining of term psychedelic, 495, 497
Osmond, Jane, 483
Oz (magazine), 316, 319, 367

Pahnke, Walter, 107, 366
Paik, Nam June, 333–334, 345–347
Pakistan, 13, 473–487
Panama, 193
Parapsychology, 8, 264–265, 271–278, 384
Pavlov, Ivan, 100, 295
Pélicier, Yves, 93
Peru, 3, 247–249, 449, 459
Peticov, Antonio, 388–389

Peyote, 2, 59, 62, 169, 195, 206, 342, 413, 491, 501. See also mescaline
Phillips, Terry, 322
Pichon, Édouard, 57–58
Pichon, Marcel, 175, 178
Pierret, Janine, 92
Pinel, Philippe, 240
Piva, Roberto, 386
Playboy (magazine), 336
Poisson, Jacque, 173–174
Pollan, Michael, 500
Portella Nunes Filho, Eustáchio, 244–245
Portugal, 3
Powick Psychiatric Hospital, 9, 121–122, 125, 127–135, 285, 291, 430
Psilocybin, 1, 3, 62, 114, 228–229, 230, 232, 278, 393, 394, 479–480, 496, 498. See also mushrooms
   and psychiatry, 141, 154, 155, 270–273, 300, 359
Psychedelic renaissance, 3, 122, 133, 370, 438, 493, 500
Psychedelic Review, The (journal), 340, 366
Psychoanalysis, 52, 59, 101–102, 107, 108, 124, 194, 204–205, 207, 243, 288–289, 290, 292, 294–295, 301–302, 348, 359–360, 381–383, 408, 430
Psycholytic therapy, 102, 103–108, 111, 114, 128, 359–360
   coining of term, 128, 429
Psychotomimetic, 57, 239–241, 250–251, 253, 256n48, 262, 358, 366, 382, 400–401, 429, 495
Purkyně, Jan Evangelista, 101

Quercy, Pierre, 61–62
Quintero, Muro, 245

Radical Software (magazine), 333
Radicalism, 11, 165, 166, 309–324, 328n68, 332, 367–370, 423–425, 437. See also counterculture

Shamanism, 169, 171, 178, 195, 206–207, 266–267, 349, 459
   neo-shamanism, 450–451, 452
Shamberg, Michael, 338
Shani, Rina, 408–409
Shaughnessy, Judy, 491
Sherwood, J. N., 341
Shor, Nissan, 412
Shulgin, Alexander, 393
Shulgin, Ann, 393
Siegel, Eric, 343–345, 346
Singh, Charanjit, 492–493
Shortall, Sarah, 320, 424
Sierra Leone, 174
Silicon Valley, 11
Sillans, Roger, 196
Singapore, 300
Sisko, Bob, 196
Slovenia, 193, 195
Smythies, John, 340
Sobiecki, Jean-François, 171
Soma, 8, 23–26, 28–29, 31–40
St. Kitts, 193
Staehelin, John, 152–153
Stamm, Emma, 310
Stapf, Otto, 174–175
Stern, Rudi, 336
Stockhausen, Karlheinz, 346
Stolaroff, Myron, 334, 339–342
Stoll, Arthur, 144, 217, 220, 223–224, 239, 499
Stoll, Werner A., 144–147, 150–151, 152, 223, 239, 241, 242, 243, 499
Strate, Lance, 336, 347
Stresser-Péan, Guy, 262
Świderski, Stanisław, 196
Switzerland, 9, 10
   LSD research in, 141–142, 144–155, 223–224
   ergot production in, 215–222, 224–227, 230–232
Syrian rue (*Peganum harmala*), 25, 26, 28
Szára, Stephen, 263

Tallaferro, Alberto, 244, 249–250
Tantra, 25, 28, 38, 42n8, 44n29
Taylor, Charles, 450
Technology, 333–348. *See also* LSD, and creativity
Tehreek, Sindhiyani, 478
Teilhard de Chardin, Pierre, 334–335, 337, 338
   Phenomenon of Man, The (1955), 335
Téllez Meneses, Agustín, 241–243, 244
Thévenard, Pierre, 274
Thompson, Willie, 310
Thullier, Jean, 76, 78
Tillich, Paul, 297
Tīrthanāth, Ānanda, 28–29, 31–38, 40
Tobacco, 368, 389, 484, 500
Toledo, Luísa de Alvarez, 382
Tosar, Rey, 250, 253
Trepanation, 369–370
Turner, Fred, 334, 343

UN Convention on Psychotropic Substances, 110–111
União do Vegetal, 384, 455
United Nations, 5
United States (US), 1–4, 6, 7, 9, 100, 122, 130, 154, 168, 170, 174, 222, 501
   ibogaine use in, 190, 192–193, 198–199, 202–203, 207–208
Uruguay, 10, 249–251, 253

Varney, Edwin, 333
Vassi, Marco, 333
Vasulka, Woody, 344
Vedas, 24–25, 28, 33, 34, 39 (Vedic)
Veloso, Bahians Caetano, 386
Venezuela, 169, 243, 245
Video, 339, 343–348. *See also* LSD, and creativity
Village Voice (newspaper), 431
Vinkenoog, Simon, 364–366, 367, 369
Voacanga africana, 167–168, 172, 173–179